Practical Cases in
OBSTETRICS AND GYNECOLOGY

Practical Cases in
OBSTETRICS AND GYNECOLOGY

Second Edition

Editor

Kanan Yelikar MBBS MD MICOG FICMCH FICOG
Professor and Head
Department of Obstetrics and Gynecology
Government Medical College and Hospital
Aurangabad, Maharashtra, India

Vice President Elect, FOGSI (2007)
Chairperson, Clinical Research Committee (FOGSI) (2004–2008)

Foreword
CN Purandare

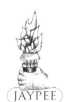

JAYPEE *The Health Sciences Publisher*
New Delhi | London | Philadelphia | Panama

Jaypee Brothers Medical Publishers (P) Ltd.

Headquarters
Jaypee Brothers Medical Publishers (P) Ltd.
4838/24, Ansari Road, Daryaganj
New Delhi 110 002, India
Phone: +91-11-43574357
Fax: +91-11-43574314
Email: jaypee@jaypeebrothers.com

Overseas Offices

J.P. Medical Ltd.
83, Victoria Street, London
SW1H 0HW (UK)
Phone: +44 20 3170 8910
Fax: +44 (0)20 3008 6180
Email: info@jpmedpub.com

Jaypee-Highlights Medical Publishers Inc.
City of Knowledge, Bld. 237, Clayton
Panama City, Panama
Phone: +1 507-301-0496
Fax: +1 507-301-0499
Email: cservice@jphmedical.com

Jaypee Medical Inc.
The Bourse
111, South Independence Mall East
Suite 835, Philadelphia
PA 19106, USA
Phone: +1 267-519-9789
Email: jpmed.us@gmail.com

Jaypee Brothers Medical Publishers (P) Ltd.
17/1-B, Babar Road, Block-B
Shaymali, Mohammadpur
Dhaka-1207, Bangladesh
Mobile: +08801912003485
Email: jaypeedhaka@gmail.com

Jaypee Brothers Medical Publishers (P) Ltd.
Bhotahity, Kathmandu, Nepal
Phone: +977-9741283608
Email: kathmandu@jaypeebrothers.com

Website: www.jaypeebrothers.com
Website: www.jaypeedigital.com

© 2015, Jaypee Brothers Medical Publishers

The views and opinions expressed in this book are solely those of the original contributor(s)/author(s) and do not necessarily represent those of editor(s) of the book.

All rights reserved. No part of this publication may be reproduced, stored or transmitted in any form or by any means, electronic, mechanical, photocopying, recording or otherwise, without the prior permission in writing of the publishers.

All brand names and product names used in this book are trade names, service marks, trademarks or registered trademarks of their respective owners. The publisher is not associated with any product or vendor mentioned in this book.

Medical knowledge and practice change constantly. This book is designed to provide accurate, authoritative information about the subject matter in question. However, readers are advised to check the most current information available on procedures included and check information from the manufacturer of each product to be administered, to verify the recommended dose, formula, method and duration of administration, adverse effects and contraindications. It is the responsibility of the practitioner to take all appropriate safety precautions. Neither the publisher nor the author(s)/editor(s) assume any liability for any injury and/or damage to persons or property arising from or related to use of material in this book.

This book is sold on the understanding that the publisher is not engaged in providing professional medical services. If such advice or services are required, the services of a competent medical professional should be sought.

Every effort has been made where necessary to contact holders of copyright to obtain permission to reproduce copyright material. If any have been inadvertently overlooked, the publisher will be pleased to make the necessary arrangements at the first opportunity.

Inquiries for bulk sales may be solicited at: jaypee@jaypeebrothers.com

Practical Cases in Obstetrics and Gynecology

First Edition: 2007

Second Edition: **2015**

ISBN 978-93-5090-536-4

Printed at Rajkamal Electric Press, Plot No. 2, Phase-IV, Kundli, Haryana.

Dedicated to

My family—Dr Avinash, Dr Ashwini and Dr Aditya

Contributors

Abha Singh
Professor and Head
Department of Obstetrics and
Gynecology
Pt Jawahar Lal Nehru Memorial
Medical College
Raipur, Chhattisgarh, India

Ashish R Kale
Consultant
Ashakiran Hospital
Pune
Assistant Professor
Maharashtra Institute of Medical
Education and Research (MIMER)
Medical College
Pune, Maharashtra, India

Ashish Zararia
Assistant Professor
Government Medical College
and Hospital
Nagpur, Maharashtra, India

Ashwini Talpe
Assistant Professor
Government Medical College and
Hospital
Aurangabad, Maharashtra, India

Ashwini Yelikar
Consultant, Obstetrician and
Gynecologist
Lotus Hospital
Pune, Maharashtra, India

Bharati Shrihari Dhore Patil
Honorary Associate Professor
Bharati Vidhyapeeth
Pune, Maharashtra, India

Chandan Gupta
Assistant Professor
Department of Obstetrics and
Gynecology
Government Medical College and
Hospital
Aurangabad, Maharashtra, India

CN Purandare
Consultant Obstetrician and
Gynecologist
St Elizabeth, Saifee and BSES Hospitals
Mumbai
Ex Hon Professor (Obs and Gyne)
Grant Medical College and JJ Hospital
Mumbai, Maharashtra, India
President FOGSI-2009
President Elect, FIGO
Dean, Indian College of Obstetricians
and Gynecologists
Editor Emeritus, FOGSI-Journal

Deepti Dongaonkar
Dean
Government Medical College
Latur, Maharashtra, India

Girija Wagh
Professor and Head
Department of Obstetrics
and Gynecology
Bharati Vidhyapeeth
Pune, Maharashtra, India

Haresh U Doshi
Associate Professor and Unit Chief
BJ Medical College
Ahmedabad, Gujarat, India

Hemant Deshpande
Professor
Department of Obstetrics and
Gynecology
DY Patil Medical College
Pune, Maharashtra, India

Jayam Kannan
Emeritus Professor
The Tamil Nadu Dr MGR Medical
University
Chennai, Tamil Nadu, India

Jayantdeep Nath
Assistant Professor
(Obstetrics and Gynecology)
Gauhati Medical College
Guwahati, Assam, India

Jayprakash Shah
Consultant (Fetal Medicine)
Rajni Hospital and Fetal Medicine Center
Ahmedabad, Gujarat, India

Jyoti Bindal
Professor
Department of Obstetrics and
Gynecology
Gajra Raja Medical College
Gwalior, Madhya Pradesh, India

Kalpana Kalyankar
Assistant Professor
Department of Obstetrics and
Gynecology
Government Medical College and
Hospital
Aurangabad, Maharashtra, India

Kalpana Mahadik
Professor and Head
Ruxmaniben Deepchand
Gardi Medical College
Ujjain, Madhya Pradesh, India

Kamini Rao
Medical Director
Bangalore Assisted Conception Center
Bengaluru, Karnataka, India

Kanan Yelikar
Professor and Head
Department of Obstetrics
and Gynecology
Government Medical College
and Hospital
Aurangabad, Maharashtra, India
Vice President Elect, FOGSI (2007)
Chairperson, Clinical Research
Committee (FOGSI) (2004–2008)

Kavita N Singh
Associate Professor
Department of Obstetrics
and Gynecology
Netaji Subhash Chandra Bose
Medical College
Jabalpur, Madhya Pradesh, India

Late Mandakini Parihar
Director
Madakini IVF Center
Mumbai, Maharashtra, India

Madhuri A Patel
Hon Clinical Associate
N Wadia Hospital, Mumbai
Ex Professor and Head
Department of Obstetrics
and Gynecology
ESIC-PGIMSR, MGMH, Mumbai
Ex Associate Professor
Government Medical College
Mumbai, Maharashtra, India
Treasurer FOGSI
Joint Secretary FOGSI-2009
First Assistant Editor
Journal OBGYN of India

Manjusha Yetalkar
Ex Lecturer
Grant Medical College and
Sir JJ Group of Hospitals
Mumbai, Maharashtra, India

Manorama Purwar
Ex Professor and Head
Department of Obstetrics
and Gynecology
Government Medical College and
Hospital
Nagpur, Maharashtra, India

Milind Shah
Chairperson
Rural Obstetrics Committee of FOGSI
Solapur, Maharashtra, India

Nikhil Purandare
Specialist Registrar
Department of Obstetrics and
Gynecology
The Adelaide and Meath Hospital
Ireland

Nupur Gupta

Pankaj Desai
Associate Professor and Unit Chief
Department of Obstetrics and
Gynecology
Medical College
Vadodara, Gujarat, India

Prachi S Koranne

Pradeep Ingale
Assistant Professor
Department of Obstetrics and
Gynecology
Government Medical College and
Hospital
Aurangabad, Maharashtra, India

Pradip Sambarey
Professor
Department of Obstetrics and
Gynecology
Byramjee Jeejeebhoy Government
Medical College
and Sassoon General Hospitals
Pune, Maharashtra, India

Pralhad Kushtagi
Professor
Department of Obstetrics and
Gynecology
Kasturba Medical College and Hospitals
Mangaluru, Karnataka, India

Pushpa S Junghare
Professor
Department of Obstetrics and
Gynecology
Punjabrao Alias Bhausaheb Deshmukh
Memorial Medical College
Amravati, Maharashtra, India

Raina Chawla
Assistant Professor
Department of Obstetrics and
Gynecology
Kasturba Medical College and Hospitals
Mangaluru, Karnataka, India

Rajesh Darade
Associate Professor
Department of Obstetrics and
Gynecology
Government Medical College and
Hospital
Latur, Maharashtra, India

Sachin Khedkar
Assistant Professor
Department of Obstetrics and
Gynecology
Government Medical College and
Hospital
Aurangabad, Maharashtra, India

Sadhana M Tayade
Medical Superintendent
Cama and Albless Hospital
Mumbai, Maharashtra, India

Sanjay A Gupte
Honorary Associate Professor
Department of Obstetrics and
Gynecology
BJ Medical College
Pune, Maharashtra, India

Shaila Sapre
Dean, Professor and Head
Department of Obstetrics and
Gynecology
Gajra Raja Medical College
Gwalior, Madhya Pradesh, India

Shashikant M Umbardand

Shirish Daftary
Emeritus Professor
Department of Obstetrics and
Gynecology
Former Dean
Nowrosji Wadia Maternity Hospital
Mumbai, Maharashtra, India
Past President FOGSI

Shrinivas Gadappa
Associate Professor
Department of Obstetrics and
Gynecology
Government Medical College and
Hospital
Aurangabad, Maharashtra, India

Shyam Desai
Gynecologist/Obstetrician
Mothercare Nursing Home
Mumbai, Maharashtra, India

Sonali Deshpande
Associate Professor
Department of Obstetrics and
Gynecology
Government Medical College and
Hospital
Aurangabad, Maharashtra, India

SR Wakode
Associate Professor
Department of Obstetrics and
Gynecology
Government Medical College and
Hospital
Nanded, Maharashtra, India

Suchitra N Pandit
Consultant-Oncologist
Kokilaben Hospital
Mumbai, Maharashtra, India
President Elect FOGSI 2014

Sudha Sharma
Assistant Professor
Postgraduate Department of Obstetrics
and Gynecology
Government Medical College
Jammu, Jammu and Kashmir, India

Suguna
Ex Professor (Obstetrics and Gynecology)
Al Ameen Medical College
Bijapur, Karnataka, India

Sunita Mittal
Professor and Head
Department of Obstetrics and
Gynecology
All India Institute of Medical Sciences
New Delhi, India

Swati S Shiradkar
Professor and Head
Department of Obstetrics and
Gynecology
Mahatama Gandhi Mission's (MGM)
Medical College
Aurangabad, Maharashtra, India

Vaman B Ghodake

Vandana Nimbargi
Associate Professor
Department of Obstetrics and
Gynecology
Bharati Vidhypeeth
Pune, Maharashtra, India

Varsha Deshmukh
Associate Professor
Department of Obstetrics and
Gynecology
Government Medical College and
Hospital
Aurangabad, Maharashtra, India

Vidhya Choudhary
Assistant Professor
Department of Obstetrics and
Gynecology
Maharani Laxmibai Medical College
Jhansi, Uttar Pradesh, India

Vidya Thobbi
Professor and Head
Department of Obstetrics
and Gynecology
Al Ameen Medical College
Bijapur, Karnataka, India

Vishal R Tandon
Postgraduate Department of Obstetrics
and Gynecology
Govenment Medical College
Jammu, Jammu and Kashmir, India

Foreword

I am extremely happy to see the second edition of *Practical Cases in Obstetrics and Gynecology*, edited by Professor Dr Kanan Yelikar, who is a renowned teacher in the field of Obstetrics and Gynecology being published.

The book is very useful for viva voce for undergraduate and postgraduate students. It covers all the topics in obstetrics and gynecology and it will definitely increase the level of confidence of students appearing for the practical examination.

I appreciate the hard work put in by the editor in getting the chapters contributed from various contributors representing teachers from every corner of the country.

I admire the attitude of a teacher in her heart of imparting knowledge to everyone, whenever and wherever possible. I wish all the success to the book.

I am sure students will appreciate the book immensely.

CN Purandare
MD MA (Obs) (Ireland) DGO
DFP D.Obst RCPI (Dublin)
FICOG FRCOG (UK)
FICMCH PGD MLS (Law)
Consultant Obstetrician and Gynecologist
St Elizabeth, Saifee and BSES Hospitals, Mumbai
Ex Hon Professor (Obs and Gyne)
Grant Medical College and JJ Hospital
Mumbai, Maharashtra, India
President FOGSI-2009
President Elect, FIGO
Dean, Indian College of Obstetricians and Gynecologists
Editor Emeritus, FOGSI-Journal

Preface to the Second Edition

I am extremely happy to bring about second edition of *Practical Cases in Obstetrics and Gynecology* for MBBS and MD students. It was the demand of the students to have the book totally dedicated to practical cases.

I express my thanks to all my contributors, who have been carefully chosen, for their vast experience in teaching who were kind for their timely contribution.

I would like to take this opportunity to thank, The Dean, Government Medical College and Hospital, Aurangabad, Maharashtra, India, and The Director, Medical Education and Research, Maharashtra, India, for permitting to go ahead with my endeavor.

I am thankful Dr CN Purandare for his foreword. It would not have been possible to publish the book, without M/s Jaypee Brothers Medical Publishers (P) Ltd, New Delhi, India, especially Shri Jitendar P Vij (Group Chairman), Mr Ankit Vij (Group President), and Mr Tarun Duneja (Director–Publishing).

I am also thankful to Dr Sonali Deshpande (Associate Professor), who was a constant support; my colleagues and postgraduates from the Department of Obstetrics and Gynecology, who supported me throughout the year.

I am indebted to my family members Dr Avinash, Dr Ashwini, Dr Ashish, Dr Aditya, and my mother-in-law Smt Laxmibai Yelikar for bearing with my long absentees.

I am thankful to all my patients and my dear students past and present, who are the constant source of inspiration.

Kanan Yelikar

Preface to the First Edition

I am extremely happy to bring about my book on *Practical Cases in Obstetrics and Gynecology* for MBBS and above students. The idea of editing and publishing such a type of book, came in, when my daughter Ashwini was appearing for her III MBBS practical examinations. When she demanded that I must teach her complete syllabus of Obstetrics and Gynecology in 2 hours time, which was next to impossible. And the idea of having a book totally, dedicated to practical cases was born.

I am thankful to all my contributors, who have been carefully chosen, for their vast experience in teaching who were kind enough for their timely contribution.

I would like to take this opportunity to thank the Dean, Government Medical College and Hospital, Aurangabad, Maharashtra, India, and the Director, Medical Education, Maharashtra, India, for permitting to go ahead with my endeavor.

Thanks to Dr Nagnath Kottapale, Vice Chancellor, Dr Babasaheb Ambedkar Marathwada University, Aurangabad, Maharashtra, India, for his foreword. It would not have been possible to publish this book without M/s Jaypee Brothers Medical Publishers (P) Ltd, New Delhi, India, especially Mr Tarun Duneja (Director–Publishing), who was kind enough to accept my book.

Last but not the least, my colleagues and postgraduates from the Department of Obstetrics and Gynecology who supported me throughout the year (special mention of Dr Sonali Deshpande, Dr Ajeet Deshmukh, Dr Kapil and Dr Swati).

I am indebted to my family members Dr Avinash, Dr Ashwini, Dr Aditya and my mother-in-law Smt Laxmibai Yelikar for bearing with my long absentees.

I express my gratitude to all my patients and my dear students past and present, who are the constant source of inspiration.

Kanan Yelikar

Contents

1. **Abortion** — 1
   Abha Singh, Pradeep Ingale

2. **Pregnancy-induced Hypertension** — 5
   Shrinivas Gadappa

3. **Antepartum Hemorrhage** — 14
   Kanan Yelikar, Sonali Deshpande

4. **Anemia in Pregnancy: Modern Aspects of Diagnosis and Therapy** — 18
   Sunita Mittal, Nupur Gupta, Pradeep Ingale
   Approach to diagnosis *18*

5. **Heart Disease in Pregnancy** — 24
   Ashwini Yelikar, Ashish R Kale

6. **Diabetes Mellitus in Pregnancy** — 27
   Kanan Yelikar, Sonali Deshpande

7. **Antenatal Care** — 30
   Pradip Sambarey, Kanan Yelikar
   Need for antenatal care *30*
   Nonstress Test (NST) *32*
   Contraction Stress Test (CST) *32*
   Biophysical Profile (Manning Score) *32*

8. **Normal Labor** — 34
   Ashwini Yelikar

9. **Partograms** — 37
   Shyam Desai, Kanan Yelikar
   Illustrative Partogram *37*
   Interpretations *37*

10. **High-risk Pregnancy** — 41
    Manorama Purwar, Ashish Zararia

11. **Prelabor Rupture of Membranes** — 45
    Sadhana M Tayade, Chandan Gupta

12. **Prolonged Pregnancy** — 49
    Vandana Nimbargi, Hemant Deshpande

13. **Previous Cesarean Section** — 52
    Kanan Yelikar, Ashwini Yelikar
    Recent Advances/Update Changing Trends *52*

14.	**Rh-Negative Mother** *Kanan Yelikar, Sonali Deshpande*	**56**
15.	**Preterm Labor** *Jyoti Bindal, Ashwini Yelikar*	**60**
16.	**HIV Infection during Pregnancy** *Deepti Dongaonkar, Sachin Khedkar* Types of HIV Viruses *67* Prevalence and Incidence (NACO 2004–2005) *67* Types of Tests for HIV Diagnosis *67* Association of HIV and Tuberculosis *68*	**67**
17.	**Grand Multipara** *Pushpa S Junghare, Kanan Yelikar, Kalpana Kalyankar*	**72**
18.	**Occipitoposterior Position** *Ashwini Yelikar, Chandan Gupta, Kanan Yelikar*	**74**
19.	**Breech Presentation** *Sonali Deshpande*	**76**
20.	**Transverse Lie/Shoulder Presentation** *Kanan Yelikar, Ashwini Yelikar*	**81**
21.	**Obstructed Labor** *Kanan Yelikar, Ashwini Yelikar*	**82**
22.	**Third Stage Complications** *Kalpana Mahadik* Postpartum Hemorrhage (PPH) *83* Retained Placenta *84* Inversion of Uterus *85* Postpartum Shock *85*	**83**
23.	**Multiple Pregnancy** *Kanan Yelikar, Varsha Deshmukh* Diagnosis *87*	**87**
24.	**Drugs in Obstetrics and Gynecology** *Shrinivas Gadappa, Kanan Yelikar, Sonali Deshpande* Magnesium Sulfate *90* Labetalol *90* Nifedepine *91* Alpha-methyldopa *91* Oxytocin *91* MethylErgometrine *91* Misoprostol (PGE_1) *92* Dinoprostone PGE_2 *92* Carboprost 15-Methyl-PGF2-Alpha *92* Mifepristone RU-486 (Russell unit) *93*	**90**

Ethacridine Lactate 93
Oral Iron 93
Folic Acid 93
Terbutaline 93
Ritodrine 94
Isoxsuprine 94
Maternal Corticosteroids 94
Corticosteroids 94
Cefotaxime 94
Metronidazole 94
Ciprofloxacin 95
Clotrimazole 95
Clindamycin 95
Fluconazole 95
Nevirapine 95
Methotrexate 96
Metformin 96
Cabergoline 96
Tetanus vaccine 96
Anti-Rc Immunoglobulin 96
TranexAmic Acid 97
Hormones in Gynecology 97
Progestins 98

25. **Induction of Labor** 100
Kanan Yelikar, Varsha Deshmukh
Assessment before Induction 100

26. **Instrumental Vaginal Delivery: Forceps and Ventouse** 103
Shaila Sapre, Vidya Thobbi, Suguna
Operative Vaginal Delivery—Vacuum Extractor/Ventouse 107

27. **Contraception** 110
Haresh U Doshi, Sonali Deshpande

28. **Ultrasonography in Obstetrics** 122
Kanan Yelikar, Jayprakash Shah

29. **Intrauterine Growth Retardation** 125
Pankaj Desai, Kanan Yelikar
Case Study 125

30. **Maternal Mortality** 128
Milind Shah, Ashwini Talpe

31. **Gestational Trophoblastic Neoplasia** 136
Sonali Deshpande
Examination 136
Ultrasound 136

32. Ectopic Pregnancy **140**
Kamini Rao, Sonali Deshpande
Diagnosis and Treatment *140*
Definition *140*
Etiology of Ectopic Pregnancy *140*
Reasons for Increased Rates of Ectopic pregnancy *140*

33. Vaginitis **144**
Varsha Deshmukh
Different Types of Vaginitis *144*
Criteria for Clinical Diagnosis of Vaginal Discharge *144*

34. Sexually Transmitted Infections **147**
Jayantdeep Nath, Pralhad Kushtagi
Syphilis *148*
Gonorrhea *150*
Chlamydial infection *151*
Bacterial vaginosis *151*
Herpes Virus infection *152*
Human Papillomavirus Infection *152*
Trichomoniasis *153*
Candidiasis *154*
Chancroid *154*
Lymphogranuloma venereum *155*
Granuloma inguinale *156*
Viral Hepatitis *156*

35. Abnormal Uterine Bleeding **158**
Pralhad Kushtagi, Raina Chawla

36. Amenorrhea **166**
Bharati Shrihari Dhore Patil, Chandan Gupta

37. Endometriosis **170**
Sudha Sharma, Vishal R Tandon, Sonali Deshpande

38. Menopause **176**
Girija Wagh, Sanjay Gupte

39. Hormones and Allied Medications in Gynecology **184**
Shirish Daftary, Pralhad Kushtagi
Estrogens *184*
Progestogens *185*
Androgens *186*
Testosterone *186*
Danazol *186*
Gestrinone *186*
Antiestrogens *186*
Clomiphene Citrate *186*

Tamoxifen *187*
Letrozole *187*
Antiprogesterones *187*
Antiandrogens *188*
Cyproterone Acetate *188*
Spironolactone *188*
Pituitary gonadotropins *188*
GnRH and analogs *188*
Bromocriptine *189*

40. Pelvic Organ Prolapse   **190**
CN Purandare, Jayam Kannan, Madhuri A Patel, Manjusha Yetalkar, Nikhil Purandare

41. Uterine Fibroids   **197**
Suchitra N Pandit, Prachi S Koranne, Vaman B Ghodake, Shashikant M Umbardand

42. Infertile Couple   **207**
Late Mandakini Parihar, Ashish R Kale
Examination *207*

43. Ovarian Tumors   **214**
Swati S Shiradkar
Types *214*
Points to be Noted in History *214*
General Examination *215*
Per Abdomen Examination *215*
Per Speculum Examination *215*
Per Vaginum Examination *215*
Per Rectal Examination *215*
Confirmation of Diagnosis *215*

44. Cancer of Cervix   **219**
SR Wakode, Vidhya Choudhary
Symptoms *219*
Signs *219*

45. Endometrial Carcinoma   **225**
Kavita N Singh

46. Endoscopy   **229**
Ashish R Kale, Rajesh Darade

Index   *235*

PLATE 1

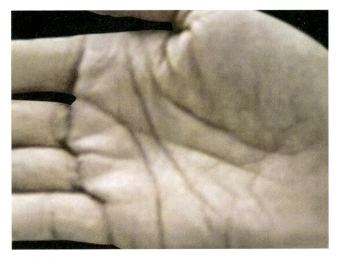

P Polyp
A Adenomyosis
L Leiomyoma
M Malignancy, endometrial hyperplasia

Fig. 35.1 Structural causes of AUB

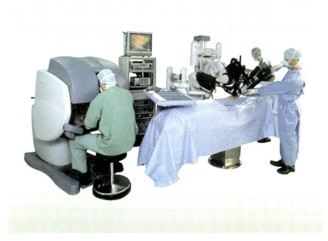

Fig. 41.2: Robotic surgery team and setup

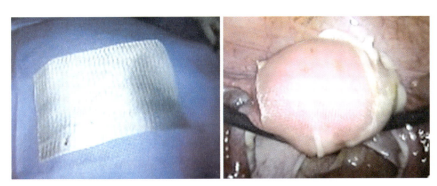

Fig. 41.3: Cloth like material being wrapped around the raw areas from surgery

Abortion

Abha Singh, Pradeep Ingale

1. What is abortion?
WHO defines abortion as induced or spontaneous termination of pregnancy before 20 weeks of gestation or with fetus weighing less than 500 g.

2. What is the incidence of abortion?
About 10–20% of all pregnancies end up in abortion, of which 3/4th occur before 16 weeks and out of these 75% before 8 weeks.

3. What are the different common types of abortion met in clinical practice?
Common varieties of abortion are:
- Threatened
- Inevitable
- Incomplete
- Complete
- Missed
- Septic.

In developing countries, incidence of septic abortions are also quite high, approximately 10% of abortions requiring admission to the hospital.

4. What is the most common cause of first trimester abortion?
Genetic factors in the form of chromosomal abnormalities in the conceptus are the most common causes.

5. What are the common chromosomal abnormalities of the conceptus?
Autosomal trisomies occur in about 50% cases. The most common trisomies are 16, 21 and 22.

6. What is blighted ovum?
Blighted ovum is the failure of development of fetal pole even after the gestational sac diameter of 2.5–3 mm or more on transabdominal sonography.

7. At what gestational age, fetal pole should appear in the gestational sac normally (it is a sonographic diagnosis)?
- 4.5 weeks by TVS (18 mm gestational sac)
- 5.5 weeks by TAS (25 mm gestational sac).

8. How will you treat a patient diagnosed to have a blighted ovum?
If the duration of gestation is confirmed, termination of pregnancy is advised after counseling, otherwise a repeat USG scan should be done after a week.

9. How will you diagnose a case of threatened abortion?
Threatened abortion is the one where process has started but has not progressed to inevitable, so clinically patients will present with bleeding per vaginum, which is bright red in color, mild to moderate in amount with some degree of lower abdominal pain and backache. Bleeding precedes the pain. On examination, the general condition is good, external os is closed and uterus corresponds to the period of amenorrhea. It is important to subject the patient to USG for confirmation of cardiac activity.

10. What are the features of inevitable abortion? How will you treat it?
Continuous contraction and dilatation of cervix is associated with inevitable abortion. Sonographically, it shows gestational sac separated from decidua and in the process of expulsion.

According to weeks of gestation, measures are used to complete the process of expulsion.
- If <12 weeks:
  - Tab misoprostol 800 mcg per vaginally single dose
  - Dilation and evacuation (D and E)
- If >12 weeks:
  - Tab misoprostol 600 mcg per vaginally followed by 400 µg per vaginally 3 hourly maximum 5 doses
  - Oxytocin 10 units in 500 mL of NS, 40–60 drops/min.

If profuse bleeding is there but os closed, hysterectomy may have to be done (very rare).

11. Which is the most important prognostic factor on USG in threatened abortion?
Presence of fetal cardiac activity. It is associated in 98% cases with continuation of pregnancy.

12. What is incomplete and complete abortion?
- When a part of conceptus is left inside the uterus, it is known as incomplete variety. It is most commonly met with and is a dangerous entity as patient may present with shock due to continuous bleeding per vaginum.
  Clinical features of incomplete abortion:
  - Continuous pain
  - Bleeding P/V (at times, profused)
  - Patulous external os.
- Complete abortion—when whole of conceptus is expelled en masse with subsidence of pain and bleeding.

13. What are the sonographic criteria for missed abortion?

- Absence of cardiac activity
- Sac diameter 25 mm or more without a yolk sac/embryo (TAS)
- Sac diameter 18 mm or more without yolk sac/embryo (TVS).

14. What are the features of septic abortion?

- Increased temperature 100.4°F per 24 hours or more
- Offensive vaginal discharge
- Lower abdominal pain and tenderness.

15. What are the common organisms associated with septic abortion?

Mixed infection is common. Organisms associated are (a) Anaerobic: *Bacteroides* group, anaerobic streptococci, *Clostridium welchii, C. tetani, C. perfringens, C. sordellii*, (b) Aerobic-*Escherichia coli, Klebsiella, Staphylococcus* and *Pseudomonas*.

16. How is severity of septic abortion classified?

It is classified in grades. Mildest and most common being grade I-endomyometritis.

- *Grade I*—Infection limited to uterus.
- *Grade II*—Infection spreads beyond uterus involving parametria, tubes, ovaries and pelvic peritoneum.
- *Grade III*—Generalized peritonitis, endotoxic shock and acute renal failure.

17. What are the complications associated with septic abortion?

- Septicemia
- Hemorrhage
- Shock
- Bowel injuries
- Uterine perforation.

18. Indications of active surgery in septic abortion?

- Hemorrhage
- Presence of foreign body
- Intestinal injury
- Unresponsive peritonitis with collection of pus.

19. What are the basic investigations in any of the varieties of abortion?

- Complete blood count
- Serum quantitative β-hCG
- Rh factor determination
- Pelvic USG.

20. How can cervical trauma be minimized?

Preoperatively:
- Consider USG assessment of the gestational age
- Appropriate cervical preparation
- Prostaglandin analogue should preferably be used.

Intraoperatively:
- Grasp the cervix with two vulsellum/tenacula
- Use graduated dilators
- Dilate against appropriate countertraction.

Management of cervical tear:
- If small and not bleeding—no action
- If large amount of bleeding—hemostatic polyglactin sutures
- May require packing and admission for overnight observation.

21. What are the causes of first trimester abortions?

- Genetic abnormalities
- Luteal phase defect
- Thyroid deficiency
- Maternal diabetes
- Polycystic ovarian syndrome
- Autoimmunity.

22. What are the causes of second trimester abortions?

- Genetic abnormalities
- Antiphospholipid antibodies (APLA) syndrome
- Incompetent cervix
- Müllerian anomalies
- Inherited thrombophilias—protein C and S deficiency, factor V Leiden mutation.

23. What is habitual or recurrent pregnancy loss?

Three or more consecutive abortions before 20 weeks are known as recurrent pregnancy loss (RPL).

24. What causes are associated with recurrent pregnancy loss?

Etiology of RPL— is most often obscure.

- *Genetic:*
  - Parental—chromosomal abnormalities (3.5-5%) Most common—balanced translocation
  - Single gene defects
  - Multifactorial
- *Endocrine abnormalities (17-20%):*
  - Luteal phase defect/progesterone deficiency
  - Serum progesterone levels less than 15 ng/mL, indicate need for progesterone supplementation
  - Thyroid disorders
  - Diabetes
  - Increased androgen
  - Polycystic ovarian syndrome
  - Prolactin disorders
- *Immunological factors (20-50%):*
  - Antiphospholipid antibody (APLA) syndrome
  - Anticardiolipin antibody
  - Lupus anticoagulant
  - Antithyroid antibody

- Antitriphoblast antibody
- Blocking antibody deficiency
- Defective cellular immunity.

Alloimmune etiology is less common.

- *Anatomical causes (12–16%):*
    - Congenital
        i. Cervical incompetence
        ii. Müllerian abnormalities
        iii. Diethylstilbestrol exposure in uterus
    - Acquired
        i. Cervical incompetence
        ii. Uterine synechiae
        iii. Leiomyoma
        iv. Adenomyosis.
- *Infections (0.5–5%)*
- *Others:*
    - Adhesion molecule defects
    - Medical illness—cardiac, renal, hepatic
    - Smoking
    - Illicit drug abuse
    - Environmental toxins
    - Unknown reasons.

25. How will you proceed to investigate a case of RPL?

a. Valuable tests:
   - Anticardiolipin and lupus anticoagulant testing
   - Thyroid function tests (TFTs)
   - Platelet count
   - Hysteroscopy, hysterosalpingography
   - Parenteral peripheral blood karyotyping
   - Thrombophilia testing—factor V Leiden mutation, serum homocysteine, protein C and protein S

b. Tests with unproven/unknown utility:
   - Ovarian reserve testing
   - FSH, LH, serum androgen
   - Antithyroid antibody testing
   - Cellular immunity dysregulation testing
   - Cervical cultures

c. Tests with no utility:
   - Parental HLA
   - Mixed lymphocyte culture
   - Suppressor cell factor determination.

26. What is antiphospholipid antibody syndrome?

Antiphospholipid antibody syndrome (APLA) is defined using Sapporo criteria, presence of one or more clinical and laboratory criteria must be present.

Clinical:
- One or more episodes of confirmed vascular thrombosis–venous, arterial, small vessel
- Pregnancy complications:
    - 3 or more spontaneous pregnancy loss at <10 weeks
    - 1 or more fetal deaths >10 weeks
    - 1 or more preterm births at <34 weeks secondary to severe pre-eclampsia or placental insufficiency

Laboratory:
- Positive anticardiolipin antibodies (ACAs) at medium to high levels
- Positive lupus anticoagulant (LAC).

27. How will you manage a case of RPL with APLA syndrome?

Treatment of antiphospholipid antibody syndrome consists of prophylactic heparinization and low dose aspirin. For unfractionated heparin, the initial dose is 5000 units subcutaneous twice daily, and may be increased to 7500–10,000 units. Another choice is of low molecular weight heparin (LMWH) 40 mg subcutaneous twice daily. Low molecular weight heparin has advantage of reducing chances of heparin-induced thrombocytopenia and spontaneous bleeding episodes. The usual dose of aspirin is 60–80 mg orally daily.

28. What is the percentage of risk of abortion with increasing number of abortions?

No. of abortions	Subsequent risk (%)
0	15
1	19
2	35
3	47

29. What is cervical incompetence?

Cervical incompetence or insufficiency is a condition characterized by the inability of the cervix to retain a pregnancy in absence of uterine contractions.

30. What are the surgical options for the treatment of cervical incompetence?

Name the commonly used operations: Commonly used surgical procedures are Shirodkar and McDonald. Other surgical procedures—Lash and Lash, Page's procedure, Arias operations, Baden and Baden, Wurm procedure, Ritter and Ritter, etc.

31. What is the success rate of McDonalds vs Shirodkar operation?

Both varieties—80–90%.

32. Which one is preferred and why?

McDonalds, because it is technically easy.

33. When will you remove the stitch?

At 37 completed weeks of gestation or if patient goes in labor, whichever is earlier.

34. What is the optimal timing for circlage operations?

It should be done preferably in 2nd trimester at 14-16 weeks, two weeks prior to the wastage of previous pregnancy.

35. What are the contraindications of encirclage operation?

- IUD
- Congenitally abnormal fetus
- Bleeding P/V
- Intrauterine infections
- Uterine contraction
- Ruptured membranes
- Cervical dilatation >4 cm effacement >50%
- GA >32 weeks.

36. Discuss Medical Termination of Pregnancy Act (MTP Act, 1972).

In India MTP is legal up to 20 weeks of gestation and is governed by MTP Act, 1972. The law was revised in 1975; latest revision has been done in June 2003.

The following provisions are laid down:
- The continuation of pregnancy would result in serious risk of life or cause grave injury to physical or mental health of the pregnant woman
- There is substantial risk of the child being born with serious physical or mental abnormalities so as to be handicapped for life
- When the pregnancy is caused by rape, both in minor and major girls and in mentally imbalanced women
- Pregnancy caused as a result of failure of contraception. The law recommends that MTP should be done only by a registered medical practitioner, in government hospitals/hospitals approved by government, only after written consent of woman and only up to 20 weeks.

The abortion is to be kept confidential and reported only to the Directorate Health Services (DHS) of State.

A registered medical practitioner should have:
- Diploma or degree qualification in obstetrics and gynecology, or
- 6 months house officer training in obstetrics and gynecology, or
- Having certificate of assisting 25 MTP at registered center.

Opinion of 2nd Registered Medical Practitioner (RMP) is required for second trimester pregnancy termination (12-20 weeks).

37. What are the different forms used under MTP Act?

- *Form A:* Form of application for approval of MTP center
- *Form B:* Certificate of approval
- *Form C:* Consent form
- *Form I:* Opinion form for second trimester MTPs
- *Form II:* Monthly report form
- *Form III:* Admission register.

38. What are the investigations recommended prior to performing MTP?

- Hemoglobin
- Urine—albumin, sugar
- ABO and Rh type
- USG—optional.

39. What are the different methods of termination of pregnancy?

First trimester MTP	Second trimester MTP (< 20 weeks)
Manual vacuum aspiration (MVA)	Dilatation and evacuation (13-14 weeks)
Suction and evacuation/curettage	Extra-amniotic instillation of ethacridine lactate
Medical methods (Mifepristone 200 mg + Misoprostol 800 µg up to 9 weeks)	Prostaglandins PGE_1 (misoprostol) PGF_2-alpha, PGE_2 (not approved in India)
	Hysterotomy

40. Discuss Preconception and Prenatal Diagnostic Techniques Act, 1994.

- The Preconception and Prenatal Diagnostic Techniques (Prohibition of Sex Selection) Act (PCPNDT) was passed in 1994 and amended in 2002
- It prohibits the use of preconception and prenatal techniques for sex determination and sex selection
- While prenatal diagnostic tests like ultrasound or amniocentesis can be used for purposes defined under the Act; to reveal the sex of the fetus is illegal
- Act defines the conduct and codes while performing procedures, which have ability to reveal the sex of fetus
- Imaging center/genetic center needs approval by district appropriate authority
- All records are preserved for period of 3 years
- Information is to be sent to district appropriate authorities prior to 5th of every month
- Offences under the Act are cognizable, nonbailable and noncompoundable.

MUST REMEMBER

- Ten to twenty percent of all pregnancies end up in abortion.
- Chromosomal abnormalities in the conceptus are the most common cause.
- Septic abortion still continues to be associated with 7% of all maternal deaths in India.
- Endocrine abnormalities and anatomical abnormalities contribute to bulk of RPL, which are usually correctable.
- Cervical encirclage procedure has proven role in women with incompetent cervix.
- Legalizing MTP has helped us to curb the maternal morbidity and mortality associated with illegal abortions.
- PCPNDT Act governs the use of preconception and prenatal diagnostic techniques.

Pregnancy-induced Hypertension

Shrinivas Gadappa

1. What are salient features in history taking in patient of hypertensive disorders in pregnancy?

The important facts must to be included in all cases of hypertensive disorders in pregnancy are following:

Mrs. _____ a _____ years old lady, married for _____ residing at _____ GPA with _____ months amenorrhea presents with a complaint of edema feet, face, fingers (specify the site) for ___ days. Her LMP was on _____ EDD is on _____ her past cycles were every 28 days.

- No history suggestive of heart disease
- No history suggestive of liver disease
- No history suggestive of deep vein thrombosis
- No history suggestive of renal disease
- No history suggestive of chronic hypertension
- History of headache, visual disturbances, auditory disturbances, epigastric pain (suggestive of severe pregnancy-induced hypertension and impending eclampsia)
- History of pregnancy induced hypertension in mother of the patient (inherited as an autosomal recessive trait)
- History of suggestive of diabetes mellitus (predisposing factor)
- History of excessive enlargement of the uterus, suggestive of multiple pregnancies/molar pregnancy
- History of pregnancy induced hypertension in past pregnancy
- History of diminished fetal movements (suggestive of fetal compromise).

Examination

General examination is done as usual, with stress on the distribution and severity of edema, presence of pallor and its severity, and icterus, if any. The blood pressure is checked in right upper limb in 15° lateral position and sitting posture. The mean arterial pressure is calculated by using the formula:

$$\text{Mean arterial pressure} = \frac{\text{Systolic pressure} + 2 \times \text{diastolic pressure}}{3}$$

Obstetric examination is done as usual. Special attention is given to the number of fetuses present and evidence of intrauterine growth retardation.

Calculation

Symphisofundal height (SFH), abdominal girth, height and weight of the patient, Ponderal index.

Investigations

- Hemoglobin
- Blood group, VDRL, HIV
- *Urine analysis:* Albuminuria, glycosuria, evidence of chronic renal disease
- *Renal chemistry:* Blood urea nitrogen, serum creatinine, serum electrolytes serum uric acid (more than 4 mg/dL is suggestive of poor prognostic value, the fetal prognosis being inversely related to the level of uric acid)
- *Fundoscopy:* To be repeated every week (for evidence of chronic hypertension as well as to grade the changes due to pregnancy-induced hypertension)
- Platelet count
- Serum fibrinogen, fibrinogen-fibrin degradation products (to detect chronic intravascular coagulation)
- Investigations to detect fetal growth retardation
- Investigations to assess fetal well-being.

2. How are hypertensive disorders in pregnancy classified?

In 2000, the National High Blood Pressure Education Program Working Group revised the classification system for this set of conditions. Four categories are now recognized for hypertension in pregnancy: (1) Chronic hypertension (2) Gestational hypertension (3) Pre-eclampsia and eclampsia and (4) Chronic hypertension with superimposed pre-eclampsia.

3. Define gestational hypertension.

Gestational hypertension is defined as per following criteria:

- BP > 140/90 mm Hg without proteinuria for first time during pregnancy.
- BP returns to normal within 12 weeks of postpartum. Final diagnosis made only postpartum. May have other signs or symptoms of pre-eclampsia; for example, epigastric discomfort or thrombocytopenia.

4. Who are prehypertensives?
Individuals with systolic blood pressure 120–139 mm Hg or diastolic 80–89 mm Hg are considered as prehypertensives.

5. How is chronic hypertension defined?
BP >140/90 mm Hg before pregnancy or diagnosed before 20 weeks gestation not attributable to gestational trophoblastic disease.
or
Hypertension first diagnosed after 20 weeks gestation and persistent after 12 weeks postpartum is defined as chronic hypertension.

6. Are women with chronic hypertension considered high-risk pregnancies?
Yes. Because of poor placental vascular development and ongoing elevations of blood pressure, the pregnancy is at risk for intrauterine growth restriction, abruption and stillbirth. From a maternal perspective, the patient may develop superimposed pre-eclampsia and all of the associated consequences.

7. How will you define superimposed pre-eclampsia on chronic hypertension?
New onset proteinuria >300 mg/24 hours in hypertensive women without proteinuria before 20 weeks of gestation.

A sudden increase in proteinuria or blood pressure or platelet count <100,000/mm³ in women with hypertension and proteinuria before 20 weeks' gestation is defined as superimposed pre-eclampsia on chronic hypertension.

8. What is the definition of pre-eclampsia?
Pre-eclampsia is defined by hypertension and proteinuria. For women who do not have chronic hypertension, an elevation of BP above 140 mm Hg systolic or 90 mm Hg diastolic meets the criteria. Proteinuria is defined as more than 300 mg of protein in a 24-hour urine collection.

9. What are the amendments made in new definition of pre-eclampsia?
In the past, an increase in blood pressure above baseline (a 30 mm Hg increase in systolic BP or a 15 mm Hg increase in diastolic BP) also met the blood pressure definition of pre-eclampsia, but this relative definition has been discarded in favor of the absolute definition of 140 mm Hg systolic BP or 90 mm Hg diastolic BP Proteinuria is technically defined by the outcome of a 24-hour urine collection. In practice, however, the consistent presence of more than trace protein on urine dipstick correlates well with proteinuria of 300 mg in 24 hours. Therefore, the diagnosis is commonly made without a formal 24 hours evaluation.

10. How often does pre-eclampsia occur? Which women are at greater risk?
Pre-eclampsia occurs in 6–8% of all live births. Risk factors include nulliparity, extremes of reproductive age (<15 and >35 years of age), history of pre-eclampsia in a first-degree female relative, history of pre-eclampsia in a prior pregnancy, diabetes, chronic vascular or renal disease, chronic hypertension and multiple gestation.

11. Do we know what causes pre-eclampsia?
No. Pre-eclampsia has been described since the time of the ancient Greeks. However, the cause remains unknown. We know that hypertension, proteinuria, and the other signs and symptoms of the illness are merely the outward manifestations of a systemic illness characterized by vasoconstriction and hypovolemia. All organs, including the fetoplacental unit show evidence of poor perfusion.

12. What are some of the theories of the cause of pre-eclampsia?
Immunologic response: Inappropriate maternal antibody response to the fetal allograft results in vascular damage from the circulating immune complexes. This theory is supported by an increased prevalence of the disease in pregnancies with limited prior antigen exposure (young nulliparas) and in situations with increased fetal antigen (twins, molar pregnancy, hydropic pregnancies, and diabetics with large placentas). Actual measurement of immune complexes has been inconsistent.

Circulating toxins: Vasoconstrictive substances reportedly have been extracted from blood, amniotic fluid, and the placenta in women with pre-eclampsia. Symptoms have been reproduced in some but not all animal studies.

Endogenous vasoconstrictors: Increased sensitivity to vasopressin, epinephrine and norepinephrine has been reported. Loss of normal third-trimester resistance to angiotensin II has also been noted.

Endothelial damage: Primary endothelial damage results in a decrease in prostacyclin production (potent vasodilator) and a relative increase in thromboxane A2 (relative vasoconstrictor). Low-dose heparin or low dose aspirin may play a role in prevention, but the cause of the endothelial damage, and prostaglandin change is unclear.

Primary disseminated intravascular coagulation: Microvascular thrombin formation and deposition have been noted, producing vessel damage especially in the kidney and in the placenta.

Abnormal trophoblastic invasion of uterine vessels.

Dietary deficiency: Genetic factor—HLA DRW4–Maternal maladaptation to cardiovascular or inflammatory changes of normal pregnancy.

13. How is pre-eclampsia classified? What are the implications of the classification?

Pre-eclampsia is classified as mild and severe. Any of the following parameters classify a woman's pre-eclampsia as severe:
- Systolic blood pressure >160 mm Hg or diastolic blood pressure >110 mm Hg on two occasions at least 6 hours apart
- Proteinuria >5 g/24 hours
- Oliguria <500 cc/24 hours
- Cerebral or visual symptoms
- Epigastric or right upper quadrant pain
- Low platelets
- Elevated serum creatinine
- Elevated liver function tests
- Fetal growth restriction
- Pulmonary edema or cyanosis.

The definition of mild pre-eclampsia is any pre-eclampsia that is not considered severe. There is no category of moderate pre-eclampsia.

The classification of severity is directly related to management and the decision about when to deliver the baby.

14. Enumerate the predictive tests for pre-eclampsia.

Currently there are no screening tests for pre-eclampsia that are reliable, valid and economical. Few selected tests are enumerated below:
1. Roll over test (Gant and colleagues 1974). Predictive value (true positive) 33%.
2. *Uric acid:* Elevated uric acid levels >5.9 mg/dL at 24 weeks: Positive predictive value 33%.
3. *Fibronectin:* Elevated serum cellular fibronectin at 12 weeks. Positive predictive value 29%, negative predictive value 98%.
4. *Coagulation activation ratio of plasminogen activator inhibitor-1 (PAI-1):* PAI-2 is predictive (Chappell, 2002).
5. Oxidative stress increases levels of malondialdehyde, increased levels of homocystine.
6. *Cytokines:* Over 50 cytokines are present of these, few are elevated in pre-eclampsia which include—interleukins, tumor necrosis factor-α (TNF-α).
7. *Placental peptides:* Elevated levels of soluble fms–like tyrosine kinase 1 (sFlt1).
8. *Fetal DNA:* Fetal DNA in maternal serum.
9. *Uterine artery Doppler velocimetry:* Evaluation at 12–18 weeks.
   Sensitivity for prediction is 78%.
   Positive predictive value is 28%.

Combined with inhibin A and activin A the predicative value is 86% if both are abnormal and 17% if both are unaltered.

15. What fetal and maternal risks are associated with pre-eclampsia?

Fetal risks include:
- Growth restriction
- Oligohydramnios
- Placental infarction
- Placental abruption
- Consequences of prematurity (when maternal disease necessitates delivery remote from term)
- Perinatal death.

Maternal risks include:
- Central nervous system manifestations, including seizures and stroke
- Disseminated intravascular coagulation (DIC) and its complications
- Increased likelihood of cesarean delivery
- Renal failure
- Hepatic failure or rupture
- Death.

16. What are the basic management objectives for pregnancy complicated by pre-eclampsia?

Basic management objectives are:
- Termination of pregnancy with least possible trauma to the mother and the fetus
- Birth of the infant who subsequent thrives
- Complete restoration of health of the mother.

17. How will you monitor the patients of hypertension after hospitalization?

A systematic evaluation is instituted which includes the following:
- Detailed examination followed by daily scrutiny for clinical findings, such as headache, visual disturbances, epigastric pain and rapid weight gain
- Blood pressure reading in sitting position every 4 hours, except between midnight and morning
- Measurement of proteinuria daily, at least every 2 days
- Daily weight record
- Measurement of serum creatinine, hematocrit, platelets and serum liver enzymes, the frequency to be determined by the severity of hypertension
- Fetal growth and amniotic fluid index (AFI), Doppler if required.

18. Describe the management of pre-eclampsia.

Delivery of the fetus "cures" pre-eclampsia. With delivery, signs and symptoms of pre-eclampsia resolve, although the time required for resolution is variable. The difficulty in therapy is deciding when to deliver the baby.

Traditionally, all term pregnancies with pre-eclampsia—mild or severe—were delivered. For preterm pregnancies, those with severe disease were delivered and those with mild disease were managed conservatively with bed rest, antihypertensives and close fetal and maternal surveillance.

Recently, there have been efforts to extend preterm pregnancies complicated by severe pre-eclampsia rather than proceeding with immediate delivery. Administration of a short course (48 hours) of steroids to the mother confers significant benefit to premature newborns. Therefore, if pre-eclampsia develops before 32 weeks, even a short period of conservative management prior to delivery may be beneficial. Conservative management of severe pre-eclampsia, in order to gain greater fetal maturity, should only be attempted in carefully selected patients and should be managed by experienced obstetrician. These women should be hospitalized and must be observed closely for signs of worsening maternal disease or evidence of fetal compromise.

Obviously, at-term the decision is easy to make, whether the pre-eclampsia is mild or severe. The difficulty arises when pre-eclampsia is remote from term. The degree of severity and the fetal gestational age are taken into consideration, and either the patient is delivered or is placed at bed rest. With bed rest therapy, close maternal and fetal surveillance is performed until the pregnancy reaches term or the degree of severity worsens, dictating the need to deliver.

19. What is the role of expectant management in severe pre-eclampsia?

Women with severe PIH are usually delivered without delay. This approach advocates conservative or "expectant" management in selected group of women with the aim of improving infant outcome without compromising safety of mother. Expectant management includes treatment with labetolol, nifedipine and $MgSO_4$, with vigilant monitoring. Indications for delivery include uncontrollable BP, fetal distress, placental abruption, renal function deterioration, HELLP syndrome, persistent severe symptoms or an attainment of 34 weeks of gestation. Average pregnancy prolongation in different studies were 8–15 days with neonatal morbidity and few maternal complications; no maternal death. This expectant management has to be thought twice before implementing, should be strictly in expert judicial high tech institutes with 24 hours emergency services available.

20. How should delivery be accomplished in patients with pre-eclampsia?

There is no advantage of cesarean delivery over vaginal delivery for pre-eclampsia. Therefore, delivery route should be based on obstetric indications. An indication for cesarean section may be the inability to accomplish a vaginal delivery within a fixed, specified time, governed by maternal condition.

21. What is home healthcare in pre-eclampsia?

Further hospitalization is not warranted if hypertension abates within few days. Most women with mild hypertension without proteinuria are managed at home. These women should be instructed in detail about reporting symptoms. Home blood pressure and urine protein monitoring and frequent evaluation by a visiting nurse are mandatory, commonly practiced in well, intelligent groups.

22. What are the predictors for declining/worsening maternal well-being and fetal well-being?

Indicators for declining maternal well-being are:
- Increased BP
- Worsening symptoms (i.e. WS)
- Hemoconcentration (increased creatinine, urea, uric acid)
- Increasing proteinuria
- Worsening of disseminated intravascular coagulation (DIC) profile.

Indicators of declining fetal well-being are:
- Nonreactive nonstress test (NST)
- Positive contraction stress test
- Declining biophysical profile (BPP)
- Serial USG shows growth parameter slowing or arrest of growth
- Decreased fetal movement.

23. What is the role of antihypertensives in pre-eclampsia?

Mild elevations in blood pressure usually are not treated with antihypertensive. With more marked elevations (diastolic >110 mm Hg or a mean arterial pressure >125 mm Hg), medications with rapid onset, such as hydralazine and labetalol, are used intravenously (generally such management is undertaken while also proceeding with delivery, due to the severity of the disease).

Diuretics are generally not used as first-line treatment because pre-eclampsia is characterized by vasoconstriction and intravascular depletion, which are worsened by diuretics. As for other antihypertensive agents, work has shown that treatment of patients with mild-to-moderate hypertension (i.e. 90–110 mm Hg diastolic pressure) does not decrease perinatal morbidity or mortality. Therefore, antihypertensive therapy is not usually used. In severe hypertension (>110 mm Hg diastolic pressure), alpha methyl dopa 1–2 g/day, nifedepin 10 mg tid, max dose of 120 mg. Labetalol 100 mg bid is used. Maximum dose is 300 mg in 24 hours. More than likely, delivery needs to be undertaken in this circumstance, and rapid-acting antihypertensive agents (i.e. intravenous hydralazine or labetalol) are used to control severe hypertension during labor.

In a patient with known chronic hypertension whose elevated blood pressure is believed to be due to underlying disease rather than pre-eclampsia, an increase in antihypertensive therapy may be appropriate.

24. What is the role of labetalol in treatment of pre-eclampsia?

Women on labetalol have significantly lower MAP. But there is no difference between two groups in the form of prolongation of pregnancy and gestational age at birth. However, incidence of growth restriction is twice in labetalol group compared to other antihypertensive agents. It is a good drug to control acute hypertensive crisis.

25. How will you start seizure prophylaxis in severe pre-eclampsia?

Prevention of seizures done by following regimen are as follows: *Pritchard regimen* 4 g $MgSO_4$ as a 20% solution intravenously at a rate not to exceed 1 g/min.

Followed promptly with 10 g of 50% $MgSO_4$ one-half (5 g) injected deeply in upper outer quadrant of both buttocks through a 3 inch long, 20 gauge needle.

Every 4 hours thereafter 5 g of 50% solution of $MgSO_4$ injected deeply in upper outer quadrant of alternate buttock but after careful monitoring. Zuspan regimen, 4 to 6 g $MgSO_4$ IV bolus slowly followed by 2 g/hour maintenance for 24 hours after delivery after ensuring that:
- Patellar reflex present
- Respiratory rate >14/min
- Urine output > 30 mL/hours or 100 mL in 4 hours.

26. Should all women with gestational hypertension or pre-eclampsia be treated with $MgSO_4$ for seizure prophylaxis?

The purpose of $MgSO_4$ is to reduce the likelihood of seizures. Seizures occur less frequently in women with gestational hypertension and mild pre-eclampsia compared to women with more severe disease. In addition, like any medication, $MgSO_4$ can have side effects, the most significant of which is respiratory compromise due to respiratory suppression and pulmonary edema. Because of this risk and given the lower risk of seizures in women with mild disease, many clinicians reserve anticonvulsive prophylaxis for women with severe pre-eclampsia, HELLP syndrome, or eclampsia.

27. What are the serum magnesium levels and their effects?

Dose	Effect
5–8 mg/dL	Therapeutic level
10 mg/dL	Loss of DTR
15 mg/dL	Respiratory paralysis
25 mg/dL	Cardiac arrest

Intravenous calcium gluconate is the antidote for $MgSO_4$ toxicity.

28. Is there a way to prevent pre-eclampsia?

Numerous interventions have been attempted. Dietary manipulation with decreased sodium intake or increased calcium intake and pharmacologic therapy with prophylactic low-dose aspirin have been extensively studied with randomized controlled trials. Unfortunately neither of these interventions have been able to reduce the incidence of pre-eclampsia.

29. Does pre-eclampsia recur in subsequent pregnancies?

Yes. If pre-eclampsia occurs in the first pregnancy there is a 25% chance of recurrence in subsequent pregnancies. The recurrence rate appears to be affected by gestational age at onset in the first pregnancy, severity, underlying maternal diseases and underlying obstetric diseases. Women who develop pre-eclampsia early in pregnancy, or who develop severe pre-eclampsia, those with chronic medical conditions (e.g. chronic hypertension, renal disease) and those with no apparent fetal contribution (such as fetal aneuploidy) are at greater risk to develop pre-eclampsia in the future.

Multiparous patients who have had pre-eclampsia have a recurrence rate of up to 50% in subsent pregnancies.

30. Can women with a pregnancy complicated by pre-eclampsia take birth control pills after delivery?

Yes. pre-eclampsia, especially in a primiparous patient, does not contraindicate the use of oral contraceptives after delivery.

31. How will you define eclampsia?

Seizures that cannot be attributed to other causes in women with pre-eclampsia is defined as eclampsia.

32. What is the management of a patient during convulsion?

Management during convulsion:
- In the premonitory stage, a mouth gag is placed in between the teeth to prevent tongue bite and should be removed after the clonic phase is over
- The air passage is to be cleared off the mucus with a mucus sucker. The patient's head is to be turned to one

side and the pillow is taken off. Raising the footend of the bed facilitates postural drainage of the upper respiratory tract
- Oxygen is given until cyanosis disappears
- Institution of anticonvulsants and other medication.

33. How is delivery accomplished in eclamptic patients?

As with pre-eclampsia, obstetric indications are used to determine route of delivery. It is not unusual to encounter evidence of fetal compromise in eclamptic patients, but this is not necessarily an indication for cesarean delivery. In general, fetal resuscitation is best accomplished *in utero* by controlling the maternal state. Stabilizing the patient (i.e. airway, oxygen, circulation and control of seizure activity) improves fetal status and subsently neonatal outcome. Labor can then be initiated and vaginal delivery accomplished, assuming no obstetric indications for a cesarean delivery.

34. Is MgSO$_4$ used for eclamptic patients?

In the past, there have been advocates for other agents, particularly phenytoin. However, a randomized controlled trial in women with eclampsia clearly favored MgSO$_4$ over phenytoin for recurrent seizure prophylaxis.

35. What is HELLP syndrome?

HELLP is an acronym for a syndrome of hemolysis, elevated liver function tests and/or low platelets. HELLP syndrome is thought to be a subcategory of severe pre-eclampsia. Patients may or may not have other signs of pre-eclampsia. HELLP syndrome often has a rapidly decelerating downhill course. Most clinicians deliver infants expeditiously regardless of the gestational age.

36. What are the causes of midepigastric pain in HELLP syndrome?

Liver capsule distention produces midepigastric pain, often with associated nausea and vomiting. Liver capsule distention can lead to hepatic rupture with poor maternal and fetal outcome.

37. What are the Eden's prognostic criteria of eclampsia?

Immediate: Once the convulsion occurs, the prognosis becomes uncertain. Prognosis depends on many factors and the ominous features are:
- Long interval between the onset of fit and commencement of treatment (late referral)
- Antepartum eclampsia specially with long delivery interval
- Number of fits more than 10
- Coma in between fits
- Temperature over 102°F with pulse rate above 120/minute
- Blood pressure over 200 mm Hg systolic
- Oliguria (<400 mL/24 hours) with proteinuria >5 g/24 hours
- Non-response to treatment
- Jaundice.

38. What are the criteria for diagnosis of aggressive inpatient management?

Aggressive inpatient management includes:

Diagnostic criteria
- Mild or severe pre-eclampsia >37 weeks' gestation
- Severe pre-eclampsia <26 weeks' gestation
- Severe pre-eclampsia 26–34 weeks' gestation, when associated with maternal jeopardy:
  – Severe persistent headache
  – Persistent visual changes
  – Hepatocellular injury
  – Thrombocytopenia or other evidence of DIC
  – Pulmonary edema
  – Abruptio placentae.
- Severe pre-eclampsia 26–34 weeks' gestation, when associated with fetal jeopardy:
  – Repetitive severe variable decelerations
  – Repetitive late decelerations
  – Repetitive BPP <4
  – Oligohydramnios [amniotic fluid index (AFI) <4 cm]
  – IUGR (estimated fetal weight < fifth percentile)
- Chronic hypertension with superimposed pre-eclampsia at any gestational age
- Eclampsia or HELLP syndrome at any gestational age.

39. What are the guidelines for aggressive inpatient management?

Guidelines:
- Maintenance of diastolic BP between 90 and 100 mm Hg. Further reduction of BP jeopardizes placental blood flow. Appropriate antihypertensive medications include:
  – Hydralazine (direct arteriolar vasodilator), which causes baroreceptor sympathetic stimulation [increasing heart rate (HR) and cardiac output (CO)], thus preserving placental blood flow
  – Labetalol (nonselective β-blocker), which preserves uteroplacental blood flow.
- Prevention of convulsions with intravenous (IV) magnesium sulfate:
  – Administration of loading dose of 5 g IV over 20 minutes, and maintenance infusion at 2 g/hour. The maintenance IV infusion should be given for 24 hours after delivery.

- Watching for clinical evidence of magnesium toxicity
- Absence of toxicity is ensured as long as deep tendon reflexes are obtainable
- Intravenous calcium gluconate is the antidote for magnesium toxicity
- *Initiation of labor:* Labor can be induced anticipating vaginal delivery if the patient is stable and there are no contraindications. Otherwise, cesarean delivery is indicated.

40. What are the diagnostic criteria and treatment modality for conservative inpatient management?

Conservative inpatient management is appropriate in the following cases:
- Mild pre-eclampsia that is remote from term (<37 weeks).
  Guidelines include:
  - Monitoring BP every 4 hours
  - Performing a daily urine dipstick for protein
  - Performing twice-weekly 24 hour urine protein measurements
  - Performing weekly liver function tests and electrolyte levels
  - Initiating delivery if criteria for severe pre-eclampsia are met.
- Severe pre-eclampsia in carefully selected cases.
  - All of the following criteria must be met:
    - Gestational age > 26 weeks but <34 weeks
    - BP persistently >160/110 mm Hg
    - Absence of fetal jeopardy
    - Absence of maternal jeopardy.
  - Guidelines include:
    - Intensive maternal and fetal monitoring in a tertiary perinatal center
    - Cautious volume expansion
    - Aggressive antihypertensive therapy (e.g. hydralazine, labetalol)
    - Anticonvulsant therapy (e.g. magnesium sulfate)
    - Corticosteroids to enhance fetal lung maturity
  - Initiation of delivery if maternal or fetal deterioration occurs.

41. What are the diagnostic criteria and treatment modality for conservative outpatient management?

Diagnostic criteria and treatment modality for conservative outpatient management.
- Patient selection criteria:
  - Transient hypertension (i.e. BP in the mildly elevated range, no proteinuria)
  - Uncomplicated chronic hypertension (without superimposed pre-eclampsia).
- Guidelines include:
  - Bed rest in the left lateral position
  - Home BP monitoring
  - Twice-weekly outpatient visits
  - Initiation of delivery if maternal or fetal deterioration occurs.

42. What are the causes of maternal deaths in eclampsia?

Causes of maternal death are:
- Cardiac failure
- Pulmonary edema
- Aspiration and/or septic pneumonia
- Cerebral hemorrhage
- Anuria
- Pulmonary embolism
- Postpartum shock
- Puerperal sepsis.

43. What are the causes of perinatal mortality in eclampsia?

Fetal: The perinatal mortality is very high to the extent of about 30–50%.

The causes are:
- Prematurity—Spontaneous or induced
- Intrauterine asphyxia due to placental insufficiency arising out of infraction, retroplacental hemorrhage and spasm of uteroplacental vasculature
- Effects of the drugs used to control convulsions
- Trauma during operative delivery.

44. Does pre-eclampsia have risk of hypertension in later life?

No pre-eclampsia does not increase the risk of hypertension later in life. An exception may be women who have recurrent pre-eclampsia, which may suggest unrecognized chronic hypertension or other underlying maternal diseases.

45. Case Study

For each of the following cases, select the most appropriate management option.

Case 1: A 38-year-old woman primi gravida presents for a routine visit at 39 weeks gestation. Blood pressure is noted to be persistently 140/90 mm Hg, and urine protein is +2. She is completely asymptomatic and her physical examination is otherwise unremarkable. Cervix is 2 cm dilated, 90% effaced, with the fetal vertex at 0 station.

Case 2: A 25-year-old woman 2nd gravida, presents at 33 week's gestation for a routine visit. In the office, her blood pressure is noted to be 150/100 mm Hg, and urine protein + 3. She is otherwise asymptomatic.

Options:
a. Immediate cesarean section
b. Induction of labor

c. Admission to hospital for observation
d. Outpatient observation.

Ans. The answers are Case 1-b, Case 2-c.

The first patient has a diagnosis of mild pregnancy-induced hypertension (PIH) at term. Because she does have proteinuria, she may be further classified as pre-eclampsia, she may be further classified as pre-eclamptic. The indicated treatment of PIH of any severity at term is delivery. Because her cervix is favorable, induction of labor is the preferred method of delivery. Induction can be started with intravenous oxytocin, and parenteral magnesium sulfate should be used for seizure prophylaxis.

The second patient presents with a more difficult problem, because she is preterm. She appears to have PIH on examination, but does not at this point meet criteria for severe disease. With mild disease in a preterm patient, observation and evaluation for severe disease is indicated. Because of the serious complications that can occur, the patient is best managed in the hospital until sufficient evaluation to exclude severe PIH is completed. If further evaluation reveals severe disease, delivery is indicated.

46. What is two stage disorder in pre-eclampsia?

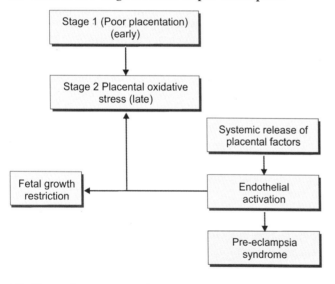

47. Describe systemic changes seen in pre-eclampsia.
- CVS—Increase afterload
  Cardiac preload affected by diminished hypervolemia of pregnancy. Endothelial activation with extravasation of intravascular fluid into ECF.
- Hemodynamic—hemoconcentration
- Coagulation—thrombocytopenia
  HELLP syndrome
- Endocrine—less rise in level of rennin, angiotensin, aldosterone as compared to that in normal pregnancy.
- Renal — Increased urinary sodium
  - Mild increase in GFR
  - Increase in serum uric acid
  - Hepatic – increase AST/ALT
- CNS—PRES, retinopathy, cerebral edema.

48. What is definitive management of eclampsia?
- Control of convulsions usilng $MgSO_4$
- Control of hypertension
- Delivery of fetus.

49. What is Magpie trial?

It is the largest multicentric study for prevention of elcampsia using $MgSO_4$. The study proved that women with pre-eclampsia given $MgSO_4$ had 58% lower risk of developing eclampsia than placebo.

50. What is PRES syndrome?

Posterior reversible encephalopathy syndrome (PRES), also known as reversible posterior leukoencephalopathy syndrome (RPLS), is a syndrome characterized by headache, confusion, seizures and visual loss. It may occur due to a number of causes, predominantly malignant hypertension, eclampsia and some medical treatments. On magnetic resonance imaging (MRI) of the brain, areas of edema (swelling) are seen. The symptoms tend to resolve after a period of time, although visual changes sometimes remain. It was first described in 1996.

51. What are the predictors of PIH?
- *VEGF, sFlt-1, sVEGFR-2, sEng PIFG:* Elevated levels in maternal serum are seen five weeks before clinical symptoms appeared. Low levels of free PIGF have been reported in the 1st and 2nd trimesters in women developing pre-eclampsia
- PAPP-A is a IGFBP protease, maternal serum PAPP-A was measured between 11 and 13 weeks' gestation, as part of the first trimester screening of aneuploidies. PAPP-A multiples of gestation specific median (MoM) value <0.8 predict PIH
- *Placental protein 13:* It is expressed as MoM (multiples of gestation specific median) PP13 is measured using sandwich based ELISA. In PIH:
  - low multiples of gestation specific median (MoM) in 6–10 weeks of gestation
  - high multiples of gestation specific median (MoM) in 16 to 20 weeks of gestation PP13 is useful in detecting preterm pre-eclampsia between 11 and 14 weeks of gestation, maternal plasma concentrations of PTX3 were higher in women who subsequently developed pre-eclampsia

- Reduced levels of IGF-1 and IGFBP-1 during the late 1st trimester predict PE.
- Inhibin A and activin A are glycoproteins belonging to the growth factor superfamily and are localized in cyto- and syncytotrophoblast. They regulate synthesis of hCG and steroids. Elevated levels have been reported both in the 1st and 2nd trimesters, but with quite moderate sensitivities for other than early onset PE
- Increased level of cytokine receptor for IL-2 in the 1st trimester
- Neurokinin B is increased in PE pregnancies already in 9-13 weeks of gestation
- *Cell-free circulating DNA:* Using PCR free DNA levels in the serum can be detected. In PIH there is increase in free DNA levels because of increase in apoptosis of cytotrophoblasts
- In PE, PA1-1 is increased because of endothelial dysfunction
- Fibronectins are released from endothelial cells and ECM in response to endothelial injury
- Hyperhomocysteinemia causes oxidative stress and endothelial injury. Increased levels of homocystein 3-4 fold in mid-trimester is an indicator of PE.

Renal function tests:
Serum uric acid— > 5.59 mg/dL at 24 weeks.

Microalbuminuria
- Sensitivity—7-90%
- Specificity—29-97%.

Urinary calcium
Urinary calcium levels less than 12 mg/dL in 24 hours.

Ratio of urine calcium: creatinine
- Normotensive = 0.44
- Chronic hypertension = 0.2
- Pre-eclampsia = 0.03.

MUST REMEMBER
- Korotkoff 5 sound is used to determine diastolic blood pressure.
- To establish diagnosis of chronic HT—it is necessary to document HT before pregnancy or before 20 weeks GA.
- Most frequent hemodynamic finding in pre-eclampsia—increase peripheral vascular resistance.
- Characteristic renal lesion in pre-eclampsia—glomerular endotheliosis.
- Combination of prazosin and diuretic is extremely effective for HT resistant to other drugs.
- Contrary to other beta blockers—labetalol decreased BP by decrease PVR with little change in cardiac output. The main indication of Labetalol is to rapidly decrease BP in patients with severe pre-eclampsia.
- In selected patients with severe pre-eclampsia between 24 and 34 weeks delivery may be postponed for 48-72 hours for the purpose of giving maternal steroids to prevent neonatal RDS and IVH.
- The most common cause of maternal death in eclampsia are intracranial bleeding and acute renal failure.
- The most common cause of fetal death in eclampsia—prematurity and fetal asphyxia.

Antepartum Hemorrhage

Kanan Yelikar, Sonali Deshpande

Hemorrhage is the most common cause of maternal mortality in India. Common causes of antepartum hemorrhage (APH) are placenta previa and abruption placenta. Adequate fluid replacement and blood transfusion in time will help to reduce maternal mortality.

1. What is APH?

Antepartum hemorrhage is defined as any bleeding from and into the female genital tract between fetal viability (28 weeks) and delivery of the fetus.

2. What is perinatal death?

Perinatal death is late fetal and early neonatal death.

3. What is the incidence of APH?

Two to five percent is the incidence of APH.

4. What are the causes of APH?

- Placenta previa 31%
- Abruptio placenta 22%
- Undetermined 47%.

5. Define placenta previa.

Placenta that is implanted entirely or in part in the lower uterine segment.

6. What are the different types of placenta previa?

- Major (Type 2 posterior 3 and 4)
- Minor (Type 1 and 2 anterior).

Type	Description
Low lying placenta previa	Placenta is in the lower uterine segment but the lower edge does not reach the internal OS (Stops short by 3 cm)
Marginal placenta previa	Lower edge of the placenta reaches internal OS but does not cover it
Partial placenta previa	Placenta covers the internal OS asymmetrically
Total placenta previa	Placenta covers the cervix (OS) symmetrically

7. What are the etiological factors of placenta previa?

- Damage to the endometrium or the myometrium predisposes a low implantation and subsequent development of placenta previa, e.g. previous uterine surgery or uterine infection
- Increased risk of placenta previa 1.2% after one or more lower segment cesarean section (LSCS) as compared with nonscared uterus
- Abnormal fetal presentation and congenital malformations are strongly associated with placenta previa
- Increasing maternal age, parity multiple gestation, anemia, closely associated with placenta previa.

8. What are the theories to explain placenta previa?

- Drooping down theory—Fertilized ovum drops and is implanted in the lower segment may be the cause
- Persistence of chorionic activity in the decidua capsularis
- Defective decidua
- Big surface of placenta

9. What is the clinical presentation of placenta previa?

The two classical presentation of placenta previa are:
i. Painless, sudden onset, causeless and recurrent bleeding. The 1st episode is usually not severe but on some occasion it may be severe.
ii. Fetal malpresentation in late pregnancy.

10. How will you diagnose placenta previa?

In current obstetrics the diagnosis of placenta previa is made on the basis of a routine ultrasound scan. In symptomatic patients sudden onset, painless bleeding may be affecting the general condition of the patient.

Obstetric examination: Uterus soft and nontender. There is typically high floating head or malpresentation and the fetal heart rate is usually normal.

- Per speculum (P/S) exam is done to rule out local causes of APH
- Per vaginum (P/V) exam is contraindicated
- Transvaginal USG is superior to transabdominal and do not report any hemorrhagic complication due to the use of transvaginal sonography (TVS)
- *Magnetic resonance imaging (MRI)*: Expensive but excellent method as both placental edge and cervical canal can be readily visible.

11. What are the management options for placenta previa?

Management depends on the stage of pregnancy and extent of hemorrhage.

Expectant management

Care comprises judicious noninterference and intensive monitoring and is called Johnson and McAfee protocol.

The prerequisites are:
- Gestation less than 37 weeks
- Maternal and fetal condition stable
- Patient not in labor

Protocol:
- Complete bed rest with bedside toilet facilities. IV diazepam 5 mg to improve compliance
- Blood should be grouped, cross-matched and reserved for the patient at all times
- Iron, calcium supplementation should be continued. Laxative may be given to avoid straining at stools
- The patient's pulse rate, BP and fetal heart rate (FHR) are monitored till her condition is stable. Hb estimation at regular interval

The expectant management should extend for more than 1 week in duration to call it successful.

Definitive management

Indication:
- First bout of bleeding after 37 completed weeks
- Successful conservative treatment brings the patient up to 37 weeks
- Bleeding that makes vitals unstable
- Fetal distress/fetal death.

Protocol—Resuscitation of patient with:
- Type 1 to Type 2 anterior → artificial rupture of membrane (ARM) + pitocin (enhancement of labor)
- Type 2—posterior and Type 3 and Type 4—CS.

12. What are the different difficulties encountered during LSCS?

- As the lower segment is vascular, the dilated vessels should be ligated and incised in between when the incision is made
- In anteriorly situated placenta, the placenta may have to be cut or separated to deliver the baby. All these manipulation require great dexterity and speed
- Placental bed oozing requires compression and placental bed hemostatic sutures
- Postpartum hemorrhage (PPH)—Obstetric hysterectomy may be required
- Lateral extension of incision
- Removal of placenta may be difficult due to placenta-accreta.

13. What is Stallworthy's sign?

Slowing of fetal heart rate (FHR) on pressing the head down into the pelvis which soon recovers promptly when the pressure is released, which is suggestive of the presence of low lying placenta especially of posterior type.

14. What are the different complications of placenta previa?

Maternal:
- APH with shock
- Preterm labor
- Malpresentation
- Cord prolapse
- Increased operative interference
- Postpartum hemorrhage (PPH)
- Sepsis
- Anemia
- Fetal
- Prematurity
- Asphyxia
- Intrauterine fetal demise (IUFD)
- Birth injuries.

15. Why antipartum hemorrhage (APH) is more prone for postpartum hemorrhage (PPH)?

- Interfere with retraction of lower uterine segment (LUS) on which placenta is situated
- Trauma to lower uterine segment (LUS) and cervix due to extreme softness.
- Occasional morbidly adherent placenta.

16. What do you mean by migration of placenta?

Early in pregnancy the placenta appears to cover the internal cervical OS but as the uterus enlarges, the lower uterine segment develops and placenta moves in cephalad direction. This is called migration of placenta. Repeat USG at 30 weeks of gestation will give the complete idea about the migration.

17. What is double set up examination?

- In some symptomatic patient after 36 weeks when transabdominal USG is not capable of accurately diagnosing placenta previa, this double set up examination is used
- Keeping everything ready for LSCS, P/V examination is performed to determine the placental localization
- But because of transvaginal sonography (TVS), this procedure is obsolete in modern obstetrics.

18. How to evaluate the severity of bleeding?

- In mild bleeding (patient had lost less than 15 percent of her intravascular volume), no change in vitals and urine output.

- In moderate bleeding (blood loss between 15–30%), there is tachycardia, hypotension and inadequate circulatory volume (pallor thirst clammy extremities).
- In severe bleeding (>30–40% of her blood volume), there is hypovolemic shock oliguria, anuria apathy, agitation.

19. What is the choice of tocolytics in placenta previa?

T. Nifedipine, 10 to 20 mg 8 hourly for four to six weeks.

20. What do you mean by abruptio placenta?

Complete/partial separation of the normally situated placenta prior to the birth of the fetus.

21. How will you classify abruptio placenta?

Grade I:
- Retrospectively diagnosed
- Blood loss 150–500 mL
- Fetus is not at risk.

Grade II:
- APH is accompanied by the classic features of the abruption placenta
- Blood loss may be more than 500 mL
- Fetus at risk.

Grade III:
- APH accompanied with classic features of the abruption placenta
- Fetus death
- Presence/absence of coagulopathy.

22. What are the clinical features of abruptio placentae?

Painful uterine bleeding associated with features of toxaemia and maternal condition is out of proportion to the visible blood loss in concealed variety.

Height of uterus may be more than period of amenorrhea uterus tense, tender, rigid fetal heart rate (FHS) usually absent.

On USG, there is separation of placenta situated in upper segment.

23. What are the different etiological factors of abruptio placentae?

- Maternal hypertension and vascular disease
- High parity, poor nutrition especially folic acid deficiency (not proved)
- Maternal drug abuse—cocaine smoking
- Sudden decrease in the height of uterus (in hydramnios)
- Trauma, kick, external cephalic version (ECV).

24. What are the different varieties of abruption placenta?

- *Revealed*: Following separation of placenta, the blood insinuates downwards between the membranes and the deciduas. Ultimately the blood becomes visible in the cervical canal.
- *Concealed*: The blood is collected in between the membranes and decidua. Blood is prevented from coming out of the cervix by presenting part. Blood percolates in the amniotic sac after rupturing the membranes.
- *Mixed*: Part of the blood is collected inside and a part is expelled out.

25. What is couvelaire uterus?

This condition is associated with severe variety of abruptio placentae. The uterus becomes dark port wine color which may be patchy or diffuse due to sequestration of blood in uterine myometrium.

26. What are the investigations that you should perform in case of abruptio placentae?

Hb percent, urine, platelet count, blood group and Rh typing, coagulation profile, liver function test (LFT), kidney function test (KFT).

27. What is the role of USG in abruptio placentae?

- It may help to locate retro-placental (RP) clot in slight vaginal bleeding when patients general condition is stable
- May show fetal heart activity (FHA) and presentation in severe abruption.

28. How to estimate the blood loss in abruptio placentae?

Blood loss is calculated by formula (weight of RP clot in gram × 3)

29. What are the objectives in the treatment of abruptio placentae?

According to Pritchard's:
- Keep hematocrit of at least 30 percent and
- Urinary output of at least 30 mL/hr.

30. What are the complications of abruptio placentae?

Maternal:
- Hemorrhagic shock
- Disseminatal intravascular coagulation (DIC)
- Acute renal failure (ARF)
- Postpartum hemorrhage (PPH)
- Sepsis

Fetal:
- Intrauterine fetal death (IUFD)
- Prematurity
- Fetal distress.

31. What are the bedside tests for monitoring blood coagulation disorders?

a. Clot observation test (Weiner) 5 mL of venous blood is placed in a 15 mL dry test tube and kept at 37°C. Usually, clot forms in 12 to 30 min and clot retract and remain firm at the end of one hour.

b. No clot after 30 minutes → Fibrinogen <100 mg/dL
c. Clot formed but disintegrated within 30 minutes clot lysis → Excessive fibrinolytic activity
d. Clot retraction denotes adequate functioning of intact platelets and divalent cations. Normal clot should remain intact for at least 48 hours. If it dissolves within 24 hours fibronolysis is more. It means plasma fibringen level is less than 100 mg/dL.

32. Why DIC is common in abruptio placentae?

Due to abruption, liberation of thromboplastin leading to the consumption of platelets and coagulation factors (consumptive coagulopathy) and intravascular coagulation.

$$\text{Abruption} \xrightarrow[\text{Intravascular coagulation}]{\text{Thromboplastin}} \text{Consumptive coagulopathy}$$

The fibrin may be converted to fibrin degradation products (FDP) with plasmin causing defective hemostasis.

Thus, depending on the extent of placenta separation, disseminatal intravascular coagulation (DIC) can cause coagulation failure, renal cortical/tubal necrosis and microangiopathic hemolysis.

33. For fetal demise, how much placenta needs to be detached?

For fetal demise, the placental detachment is usually greater than 60%.

34. What is the cause of severe abdominal pain in abruptio placentae?

Abdominal pain is due to the retroplacental (RP) clot causing intravasation of blood and disruption of myometrial fibers.

35. How will you manage abruptio placentae?

The following flow chart depicts the management of abruptio placentae:

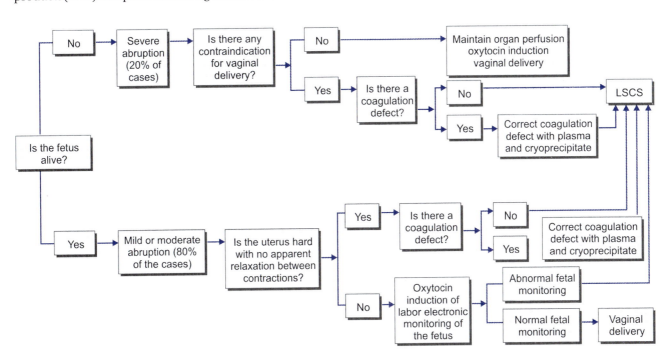

MUST REMEMBER
- Dangerous placenta previa—Marginal placenta previa implanted over posterior uterine wall.
- Stallworthy sign—When marginal placenta previa located on posterior uterine wall, slowing of fetal heart rate with decent of head in pelvis due to compression of placenta.
- Vasa previa—Umbillical vessels traverse the membrane in lower uterine segment in front of presenting part.
- Per vaginal examination is contraindicated, double set up examination should be done.
- Per vaginal examination is contraindicated.
- McAfee and Johnson's regime—Delay pregnancy until fetal maturity.

Anemia in Pregnancy: Modern Aspects of Diagnosis and Therapy

Sunita Mittal, Nupur Gupta, Pradeep Ingale

APPROACH TO DIAGNOSIS

History

Related to underlying disorders are poor dietary history, gastrointestinal bleeding or hematuria, previous history of anemia, worms, malaria, kala-azar, repeated blood donations (>3 per year), intrauterine device usage, non-steroidal anti-inflammatory drugs (NSAIDs) abuse, family history of thalassemia, pica, etc.

Symptoms

Dyspnea on exertion, weakness, palpitation, ankle swelling, headache, worsening of pre-existing angina, tinnitus, taste disturbances, dysphagia, skin and nail changes, lack of appetite, etc.

Family history: Thalassemia, sickle cell disease.

Obstetrical history: Frequent child births, postpartum hemorrhage (PPH).

Menstrual history: Heavy flow during menses.

Examination

Signs

Pallor of skin, mucous membranes and palms, koilo/platynychia, cheilosis, glossitis, etc. and clinical decompensation is associated with altered mental state, apathy, pallor, tachycardia, tachypnea, increased jugular venous pressure (JVP), heart murmurs, ankle edema, postural hypotension, etc.

1. Define anemia:

- WHO defines anemia as hemoglobin concentration of less than 11 g% and hematocrit of less than 0.33 g/dL.
- Centers for Disease Control (CDC) defines anemia as hemoglobin concentration of less than 11 g% in first and third trimester and less than 10.5 g% in second trimester.
- Indian Council of Medical Research (ICMR) categories of anemia based on hemoglobin level.

Category	Severity of anemia	Hemoglobin level (g/dL)
1.	Mild	10.0–10.9
2.	Moderate	7.0–10.0
3.	Severe	<7.0
4.	Very severe (decompensated)	<4.0

2. What is physiological anemia of pregnancy?

Anemia which results from hemodilution secondary to an increase in plasma volume, where hematocrit drops by 3 to 5 percentage points, plasma volume expands by 46 to 55% whereas red cell volume expands by 18 to 25%. Although the maternal red blood cell mass also increases during gestation, its expansion and the expansion of the plasma volume are not synchronous. Thus, hemoglobin concentrations and hematocrit decline throughout the first and second trimesters, reach a nadir early in the third trimester, and then rise again nearer to term.

3. What is the impact of anemia on pregnancy?

Anemia is a risk factor for both mother and fetus.

- *Maternal hazards:*
  - The second most common cause of maternal deaths, accounting for 20% of total maternal deaths. Deaths from severe anemia result from heart failure, shock, or infection
  - Increased susceptibility to infection—asymptomatic bacteriuria, urinary tract infection (UTI) with megaloblastic anemia.
  - Thromboembolism.
- *Fetal hazards:*
  - Anemia early in pregnancy is associated with low birth weight (LBW), preterm delivery
  - Moderate anemia before 28 weeks of gestation is associated with an increased risk of stillbirth
  - Low intake of dietary folate <240 pg/day leads to 2 fold increase in preterm labor (PTL) and 10 fold increase in LBW infants

- Megaloblastic anemia may manifest as abortion, prematurity, dysmaturity and fetal malformations.

4. Describe the iron requirements in pregnancy.
- The overall iron requirement in pregnancy is 1030 mg (800–1650 mg)
- Overall daily requirement is 4 mg/day
- 2.5 mg/day in early pregnancy
- 5.5 mg/day from 20 to 32 weeks
- 6.6 to 8.4 mg per day from 32 weeks onwards.

5. What is the differential diagnosis of hypochromic anemia?
- Iron deficiency anemia (IDA) is the commonest type of nutritional anemia in pregnancy
- Thalassemia
- Sideroblastic anemia
- Chronic disease anemia.

6. Describe the sources of dietary iron.
- Heme iron:
  - Meat, fish and poultry and blood products
  - Accounts for 10–15% of iron intake in developed countries and <1% in developing countries
  - High bioavailability and 20–30% absorption rate.
- Non-heme iron:
  - Cereals, tubers, vegetables and pulses
  - Forms a part of exogenous iron originating from the soil, dust, and water or cooking vessels
  - Another source—Fortified iron present in sugar, salt and flour
  - Absorption of non-heme iron is highly variable.

7. Desribe the bone marrow changes in anemia.
- *Iron deficiency anemia:* Hypercellular bone marrow, erythroid hyperplasia, normoblastic cell reaction, hemosiderin storage nil.
- B_{12}/*folate deficiency anemia:* Hypercellular bone marrow, giant metamyelocytes, dysplastic megakaryocytes, hemosiderin normal.
- *Hemolytic anemia:* Hypercellular bone marrow, normoblastic cell reaction, hemosiderin increased.
- *Hypoplastic anemia:* Hypocellular bone marrow, scanty cells with adipose tissue, hemosiderin normal.

8. What are the instructions given to a women taking oral iron?
One should explain patients about possible side effects and reassure that they will usually settle along the course of therapy. Iron tablet should be taken half to one hour after meals.

Tea, coffee and calcium supplements with or within one hour of intake of iron tablet should be avoided. Foods rich in vitamin C may be taken to enhance dietary iron absorption. The frequency of side effects is directly related to the dose of iron. Tolerance improves if taken with meals. Also, the slow release preparations have better tolerance.

9. What are Government of India recommendations about iron supplementation?
Government of India, Ministry of Health and Family Welfare has recommended routine iron supplementation in a dose of 100 mg of elemental iron with 500 µg folic acid for a period of 100 days in pregnancy (GOI, 2000). To be started from second trimester when nausea and vomiting of pregnancy have subsided and it is to be continued 100 days after delivery.

Side effects: The oral administration of iron can cause gastrointestinal side effects such as epigastric discomfort, nausea, vomiting, constipation and diarrhea.

10. How is the response to iron therapy?
There is an increase in reticulocyte count within 5–10 days of start of therapy. Rise in hemoglobin is 0.3 to 1 g per week (same for oral and parenteral therapy). Response is also indicated by a feeling of well-being and an improvement in appetite.

11. What are the causes of nonresponse to oral iron therapy?
When there is no increase in hemoglobin levels after four weeks of oral therapy, then cause of resistant iron deficiency should be evaluated.

Possibilities are:
- Inaccurate diagnosis
- Ineffective oral intake, poor compliance, side effects and antacid intake
- Ineffective absorption, malabsorption states, gastric surgery, etc.
- Continuing blood loss, worm infestations, bleeding piles, NSAID abuse, occult malignancy, etc.
- Coexisting infection
- Other types of anemia, aplastic anemia, myelodysplastic syndrome, anemia of chronic disease, etc.
- Concomitant folate deficiency.

12. What are the indications of blood transfusion in anemia?
- Severe anemia beyond 36 weeks
- Anemia due to acute blood loss
- Patients not responding to oral or parenteral iron
- Packed cells are preferred for transfusion to prevent cardiac overload.

13. What are the different salts of iron available?

- Ferrous sulfate—Least expensive and most commonly used preparation
- Ferrous gluconate—Preparation with least gastrointestinal side effects
- Ferrous ascorbate
- Ferrous succinate
- Ferric ammonium citrate
- Carbonyl iron is the purest form of iron containing 98% of elemental iron
- Iron polymaltose complex (IPC)—contains nonionic iron and polymaltose in a stable complex. There are several reports of inadequate or slow rise in hemoglobin; therefore, it should not be used for oral iron therapy in human.

14. What are the indications of parenteral iron therapy?

It has no advantage over oral iron if the latter is well-tolerated. Indications for use are:

- Inadequate gastrointestinal iron absorption
- Intolerance to requisite dose of oral iron
- Chronic blood loss exceeding the oral replacement
- Combination with recombinant human erythropoietin
- Potential contraindication to blood transfusion.

15. Which are the available parenteral iron preparations?

- Jectofer (iron-sorbitol citrate complex) is only used by intramuscular route.
- Imferon (iron-dextran) can be given by both intramuscular and intravenous route.

Both are given deep into the upper outer quadrant of the buttock; skin is laterally displaced before injection (Z track technique) to prevent staining of the skin.

Each ampoule contains 50 mg/mL of elemental iron and its test dose is 0.5 mL on day 1.

Daily dose should not exceed 5 mL (250 mg of iron).

Iron dextran and recently iron sucrose (Venofer, Ancifer) are the intravenous preparations of choice for parenteral therapy. Iron dextran can also be given intravenously in the form of a drip. In this manner, total requirement of iron can be given in a single sitting. It is essential to give a small test dose intravenously before giving the total dose. Adrenaline should be kept ready in a syringe to counter anaphylactoid reactions. Iron sucrose complex therapy is a valid first line option for safe and rapid reversal of iron deficiency anemia.

16. How to determine the total dose of iron replacement required?

- Total dose = 0.3 WD + 50 percent for replenishment of body stores

W = Patient's weight in pounds
D = (100 Hb%) = observed hemoglobin concentration in percentage

- The simplest formula is:
Total dose of elemental iron (mg) = weight (kg) × Hb deficit
(Normal Hb[14]–Patient Hb) × 2.21 + 1000
- Total dose = 250 mg per gram of Hb below normal.

It is customary to add 1000 mg or above to replenish iron stores. Oral iron should be stopped at least 24 hours prior to avoid reaction.

17. What are the side effects of parenteral iron therapy?

- *Local reaction:* Skin staining, pain and abscess formation.
- *Systemic:* Fever, arthralgias, myalgia, nausea, vomiting, diarrhea, body ache, skin rash, chest pain, abdominal pain, lymphadenopathy, angioneurotic edema.
- Anaphylactic shock which has even led to death in a few cases.

18. What is megaloblastic anemia?

Anemias that are associated with enlargement of proliferating erythroid precursor cells as megaloblasts, megalocytes and macrocytes.
Cause: Folate and vitamin B_{12} deficiency.

19. What are the predisposing factors that may lead to folic acid deficiency anemia in pregnancy?

- Increased requirement
- Multiple pregnancy
- Underlying hemolytic anemia (e.g. sickle cell anemia)
- Inadequate diet
- Urinary tract infection
- Drugs that impair folate metabolism, absorption or utilization (e.g. trimethoprim, phenytoin, ethanol, nitrofurantoin, barbiturates)
- Seasonal (more likely in winter in some geographical areas secondary to decreased availability of fresh products).

20. How to evaluate macrocytic anemia (folate and vitamin B_{12} deficiency)?

- *Hemoglobin and peripheral smear:* In both folic acid and vitamin B_{12} deficiency, there is presence of macrocytic red cells mean corpuscular volume (MCV) >100 fL, mean corpuscular hemoglobin (MCH) >33 pg, mean corpuscular hemoglobin concentration (MCHC) normal), which appear large and oval. Hypersegmented neutrophilic leukocytosis—the earliest morphological change to appear in blood.
- Low reticulocyte count, nucleated RBC, Howell-Jolly bodies, pancytopenia are also seen.

- *Serum folate concentration* is not a reliable test in pregnancy.
- *Red cell folate:* More reliable indicator of the folate status as it does not reflect the daily and short-term variations of plasma folate. The test, however, lacks specificity, because red cell folate level is decreased in over half of the cases with vitamin B_{12} deficiency.
- *Excretion of formiminoglutamic acid (FIGLU):* No longer recommended as a screening test in pregnancy.
- Serum vitamin B_{12}.
- Liver and kidney function tests.
- Stool for occult blood and analysis.
- Upper and lower GI endoscopy and/or barium studies of gastrointestinal tract.
- Pelvic ultrasound, if required.
- *Bone marrow:* Megakaryocytes may be abnormally large with decreased granulation and bizarre nuclear appearance. Look for metamyelocytes, RBC precursors, pronormoblasts and nuclear cytoplasmic asynchrony.

21. What is the treatment of folate deficiency anemia?

One mg folic acid OD orally replenishes body stores in three weeks. In the presence of malabsorption, doses up to 5 mg/day may be required. Vitamin B_{12} deficiency must be excluded in patients on folic acid therapy as such treatment may result in progressive neurological deterioration.

22. What is the treatment of vitamin B_{12} deficiency anemia?

Parenteral: Injection of hydroxycobalamin 1000 µg daily intramuscularly for one week, then weekly for one month and then monthly thereafter. Response to therapy is characterized by reticulocytosis which occurs within one week of initiation of therapy.

Oral: 1000 to 2000 µg/day is found to be as effective as parenteral route.

Intranasal gel: Containing cyanocobalamin has recently been labeled for maintenance therapy.

23. What is the obstetric management of anemic patients?

- *Antenatal period:* Correction of anemia.
  - See for UTI, asymptomatic bacteriuria, preterm labor
- *Management of second stage of labor:*
  - Propped up position
  - Oxygen inhalation
  - Morphine for analgesia
  - Rapid digitalization in case of cardiac failure
  - Cut short second stage of labor (forceps)
  - Antibiotic prophylaxis
  - Active management of third stage of labor
  - Oxytocin given within 1 minute of delivery of baby (10 units IV, acts in 2–3 minutes)
  - Controlled cord traction
  - Uterine massage
  - Avoid IV methergin.
- *Postpartum period:*
  - Continue iron and folic acid for 3 months
  - Energetic treatment of infection
  - Lactation failure, subinvolution and thromboembolism to be taken care of
  - Contraceptive advice.

Maternal mortality can occur in last trimester, during labor, immediately after delivery and during the postpartum period due to cardiac failure and pulmonary edema.

24. What is etiological classification of anemia in pregnancy?

- Nutritional deficiency
  - Iron deficiency
  - Folate deficiency
  - B_{12} deficiency
  - Vitamin A deficiency
  - Anemia due to protein malnutrition and scurvy
- Hemorrhagic (secondary to blood loss)
  - *Acute:* Early trimester bleeding, APH
  - *Chronic:* Piles
- Hemolytic
  Acquired: Associated with pre-eclampsia [HELLP (H–hemolysis; EL–elevated liver enzymes; LP–a low platelet count) syndrome], chronic infection
  Congenital: Congenital acholuric jaundice, sickle cell anemia
- Bone marrow suppression
- Aplastic anemia
- Secondary to chronic systemic disease
- Hemoglobinopathies
- *Infection and parasitic infestation:* Malaria, hookworm, HIV.

25. What is morphological classification of anemia in pregnancy?

- Normocytic normochromic anemia
- Microcytic hypochromic anemia
- Macrocytic normochromic anemia
- Microcytic normochromic anemia (simple microcytic).

26. What is the iron requirement in pregnancy?

- External iron loss—170 mg
- Expansion of RBC mass—450 mg
- Fetal iron—270 mg

- Iron in placenta and cord—90 mg
- Blood loss at delivery—150 mg
- Total requirement—1030 mg.

27. What are the stages in development of iron deficiency?
- Depletion of iron stores
- Impaired hemoglobin production
- Menifest iron deficiency.

28. What are the dietary factors that cause inhibition of iron absorption?
- Phytates
- Calcium
- Tannins
- Tea and coffee
- Herbal drinks
- Fortified iron supplements.

29. What are the advantages of iron sucrose complex?
- Highly safe
- Highly stable
- Low tissue accumulation and toxicity
- High availability for erythropoiesis
- Rapid incorporation (bone marrow and red cells)
- Prevents iatrogenic iron depletion (e.g. after rhEPO).

30. When is the greatest risk of physiological anemia during pregnancy?

Thirty-two weeks.

31. How will you diagnose a case of anemia?
- Screening
- Clinical feature—Hb <7–8 g/dL
- Lab investigations—Hb percent decreased, hematocrit decreased, MCV decreased
- Peripheral smear examination:
  - Microcytic and hypochromic cells in iron deficiency
  - Macrocytic cells in folate/vitamin B_{12} deficiency
  - Normocytic cells in other causes or early nutritional deficiency
  - Schisto/aniso and poikilocytes in hemolytic anemia
  - Sickle cells in sickle cell anemia
  - White blood cells hypersegmented in megaloblastic anemia
  - Target cells in thalassemia
  - Platelets may be decreased
  - Parasites such as *Plasmodium malariae* and *Leishmania* may be seen.
- Serum ferritin <12 mcg/L
- Transferritin saturation <15%
- Elevated protoporphyrin level
- Serum iron concentration <60 mcg/dL

- Transferring receptor concentration increased (promising new indicator), iron binding capacity increased
- Hb electrophoresis.

32. When you will do medical evaluation for thalassemia trait and sickle cell disease?

When with oral iron for 1 to 1.5 months, no improvement and compliance reconfirmed then, medical evaluation for thalassemia trait and sickle cell disease should be done.

33. What is the WHO recommendation for daily folate and vitamin B_{12} intake?

400 µg folate/day, 2.2 µg vitamin B_{12}/day.

34. What are the special clinical features of B_{12} deficiency?

Neurological symptoms, numbness paresthesia, weakness ataxia, poor concentration, dementia and psychosis.

35. What do you mean by hemoglobinopathy?
- A collective term for the inherited disorders of Hb synthesis
- Disorders of globin synthesis, e.g. thalassemia
- Structural Hb variants, e.g. sickle cell anemia, HbC.

36. How you will diagnose thalassemia?

Hb estimation, peripheral smear examination, decreased MCV, decreased MCH and HbA2.

37. What is sickle cell disorder?
- Structural Hb variant
- Exists in homo- and heterozygous forms
- Under hypoxic conditions, HbS polymerizes, gels or crystallizes/hemolysis of cells, and thrombosis of vessels in various organs
- In long-standing cases, multiple organ damage.

38. What is sickle cell crisis?
- Acute events that occur in individuals with sickle cell disease
- Two major types of crisis—vasoocclusive and hematologic crisis
- Most crisis during pregnancy are vasocclusive occurring in the latter half of pregnancy or in the peurperium.

39. What is prophylaxis against nutritional anemia (PANA)?

A nutritional anemia during pregnancy 100 tabs of 100 mg of elemental iron in the second-half of pregnancy.

40. Define adjuvant therapy of iron deficiency anemia.
- *Diet:* Balanced diet rich in proteins, iron and vitamins and which is easily assailable is prescribed.

- *To improve the appetite and facilitate digestion:* Preparation containing acid pepsin
- Vitamin C
- Treatment of worm infestation.

41. What is dimorphic anemia?

- This is the most common type of anemia in the tropics
- It is related to dietary inadequacy or intestinal malabsorption
- Deficiency of both iron and folic acid or vitamin B_{12}
- The red cells become macrocytic or normocytic and hypochromic or normochromic
- Bone marrow picture is predominantly megaloblastic as the folic acid is required for the development of the number of red cell precursors
- The treatment consists of prescribing both the iron and folic acid in therapeutic doses.

42. What are the other investigations for anemia?

- Urine examination
- Stool examination
- Bone marrow
- Radiograph of chest
- BUN/serum creatinine.

Special investigations
- Sickling test; (i) early, and (ii) late
- Hb electrophoresis
- Direct Coombs' test
- Indirect Coombs' test
- Enzyme studies of metabolic pathways of G6PD.

MUST REMEMBER

- Anemia is the most common medical disorder affecting pregnancy.
- Contributes significantly to maternal morbidity and mortality.
- It is responsible for 40–60% of maternal deaths.
- Dimorphic anemia is the most common form of anemia.
- Oral iron therapy should be the first-line therapy for treatment of anemia.
- Parenteral iron offers no advantage as far as the rate of rise of hemoglobin, it only ensures surety of the drug delivery.
- Routine supplements with iron and folic acid should be given to all expectant mothers and continued in puerperium.

Heart Disease in Pregnancy

Ashwini Yelikar, Ashish R Kale

1. How do you evaluate a case of heart disease?
- Symptomatology
- Clinical examination
- Investigations to decide the etiology, structures involved, severity of heart disease, heart size and cardiac rhythm.

2. What are the basic investigations required?
- Complete blood count, total leukocyte count, differential leukocyte count, urine for microscopic hematuria
- Antistreptolysin (ASO) titers
- *Chest X-ray*—to look for cardiomegaly—Straightening of the left heart border, Kerley B lines
- Electrocardiogram (ECG)
- Echocardiography.

3. What is the prognosis of heart disease during pregnancy?
Immediate prognosis depends on functional capacity of heart and antenatal care provided.

4. What are the factors which precipitate failure?
- Anemia
- Upper respiratory tract infection
- Preeclampsia
- Tachycardia of any origin, arrhythmias
- Recurrence of active rheumatic fever
- Hyperthyroidism
- Excessive weight gain
- Bacterial endocarditis (characterized by pallor, pyrexia, petechial hemorrhage, palpable spleen, positive blood culture, microscopic hematuria).

5. How will you manage a case of heart disease during pregnancy?
Antenatal care:
Frequent visits, cardiologists opinion.
Advice given—adequate rest, salt restricted diet.
- Avoid exertion, cold, infection, avoid excessive weight gain, anemia
- Advice hospital admission routinely

6. Management after hospitalization.
- Bed rest
- Sedation
- Diuretic
- Prophylactic antibiotics
- Digoxin if patient is in failure.

7. How will you manage labor?
- Grade I— two weeks prior to expected date of delivery
- Grade II—at 28 weeks
- Grade III/IV—as soon as the diagnosis is made.

Patient is preferably delivered on a comfortable bed rather than the table.
- Propped up position
- O_2 kept ready
- Drugs—sedatives, diuretics, antibiotics, digoxin, restriction of IV fluids (75 mL/hr)
- Use of prophylactic forceps to cut down the second stage of labor.

8. How does the course of labor in heart disease?
The labor is usually easy due to congestion of the pelvis.

9. What is the rule of five?
There are five occasions when patient can land up in failure
- 5 weeks of gestation
- 5 months of gestation
- 5 weeks before expected date of delivery (EDD)
- 5 hours after onset of labor
- 5 minutes after delivery.

10. How do you manage the puerperium?
Puerperium is again a critical period, since patient is likely to go in failure.
- Hospitalized for 2 weeks
- Prophylactic antibiotics
- Puerperal fever of any origin is treated vigorously
- Breastfeeding is contraindicated only in grade III to IV disease, as the exertion of BF may precipitate failure.

11. What is the ideal contraception?
Barrier method is ideal. Permanent sterilization should preferably be done, in the interval period. If the patient is not fit, husband's vasectomy is advised.

12. When should the valvotomy be done?

Preferably in the interval period. In cases of unresponsive failure and patients' strong will to continue pregnancy, valvotomy can be considered around 14 to 18 weeks.

13. What are the two types of heart failures you come across?

- The right-sided failure/congestive cardiac failure (CCF) evident by increase jugular venous pressure (JVP), palpable liver and edema feet. Seen wherever considerable myocardial damage is there. Responds to diuretics, salt restricted diet, rest and digitalis.
- The left-sided failure or pulmonary edema seen in cases of tight mitral stenosis.

Tight mitral stenosis
↓
Obstruction to blood flow from left atrium to left ventricle
↓
Left atrial pressure ↑
↓
Transmitted to pulmonary veins and capillaries
↓
Pulmonary edema

Sign and symptoms:
- Paroxysmal nocturnal dyspnea
- Cough
- Frothy sputum
- Hemoptysis
- Crepts, bronchospasm

Treated by diuretics and beta-blockers.

14. In which cases pulmonary edema is common?

Pulmonary edema is seen in:
- Young patients
- Tight mitral stenosis
- Small hearts
- Regular rhythm
- Efficient right ventricle
- Healthy myocardium.

15. What are the indications of MTP in heart disease?

- Primary pulmonary hypertension
- Eisenmenger's syndrome
- Pulmonary venoocclusive disease
- Severe lung disease, with pulmonary hypertension
- Coarctation of aorta
- Marfan's syndrome with coarctation of aorta.

16. How much is the maternal mortality and what are the causes?

The maternal mortality is about 1%.

The causes are:
- Pulmonary edema
- Congestive cardiac failure (CCF)
- Pulmonary embolism
- Active rheumatic carditis
- Rupture of cerebral aneurysm.

17. What is the effect of pregnancy on heart disease?

If the cardiac reserve is poor, cardiac failure occurs.

18. What is the effect of heart disease on pregnancy?

- Intrauterine growth restriction (IUGR)
- Preterm labor.

19. What is New York Health Association (NYHA) classification?

Class 1: Asymptomatic
Class 2: Symptomatic with heavy exercise
Class 3: Symptomatic with light exercise
Class 4: Symptomatic at rest.

20. How will you classify heart disease?

- Rheumatic heart disease (RHD)
- Congenital heart disease (CHD)
- Ischemic heart disease (IHD)
- Cardiomyopathy.

21. What is critical mitral stenosis?

Valve area less than 1 sq cm.

22. What are the indications of cesarean delivery in case of heart disease?

Apart from all obstetric indications, uncorrected coarctation of aorta is the only indication for lower segment cesarean section (LSCS) in heart disease.

23. What is the prophylactic regimen for SABE?

- Ampicillin 1 g IM/IV and Gentamicin 1.5 mg/kg body weight
- Give initial dose 30 min prior to procedure and repeat the dose every 8 hours for two doses.

24. What are the indications for digitalization?

Atrial fibrillation, left ventricular dysfunction.

25. What is peripartum cardiomyopathy?

What is the criteria for defining cardiomyopathy?

It is form of dilated cardiomyopathy in previously healthy women in whom left ventricular systolic dysfunction develops in last months of pregnancy or within 5 months of delivery common in multiple pregnancy, in lower socioeconomic group.

26. What are the grades of murmur?

Grade I: Very faint, not heard in all positions, no thrill.
Grade II: Soft, heard in all positions, no thrill.

Grade III: Loud, no thrill.
Grade IV: Loud, with palpable thrill (i.e. a tremor or vibration felt on palpation).
Grade V: Very loud, with thrill, heard with only the edge of the stethoscope touching the chest wall.
Grade VI: Loudest, with thrill, heard with the stethoscope just above the precordium, not touching the skin.

27. What is the tocolytic of choice in heart disease in pregnancy?

Atosiban (oxytocin antagonist) is tocolytic of choice in heart disease in pregnancy as it has no effect on hemodynamics. Indomethacin and nonsteroidal anti-inflammatory drugs (NSAIDs) are preferred.

28. What is the method of induction of labor in heart disease?

Prostaglandin E_2 (PGE_2) (Dinoprostone) is used with caution as it has vasodilator effect which increases the cardiac output, misoprost can be used with caution. Aminotomy deferred as increased risk of infection.

29. What is fetal prognosis in heart disease?

Increased risk of IUGR, preterm labor, recurrent abortion common in cynotic heart disease.

30. Which are the antihypertensive is contraindicated in pregnancy and why?

- Angiotensin-converting enzyme (ACE) inhibitor → Fetopathy → Renal damage (Pulmonary aplasia)
- Nifedipine (Tachycardia can precipitate heart failure.

31. What are the changes in hemodynamics in pregnancy?

- Decreased pulmonary vascular resistance (PVR)
- Decreased colloid osmotic pressure
- Increased cardiac output
- Increased pulse rate.

32. How will you manage 3rd stage of labor?

- No Inj. Methergin
- Monitor for signs of precipitate cardiac failure
- Inj. Oxytocin 10 IM
- Inj. Lasix
- Propped up O_2
- Restrict IV fluids.

MUST REMEMBER

- Valvular heart disease are the most common type of heart lesion during pregnancy, since they usually manifest during childbearing age group.
- Mitral stenosis is the most common lesion amongst all of them.
- All mid-diastolic murmurs should be considered as pathological unless proved otherwise.
- The most common complication in heart disease is congestive cardiac failure.
- Congestive cardiac failure is manifested by tachycardia, tachypnea, cough, breathlessness, etc.
- Regurgitant lesions are better tolerated than stenotic lesions.
- Fluid overload should be avoided.
- Vaginal delivery is preferred; unless there is any obstetric indication for cesarean section.
- Management of congestive cardiac failure consist of propped up position, O_2 inhalation, inj. Lasix immediately after delivery, Tab digoxin, restriction of fluids, avoid methergin.
- Second trimester termination of pregnancy is contraindicated in heart disease.
- Vasectomy is a preferred method of sterilization.

Diabetes Mellitus in Pregnancy

Kanan Yelikar, Sonali Deshpande

Diabetes mellitus (DM) is a condition of altered metabolism that is due to insulin resistance or insulin deficiency and leads to hyperglycemia. Gestational diabetes is a state of carbohydrate intolerance that develops during pregnancy and is linked with several maternal and fetal complications and results in substantial morbidity. Rigorous identification and intensive treatment of pregnant women who have diabetes is critical to minimize or avoid the complications that can arise from unrecognized or inadequately treated hyperglycemia.

1. What is the gestational diabetes mellitus (GDM)?

Glucose intolerance first diagnosed during the current pregnancy. It is diagnosed by routine or selective screening of pregnant women.

2. When do you suspect a pre-existing DM?

When fasting plasma glucose is greater than 126 mg/dL, GDM is diagnosed in first trimester or recurrent GDM in a subsequent pregnancy or random blood glucose >200 mg/dL, HbA_{1C} >6.

3. How do you screen, for GDM?

Screening is done by oral 50 g glucose without reference to food and estimation of glucose after 1 hour. If it is more than or equal to 140 mg/dL, it is considered as positive glucose challenge test (GCT).

4. When is glucose challenge test (GCT) done?

In low-risk patients routinely at 24 to 28 weeks (period of maximum diabetogenesis). If GCT is negative and all low risk factors, then do not repeat. If single high-risk factor is present and GCT is normal, repeat GCT after 4 weeks.

5. What are the high-risk factors for screening?

- Age >25 years
- Obesity (BMI >29 kg/sqm)
- Glycosuria on two or more occasions
- Polycystic ovarian disease
- Diabetes in first degree relative
- History of prior gestational diabetes mellitus (GDM)
- Previous history of congenital anomaly/macrosomia or previous unexplained stillbirth. Recurrent candidiasis/urinary tract infection/chronic hypertension/recurrent preeclampsia/recurrent pregnancy loss
- South-east Asia region
- Prior shoulder dystocia.

6. When and how will you do oral glucose tolerance test?

When GCT is positive, 100 g—3 hours oral glucose tolerance test is done. GDM is diagnosed if FBG is >95 mg/dL. Three hours post meal is 140 mg/dL.

7. What is the classification of diabetes during pregnancy?

National diabetes data group classification (2000):

Type I: Insulin dependent diabetes mellitus (IDDM). Due to beta-cell dysfunction leading to absolute insulin deficiency.

Type II: Range from predominantly insulin resistance with relative insulin deficiency to a predominantly insulin secretory defect to insulin resistance.

Type III: Gestational diabetes mellitus (GDM).

8. What are the effects of diabetes on pregnancy?

If poor glycemic control in first trimester, congenital malformations seen in 22 to 25%. Pathologic levels of glucose are potent teratogen. Anomalies involve heart, central nervous system, and genitourinary system, caudal regression syndrome and sacral agenesis.

Fetal macrosomia due to fetal hyperinsulinemia, deposition of fat in subcutaneous tissue and visceral organs leading to hypertrophy.

- Unexplained stillbirth congenital anomalies
- Abortions in uncontrolled diabetes
- Increased infection like UTI/vulvovaginitis
- Increased incidence of pre-eclampsia
- Hydramnios
- During labor shoulder dystocia due to macrosomia.

9. What are the effects of pregnancy on diabetes?

Anti-insulin hormones (progesterone, human placental lactogen, cortisol, etc.) result in increased insulin requirement. Pregnancy is diabetogenic.

- Pregnant diabetic women are more prone for ketoacidosis, due to rapid lipolysis.

- Increased insulin activity in placenta
- Altered gluconeogenesis pattern
- Accelerated ketogenesis, rapid mobilization of fat, increased ketogenesis, lower fasting glucose levels. Fasting hypoglycemia. Therefore, snacks are important to prevent hypoglycemia and ketosis.

10. How will you manage a case of diabetes?

It is divided into: (i) Medical management, (ii) Obstetric management.

11. What is the medical management of diabetes?

- Diet and nutrition (1800 to 2500 kcal/day, divided in 3 meals and 3 snacks)
- Achieving glycemia SMBG (self-monitoring blood glucose postprandial 2 hours <120 mg, 1 hour <140 mg)
- Patients should be immediately switched on to injectable insulin as soon as diagnosed.

Time of day	Capillary glucose target (md/dL)
Fasting	60–95
Before lunch, dinner, or bedtime snack	60–95
Postprandial	
2 hours postprandial	<120
1 hour postprandial	<140
2–6 AM	60–90

12. Insulin regime.

General guidelines for starting doses of insulin therapy (Flow chart 6.1):

Trimester	Total units of insulin	Twice daily	Split dose
1st	0.6–0.7 units/kg	AM: Two thirds of total	Short or rapid acting: Two thirds of AM Intermediate acting: One third of AM
2nd	0.7–0.8 units/kg	PM: One-third of total	Short or rapid acting: One half of PM
3rd	0.8–0.9 units/kg		Intermediate acting: One half of PM

13. What is the obstetric management?

Antenatal screening for birth defects. Alpha-fetoproteins at 16–20 weeks and detailed USG scanning (for open neural tube defect and other structural anomalies), glycosylated Hb in each trimester.

With good glycemic control, pregnancy can safely be carried up to 37 weeks, with fetal monitoring by daily fetal movement count (DFMC)/non-stress test (NST)/biophysical profile (BPP)/Doppler. Consider induction of labor, at 37 completed weeks of gestation.

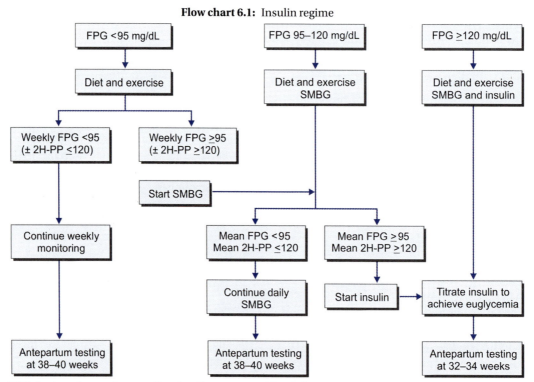

Flow chart 6.1: Insulin regime

Abbreviations: FPG, fasting plasma glucose; SMBG, self-monitoring blood glucose; 2H-PP, 2-hours postprandial

14. What is the role of steroids in preterm diabetic patient?

Steroids are better avoided since they result in sudden hyperglycemia, which is difficult to control.

15. What are the indications of cesarean delivery in a case of gestational diabetes mellitus?

- Elderly primigravida
- Multigravida with a bad obstetric history
- Diabetes difficult to control
- Obstetric complications like toxemia, fetal compromise
- Presence of large baby.

16. How to monitor intrapartum maternal blood sugar level (BSL)?

On the morning of induction of labor or cesarean delivery, patient is kept nil by mouth.
- Continuous glucose infusion (5% dextrose/lactated Ringer's solution 125 mL/hour)
- Intravenous insulin drip 0.5 to 1 unit/hour
- Glucose levels should be maintained between 100 and 119 mg/dL
- If blood glucose <100 mg/dL—insulin is discontinued
- If >150 mg/dL, glucose should be withheld
- If >180 mg/dL, then IV insulin bolus 2–4 units may be given.

17. What is the management of diabetes after delivery?

Immediately after delivery, patients do not require any insulin, as glucose levels drop down.

18. What is the ideal contraception?

Barrier method, intrauterine contraceptive device.

19. Write future precautions to be taken by diabetic woman.

- Follow a diabetic diet
- Maintain ideal body weight
- Daily exercise.

20. Enumerate neonatal complications.

- Hypoglycemia
- Respiratory distress syndrome (RDS)
- Hyperbilirubinemia
- Polycythemia
- Hypocalcemia.

21. What is perinatal mortality in gestational diabetes?

Perinatal mortality is 2 to 3 times more. Stillbirths are seen in last 4 weeks and are due to maternal ketoacidosis or fetal hypoglycemia.

22. What are the physiological effect of pregnancy on glucose metabolism?

In first-half of pregnancy, there is increased sensitivity to insulin, so accelerated fasting leads to hypoglycemia. In second-half of pregnancy (after 24 weeks of gestation), due to effect of HPL, steroids insulin resistance develops leading to hyperglycemia.

23. What is the pathogenesis of macrosomia?

Maternal hyperglycemia leads to increased blood glucose level, so extra glucose crosses the placenta and stimulates fetal pancrease leading to increased insulin production, which leads to macrosomia. This is Pederson's hypothesis.

24. What is the mnemonic for management of shoulder dystocia?

H—call for help
E—episiotomy
L—legs (McRobert's maneuver)
P—suprapubic pressure
E—enter maneuver (internal rotation)
R—remove the posterior arm
R—roll the patient.

25. What are the complications of shoulder dystocia?

- Fetal-brachial plexus injury
  - Fractured clavicle
  - Contusion
  - Brain hypoxia
- Maternal complications
  - Traumatic PPH
  - Perineal tears.

MUST REMEMBER

- *Risk factors*: Glycosuria on two occasions during antenatal period. History of diabetes in first degree relative, extreme obesity, baby weighing 4 kg or more, unexplained still birth, history of recurrent abortions, gross congenital in fetus, recurrent vulvovaginal candidiasis.
- Screening for gestational diabetes is by glucose test at 24 weeks of gestational age.
- *Maternal complications*: PIH, polyhydramnios, infection, diabetic ketoacidosis.
- *Fetal complications*: Fetal hypoglycemia, fetal hyperglycemia, fetal hypoxia.
- Caudal regression syndrome is the most common anomaly and TGA is the most specific anomaly associated with gestational diabetes mellitus (GDM).
- Multidisciplinary approach is must in treating diabetes in pregnancy.
- Insulin is the drug of choice in management of gestational diabetes mellitus (GDM).
- Combined oral contraceptives are contraindicated in gestational diabetes mellitus as they increase the risk of vascular complications which may aggravate the diabetic condition.
- Glyburide is the oral hypoglycemic agent of choice.
- Hyperglycemia and adverse pregnancy outcome (HAPO study) suggests that higher the glucose, the greater is the risk of an adverse outcome.

Antenatal Care

Pradip Sambarey, Kanan Yelikar

Health during pregnancy is directly related to health before pregnancy. Preconceptional care and counseling are integral part of prenatal care. Aim of antenatal care is to promote and maintain the health of the mother during pregnancy. Antenatal care is a periodic, regular supervision and care of a woman during pregnancy to ensure the delivery of a term *healthy baby of healthy mother* without any complication during and after pregnancy. The final goal is to decrease maternal morbidity and mortality and reduce perinatal mortality and neonatal mortality. Minimum three antenatal visits, at 16 to 20 weeks, 28 to 32 weeks and at-term are recommended, although nine antenatal visits are important to achieve the goal.

NEED FOR ANTENATAL CARE

- To screen high-risk cases likely to develop complications to mother and baby in pregnancy, labor and puerperium, and to prevent, diagnose, investigate and manage them
- Immunization for tetanus and anemia prophylaxis
- Education and counseling to prepare the woman physically and mentally for pregnancy, labor, breastfeeding, baby care and contraception
- Advice regarding hygiene, nutrition and sanitation
- Discussion with the couple for time and place of delivery
- Provide information, reassurance and support the woman
- Offer ultrasound scan for fetal viability and well-being
- Offer screening for fetal anomalies including Down's syndrome
- Offer evidence-based information to couple to make decisions.

1. How do you screen the cases initially?
Proper history taking, general and systemic examination, obstetrical examination and if required speculum and vaginal examination and routine and specific investigations.

2. When should be the first antenatal visit?
First antenatal visit should be as early as possible after missing the first menstrual period and definitely no later than second missed menstrual period.

3. What specific points are to be covered in history?
Age of marriage, previous deliveries, LMP, previous losses, surgeries done, birth weights, condition at birth, any symptoms like dyspnea, breathlessness, bleeding, edema, headache, etc. and treatment received.

4. What are the contents of obstetrical examination?
Proper inspection, overdistension, scars on abdomen, contour, lie, presentation, position, uterine irritability and tenderness, multiple fetal parts, gross fetal anomaly, liquor, scar tenderness and fetal heart auscultation.

5. How will you determine gestational age?
By last menstrual period (LMP) [Naegele's rule], any event near last period, quickening, palpation and sonography.

6. Define para.
It is the number of [delivered] pregnancies beyond period of viability, i.e. 28 weeks. Multipara is one having delivered 2 or more viable babies while she is grand multipara if she delivers five or more babies beyond viability.

7. What is the gestational age and fertilization age?
Gestational age is calculated from last menstrual period while fertilization age is calculated from the date of ovulation/fertilization (2 weeks less than gestational age).

8. What are the common causes of maternal mortality in India?
Hemorrhage, anemia, heart disease, pre-eclampsia and eclampsia, jaundice, obstructed labor, rupture uterus and sepsis are some common causes. A proper antenatal screening and care, identifying risk cases and timely proper management in labor can reduce maternal deaths.

9. What are the investigations to be done in antenatal clinic?
Hb, urine examination, blood grouping and Rh typing, VDRL (veneral disease research laboratory), sonography are to be done in first visit. Subsequently, blood sugar, thyroid function test, TORCH (toxoplasmosis, other infections, rubella, cytomegalovirus, herpes simplex virus)

may be done, if required. Doppler studies are done, when required.

10. How frequently Hb estimation is to be done?

As anemia is the most common medical disorder in pregnancy and has serious impact on pregnancy outcome, it is important to diagnose and treat anemia in pregnancy. As the most common cause of anemia is nutritional deficiency and increased demand, it can be managed with proper diet and iron therapy.

11. What is the average weight gain in pregnancy?

The overall weight gain is 11 kg with 1 kg in first, 5 kg in each second and third trimester. Less weight gain may be associated with IUGR while excessive weight gain may be a feature of pre-eclampsia.

12. What are the common causes of edema feet in pregnancy?

Edema feet are diagnosed by pressing medial malleolus or lower third of tibia with thumb for 5 seconds. The common causes are physiological, pre-eclampsia, anemia, hypoproteinemia, cardiac failure, nephrotic syndrome, etc.

13. What information is obtained from ultrasonography in pregnancy?

First trimester: Diagnosis of pregnancy, twins, abortions, hematomas, molar pregnancy, small fibroids, ectopic pregnancy, etc.
Second trimester: Growth of fetus, molar pregnancy, anomalies, twins, intrauterine death, etc.
Third trimester: Growth of fetus, intrauterine growth retardation (IUGR), liquor, abruption, placental site, major and minor anomalies, scar thickness, fetal studies, etc.

14. What are the indications for color Doppler studies?

Intrauterine growth retardation (IUGR), pre-eclampsia, chronic hypertension, APH, elderly primipara, oligohydramnios, diabetes, poor weight gain, previous losses, decreased fetal movements are common indications for Doppler studies. Uterine artery, umbilical vessels, and middle cerebral artery are considered for study.

15. What is triple test?

Triple test includes maternal serum, alpha feto-proteins, serum estriol and beta-hCG estimations. It is done at 16 to 18 weeks to diagnose Down syndrome. Low levels of alpha fetoproteins, free estriol levels with increased levels of beta-hCG and inhibin A, generate a specific risk of fetus with Down's syndrome. In addition, inhibin A is added in Quadruple test.

16. What are the indications for genetic studies?

Cases like elderly women, consanguineous marriages, previous anomalous child, gross hydramnios, diabetes, gross IUGR, etc. are subjected for genetic studies. Nuchal thickness, chorionic villous sampling, amniocentesis and cordocentesis are usually done in selected cases.

17. What is PAPPA?

PAPPA is pregnancy associated plasma protein A.
It is a glycoprotein containing zinc. PAPPA concentrations are lower in fetuses with aneuploidy. It is done between 10 and 14 weeks of pregnancy.

18. When should screening be done for gestational diabetes?

In low-risk cases, it is done at 24 to 28 weeks, while high-risk cases (family history, previous hydramnios, macrosomia, stillbirths, neonatal deaths, moniliasis, obesity) are subjected to screening as soon as pregnancy is diagnosed.

19. Is smoking and drinking alcohol advisable?

In smoking women, there is increased fetal carboxyhemoglobin, reduced utero-placental bloodflow and fetal hypoxia. The effects are abortions, low birth weight, prematurity, intrauterine growth retardation (IUGR), intrauterine fetal demise (IUFD), and abruption. Alcohol is like a potent teratogen and causes fetal alcohol syndrome characterized by growth restriction, fetal abnormalities and central nervous system (CNS) dysfunction.

20. Is HIV testing mandatory in pregnancy?

Though it is not mandatory, it is ideal to do HIV as well HbsAg during pregnancy as there are 40 percent chances of vertical transmission of HIV to the fetus. It should be done after pretest counseling and informed consent.

21. What is PCPNDT Act?

Preconceptional prenatal diagnostic tests are to be done only for specific indications and sex determination of fetus by any such technique is a crime.

22. What dietary advice is given to the pregnant woman?

Her diet should have adequate proteins, carbohydrates, important nutrients, fresh green vegetables, fruits, eggs, meat, cheese and pulses.

23. What are the social factors in improving antenatal care?

Proper health education and awareness, removing false ideas and beliefs, access to ANC clinics, dietary improvements, audiovisual aids, communication with local leaders, and health workers, holding camps and meetings, counseling, etc. will help in improvement of antenatal care and services.

24. Should air travel be done in pregnancy?
Air travel (5000 feet and above) should be avoided in first and third trimester due to hypoxic effects on fetus, preterm delivery, and possible deleterious effects on development.

25. In what cases poor fetal growth is anticipated?
In cases like pre-eclampsia, chronic hypertension, nephritis, anemia, poor nutritional status, twins, smoking, alcoholic woman, antepartum hemorrhage (APH), elderly woman, etc., poor fetal growth should be anticipated.

26. What is the importance of folic acid in pregnancy?
Folic acid deficiency is associated with abortions, abruption, PIH, neural tube defects, and poor fetal growth.

27. What symptoms are considered important in pregnancy?
Symptoms like dyspnea, palpitation, pain in abdomen, vaginal bleeding, syncope, vomiting, headache, visual symptoms, watery discharge, chest pain, breathlessness, less or absent fetal movements are important in pregnancy.

28. What are the various causes for pain in abdomen in pregnancy?
Women complaining of pain in abdomen should be examined for abortion, vesicular mole, ectopic pregnancy, retroverted gravid uterus, preterm labor, abruption, rupture uterus, torsion of gravid uterus or ovarian cyst, associated surgical and medical conditions, etc. depending on gestational age.

29. What is the importance of blood grouping and Rh typing?
Every pregnant woman should have her blood group and Rh factor known. Rh –ve woman is at risk of isoimmunization of the fetus. Cases of anemia, antepartum hemorrhage (APH), postpartum hemorrhage (PPH), V mole, ectopic pregnancy, hemoglobinopathies will require blood at anytime.

30. What are the indications for hospitalization?
All high-risk pregnancies require hospitalization as and when required. Pre-eclampsia, heart disease, antepartum hemorrhage (APH), uncontrolled diabetes, severe anemia, severe intrauterine growth retardation, etc. will require admission.

31. How will you minimize perinatal mortality?
Good antenatal care, screening for high-risk cases, prevention of prematurity, improving general condition of mothers, analyzing previous losses and investigating them, timely hospitalization, proper conduction of labor, making neonatal care facilities available contraceptive advice, immunization, etc. will help in improving perinatal outcome.

NONSTRESS TEST (NST)
Relationship between fetal movements and fetal heart rate is documented and studied. Basal heart rate of 120–160, two accelerations of 15 beats for 15 seconds, good beat to beat variability, no spontaneous decelerations are considered as reactive NST. Reactive NST means the baby is well at least for 1 week. Nonreactive NST is an indication of intrauterine hypoxia.

CONTRACTION STRESS TEST (CST)
Relationship between uterine (induced) contractions and fetal heart rate documented. It is a test for uteroplacental insufficiency. Deceleration after a uterine contraction is positive CST while no deceleration is a nonreactive CST.

BIOPHYSICAL PROFILE (MANNING SCORE)
Two points for positive and 0 points for negative findings:
- Fetal breathing movements—1 breathing for 30 seconds in 30 minutes
- Fetal gross body/limb movements—3 body/limb movements in 30 minutes
- Fetal tone—1 movement of extension followed flexion in 30 minutes
- Reactive NST
- Amniotic fluid pocket of 2 cm or more in 2 perpendicular plane
- Score of 8–10 is satisfactory, score of 6 means equivocal and needs further testing
- Score of 4 means hypoxia or compromised fetus.

Modified biophysical profile
- NST
- AFI (amniotic fluid index) <5.

Contraindications in pregnancy
All live virus vaccines [rubella, measles, mumps, varicella, yellow fever] and drugs like tetracyclines, chlorambucil, cytotoxic drugs, diethylstilbestrol (DES), lithium, valproate, alcohol, ACE inhibitors, mifepristone, radioactive iodine are not to be given.

However, influenza, rabies, hepatitis, hepatitis A and B, pneumococcal and meningococcal vaccines can be given.

Important high-risk factors
- *Social factors:* Age, height, weight, literacy, parity, socioeconomic state, nutrition

- Past pregnancy performance and losses affecting present pregnancy
- Pre-existing medical and surgical conditions
- Present pregnancy factors.

These factors are important in antenatal care and management. Antenatal care is thus a key entry point to receive broad range of health promotion and providing health services, including nutritional support, diagnosis, prevention and treatment of anemia, malaria, tuberculosis, thyroid dysfunction, sexually transmitted diseases (STDs) (bacterial vaginosis, syphilis, HIV Hepatitis B, etc.) tetanus toxoid immunization, treatment for hookworm and protection against vitamin A and iodine deficiency. Antenatal care should be woman friendly, inclusive of spouse or family member, culturally appropriate, individualized, integrated and focused and include family planning counseling. It should contain preconception counseling and advice for institutional delivery. The communication and information should be accessible to women. All facts, points, records should be well-documented and maintained.

The protocol for essential obstetric care for all include screening for anemia, pre-eclampsia, preterm birth, placenta previa and fetal growth restriction.

In addition to palpation cardiotocography, USG and Doppler studies should be done. Special consideration and care should be given to underweight and obese women, extreme age, anemia, heart disease, hypertension, renal disease, thyroid dysfunction, diabetes, epilepsy, women on drugs, asthma and respiratory disorders, HIV positive cases, and women with psychiatry, hematological and autoimmune disorders.

Women with history of recurrent pregnancy losses, previous preterm births, Rh –ve group, previous uterine surgery/MRP/stillbirths/anomalous baby should be examined and investigated thoroughly.

Antenatal care must include education on breast-feeding, infant care, contraception and birth spacing. Screening for Down's syndrome by various tests like nuchal translucency (NT), human chorionic gonadotropin (hCG), pregnancy associated plasma protein-A (PAPP-A), alpha-feto protein (AFP), unconjugated estriol (uE3) and inhibin should be offered in risk cases.

MUST REMEMBER

Essential obstetric care:
- Registration between 12 and 16 weeks.
- Antenatal visits (minimum three) at 16, 28 and 38 weeks of gestation.
- Documentation of blood pressure, weight, obstetric examination findings at each visit.
- Mandatory investigations include Hb%, ABO, Rh type, urine protein and sugar, stool and postprandial blood sugar.
- *Medications:* Oral iron, folic acid and deworming agents after 16 weeks of gestation.
- Tetanus toxoid injection, two doses/4 to 6 weeks apart.
- Timely reference for emergency obstetric care.
- Use of clean pregnancy kit for conducting delivery. The aim was to provide the auxillary nurse, midwife/skilled birth attendents to conduct safe delivery under hygienic surroundings.
- To minimize maternal deaths in rural settings.

Normal Labor

Ashwini Yelikar

1. How will you define labor?

Labor is the process by which viable fetus is expelled out of the uterus.

2. What is normal labor?

Normal labor is defined as:
- Spontaneous in onset
- With vertex presentation
- Unaided (without help of forceps/ventouse)
- Completed within 12–18 hours in primi and 8–10 hours in multi
- With a healthy mother and a healthy baby.

3. How do you calculate expected date of delivery (EDD)?

Naegele's formula EDD = 9 calendar months + 7 days or 10 lunar months or 280 days or 40 weeks from last menstrual period (LMP).

4. What percentage of patients deliver on EDD?

Only 4% deliver on the given EDD, and 80% deliver 2 weeks earlier or 1 week later.

5. What are the theories of initiation of labor?

The proposed theories are:
- *Fetoplacental contribution:* Accelerated production of estrogen and prostaglandins
- *Alteration in concentration of estrogen:* Progesterone ratio
- Triggered synthesis of prostaglandins
- Increased activity of receptors in uterus.

6. How will you differentiate between true and false labor pains?

True labor pains (TLP) are characterized by:
- TLP start as low backache and radiated towards medial side of the thigh
- The intensity, frequency, and duration of contraction increases as time passes on
- TLP is not relieved by analgesics or plain water enema
- TLP is associated with show (blood-stained mucus discharge) simultaneous dilatation of cervix and hardening of uterus
- TLP is associated with formation of bag of waters.

7. What are the stages of labor?

Labor is divided conventionally in 3 stages. Fourth stage of observation is added to it:
- *First stage* of labor starts with onset of true labor pains up to full dilation of cervix (i.e. 10 cm of dilatation). Average duration is 12–18 hours in primi and 6–10 hours in multi
- *Second stage* of labor starts from full dilation of cervix up to expulsion of fetus (1–2 hours)
- *Third stage* begins with delivery of baby up to expulsion of placenta (15–30 mins)
- *Fourth stage* stage of observation (1 hour after the expulsion of placenta).

8. What is retraction?

The muscle fibers are permanently shortened after each contraction. This shortening is called as retraction.

9. What are events in first stage of labor?
- Uterine contractions
- Cervical dilation and effacement
- Descent of the presenting part.

10. What is cervical effacement?

Taking up of the cervix in the formation of lower uterine segment (LUS). It is described as percentage of the length of the cervix, which is included in the LUS: For example, 25%, 50%, 75%, and 100% effaced is fully effaced.

11. What are the events in the second stage?

Second stage deals with the expulsion of fetus. Normal duration of second stage is up to 2 hours in primi and 1 hour in multi.

12. What are the causes of prolonged second stage of labor?

The causes could be faults in the power, passage or passenger. For example:
- Power—incoordinate uterine action
- Passage—contracted pelvis
- Unforeseen cephalopelvic disproportion
- Passenger—malposition like persistent—occipito-posterior position, malpresentations like transverse lie, hydrocephalus.

13. What are the events of third stage of labor?
Separation of placenta and expulsion of placenta along with the membranes.

14. What are the ways of separation of placenta?
- *Schultz method:* Central separation of placenta, shining fetal surface presents first (Shiny-Schultz)
- *Mathew Duncani method:* Marginal separation of placenta, maternal surface presents first (Dirty-Duncan).

15. How is the 3rd stage bleeding controlled?
- Contraction and retraction of uterine muscle fibers leads to constriction of the blood vessels, due to the "figure of eight" arrangement of fibers also called as living ligatures
- Apposition of the walls of the uterus
- Natural clotting mechanism controls the bleeding.

16. How will you manage a normal labor?
Confirm that the patient is in active labor, i.e. cervical dilatation more than 3 cm. Preliminary (PV) examination to confirm:
- Dilatation and effacement of cervix
- Status of membranes/liquor
- Position/station of vertex
- Assessment of adequacy of pelvis
- Watch for progress of labor by doing PV examination every 4 hours and plotting the partogram.

17. How will you reduce pain during labor?
Pain relief by inj. tramadol 50 mg IM at 4 cm of dilatation or inj. diazepam and fortwin (2 mg + 6 mg, IV) helps alleviate pain.

18. What is normal fetal heart rate (FHR)?
Normal fetal heart rate (FHR) ranges from 120 to 140 per minute. FHR more than 140 will be fetal tachycardia.

19. What is fetal distress?
An FHR <120 or more than 160 is called as fetal distress. Meconium-stained liquor is confirmatory of fetal distress.

20. What is caput succedaneum?
It is a soft swelling on the fetal head, which is due to serous collection beneath the scalp, due to venous congestion, due to compression of fetal head by the cervical rim (girdle of contact).

21. What is the site of formation of caput?
It is usually formed on the posterior surface of either of the parietal bone, depending on the position of the vertex. It is not limited by the sutures and hence irregular in shape.

22. What is cephalhematoma?
Cephalhematoma is a hemorrhagic collection between the pericranium and the flat bone of the skull. It is unilateral, limited by the suture lines of the skull.

23. What is the treatment of cephalhematoma?
No active treatment is necessary. Blood is absorbed within 6–8 weeks of time. Resorption of the hematoma leads to jaundice in the neonate.

24. What is prelabor?
A few days to few weeks prior to labor is called prelabor. It is associated with lightening and cervical ripening.

25. How to manage first stage of labor?
- *General management:* Ambulation, oral intake of fluids and care of bowel and bladder, emotional support
- Progress of labor should be managed by partograph and if required, continues electronic fetal monitoring in high-risk cases.

26. What are the components of active management of labor?
Special antenatal classes to prepare women for labor, strict criteria for diagnosis of labor, 4 hourly PV examination, early amniotomy, judicial use of oxytocin, labor should not be prolonged.

27. What are components of active management of third stage of labor?
1. Immediate administration of oxytocin.
2. Controlled cord traction.
3. Uterine message.

28. What are the signs of placental separation?
- Sudden gush of blood
- Uterus becomes globular firmer and harder
- Permanent lengthening of umbilical cord.

29. What is the role of artificial rupture of membranes (ARM) in labor?
- To enhance labor
- Early detection of fetal distress, to observe the color of liquor
- Invasive fetal monitoring.

30. What is asynclitism?
Asynclitism is the relation of sagittal plane of fetal head to the coronal plane of maternal pelvis. Siginificant asynclitism indicates cephalopelvic disproportion (CDP).

31. Define labor pain?
Labor pain is defined as intermittent abdominal pain radiating from back, anteriorly down toward medial side of thigh, increasing in frequency, intensity and duration,

associated with hardening of uterus accompanied by cervical changes and show and not relieved by analgesics and enema.

32. How to assess descent of fetal head per abdominally?

Descent of head can be assessed per abdominally in terms of 5th of head palpable above pubic symphysis.

33. How frequently you should do PV examination in a women in labor?

PV should be done 4 hourly in first stage and after rupture of membrane.

34. How do you assess progress of labor?

Progress of labor is assessed by cervical dilation and effacement and fetal descent.

35. What is episiotomy?

It is a deliberate incision given on perineum during contraction, after crowning in second stage of labor.

36. What are the indications for episiotomy?

- Rigid perineum
- Abnormal presentation
- Preterm delivery
- Instrumental delivery
- Shoulder dystocia
- Fetal distress in second stage of labor.

37. What are the structures cut during episiotmy?

- Skin
- Subcutaneous tissue
- Superficial and deep transverse perineal muscles
- Vaginal mucosa.

38. What are the types of episiotomy?

- Median
- Mediolateral
- Medial.
- J-shaped.

39. What are the complications of episiotomy?

- Immediate—hemorrhage, hematoma, 4th degree perineal tear
- Delayed—gaping, infections, dyspareunia.

40. What are the principal movements in mechanism of labor?

- Engagement
- Descent
- Flexion
- Internal rotation
- Crowning
- Extension
- Restitution
- External rotation.

MUST REMEMBER

- Patients in true labor and false labor should be differentiated.
- Labor should be monitored with partograph.
- Prolonged labor should be managed with labor augmentation either by ARM or oxytocin drip.
- If labor is still prolonged and crosses the action line, patient is prepared for cesarean section.
- Third stage should be managed by active management to reduce the blood loss.
- If the baby does not cry immediately after birth, needs resuscitation.

Partograms

Shyam Desai, Kanan Yelikar

INTRODUCTION

The time-honored mean cervical dilatation—time curve of Friedman (1955), constitutes the basis for partography. The descent of the presenting part normally begins well before the cervix reaches full dilatation and progresses until the presenting part reaches the perineum. The pattern is very variable and is influenced by parity as well. The sigmoid curve for cervical dilatation and the slope of fetal descent, at best, should be considered as idealized visual aids to comprehend the temporal relationships of cervical dilatation and the descent of the presenting part. The concept of the nomogram introduced by John Studd (1973) provides a basis for comparison of progress of labor in a eutocic and dystocic patient. The addition of 'alert line' and 'action line' to the partogram helps draw attention an emerging dystocia and prompt the clinician in charge of the case to take remedial actions in time or to transfer the patient to a better facility where appropriate action can be undertaken in good time to ensure satisfactory obstetric outcome. Partography forms the basis of the concept of "programmed labor" (Daftary et al., 1985) which provides close supervision of an actively managed labor, satisfactory labor analgesia, and improved obstetric outcome.

HISTORY

- Friedman E (1955)—Mean cervical dilatation time curve
- Studd J (1973)—Nomogram
- Philpott RH and Castle WM—Cervicographs and alert and action lines
- Daftary SN et al. (1977)—Cervicographs of Indian parturient primigravida
- Daftary SN et al. (2001)—Concept of programmed labor.

ILLUSTRATIVE PARTOGRAM

This represents a dynamic documentation of the events in labor as they unfold in time and provides a record of the parameters denoting maternal and fetal well-being. A constant reference of the patient's partogram to a nomogram provides markers for detecting dystocia in good time. The alert and action lines provide guideposts for judging the efficacy of interventions adopted to rectify dystocia, and lastly, alert the clinician to adopt timely obstetric interventions to achieve optimum obstetric outcome.

Contents

Besides recording cervical dilatation and the station of the presenting part with passage of time in labor, the partogram also documents the following additional information:

- Temperature—every 3-4 hours
- Pulse rate—every half an hour
- Blood pressure every half an hour
- Fetal heart rate (FHR)—every 15 minutes
- Uterine contractions every 15 minutes
- Cervical dilatation—every 2-4 hours, depending on the stage of labor and parity
- Station of the fetal head—every 2-4 hours
- Liquor and molding
- Medication and IV fluids
- Urine output—test albumin, sugar and acetone.

INTERPRETATIONS

	Diagnostic criteria			
Labor pattern	Nullipara	Multipara	Preferred treatment	Exceptional treatment
Prolongation disorder				
Prolonged latent phase	>20 hours	>14 hours	Rest and sedation	Oxytocin induction/ cesarean section (CS)
Protraction disorders				
Protracted active phase rate of cervical dilatation	<1.2 cm/hr	<1.5 cm/hr	Expectant and	CS for cephalo-pelvic disproportion (CPD)
Protracted descent	<1.0 cm/hr	<2.0 cm/hr	Supportive treatment	CS for CPD

Contd...

Contd...

Arrest disorders

Prolonged deceleration	>3 hours	>1 hour	No CPD – oxytocin	Rest if exhausted
Secondary arrest of dilatation	>2 hours	>2 hours		
Arrest of descent	>1 hour	>1 hour	Suspected CPD—CS	Cesarean section
Failure of descent	Failure of descent		With CPD-CS	

Results

- Reduced incidence of prolonged labor
- Early detection of dystocia
- Early implementation of supportive measures
- Early detection of fetal/maternal distress
- Timely transfer of difficult labor cases
- Anticipation of obstetric transfer
- Avoidance of difficult obstetric interventions
- Improved maternal morbidity and mortality
- Improved perinatal outcome
- Optimizing outcome of labor
- Promoting the concept of safe motherhood.

Programmed Labor

This concept combines:
- Partographic management of labor
- Active management of labor
- Recognizing dystocia early
- Providing timely supportive treatment
- Labor analgesia
- Timely and safe obstetric intervention
- Avoiding traumatic deliveries
- Active management of the third stage of labor to reduce blood loss and prevent PPH
- Promoting the concept of safe motherhood.

1. **Name the persons who contributed to partography.**
   - E Friedman
   - John Studd
   - Phillpott and Castle
   - Daftary SN et al.

2. **What is a partogram?**
   - It refers to the mean cervical dilatation-time curve
   - It consists of (i) latent phase (ii) active phase, and (iii) phase of deceleration.

3. **What abnormal labor patterns can you diagnose with the help of partogram?**
   - Prolongation disorder
   - Protraction disorders
   - Arrest disorders.

4. **What is a prolonged labor?**
   - Duration >20 hours in nullipara or >14 hours in multipara
   - It should be treated with immediate cesarean section
   - Rest and sedation are helpful to correct the disorder
   - Induction of labor is indicated, if pregnancy termination is desirable, if the cervix is unfavorable—consider cesarean section.

5. **What is protracted active phase of cervical dilatation? How will you treat it?**
   - Rate of cervical dilatation <1.2 cm/hr in a primigravida
   - Rate of cervical dilatation <1.5 cm/hr in a multipara
   - Consider administration of oxytocin in absence of CPD.

6. **What is secondary arrest of labor?**
   - Nonprogress in cervical dilatation for >2 hours in a nullipara
   - Nonprogress of cervical dilatation for >2 hours in a multipara
   - Consider presence of hitherto unsuspected CPD.

7. **When will you call a case as arrest of descent?**
   - Failure of descent of presenting part >1 hour
   - Under observation, the caput increases
   - In cases of occipitoposterior presentations—time required may be more
   - Deliver the baby by cesarean section if the station is low.

8. **What is a programmed labor?**
   - Monitor progress of labor on a partogram
   - Monitor fetal well-being on electronic fetal heart rate monitor
   - Provide labor analgesia
   - Active management of labor.

9. **What are the benefits of programmed labor?**
   - Provides pain relief and comfort during labor
   - Does not require active supervision
   - Reduces duration of labor
   - Improves obstetric outcome.

10. **What are the drugs used in programmed labor?**
    - Oxytocin to optimize pains
    - Morphine to relieve pain
    - Drotaverine to facilitate cervical dilatation
    - Active management of third stage of labor to reduce its duration and blood loss.

11. **What is alert line?**

Alert line is a nomogram, i.e. the course of labor followed in normal labor. Patient's partogram should always be on the left of alert line. When patient's partogram crosses the alter line on the right side, it denotes prolonged labor.

12. What is action line?

WHO has given a second line, parallel to alert line, 4 hours apart from the alert line.

13. What is to be done, when patients partogram crosses the alert line?

Refer the patient to a higher center. Reevaluate the patient. The most common cause is unforeseen CPD. Reassess the decision to rule out CPD and labor can be enhanced by ARM or oxytocic agents.

14. What will you do if the line crosses action line.

Take action, lower section cesarean section (LSCS).

15. What are the advantages of partogram?

Can be used by paramedicals:
- Early referral after detection of labor abnormalities
- Early interventions in abnormal labor patterns
- Avoid maternal morbidity and improve perinatal outcome.

16. When do you start plotting on a modified WHO partograph?

In active phase when cervix is 4 cm dilatation (Figs 9.1A and B).

17. What is partograph finding in obstructed labor?

- Arrest of dilalation and descent of fetus
- Fetal distress and maternal distress
- Grade three molding and caput
- Adequate uterine contraction
- Cervix poorly applied to presenting part
- Edematous cervix.

18. What is the most common cause of prolonged labor?

Inadequate uterine contraction.

19. what are the points to be noted in amniotic fluid during PV examination?

Clear liquor, meconium-stained liquor, and blood-stained liquor.

MUST REMEMBER

- Augmentation of labor with pitocin in intravenous drip.
- Crossing of alert line is an indication for intervention in the form of ARM/augmentation/LSCS after reevluation of the patient.
- When the patient's nomogram crosses action line, it is suggestive of prolonged labor and needs LSCS.
- Modified WHO partograph is plotted after 4 cm of cervical dilatation.
- Partogram helps detect prolonged labor earlier and early referral.
- WHO recommends use of partogram for all labors, by even paramedical staff.
- In a busy set-up, partogram should atleast be used for high risk labors.

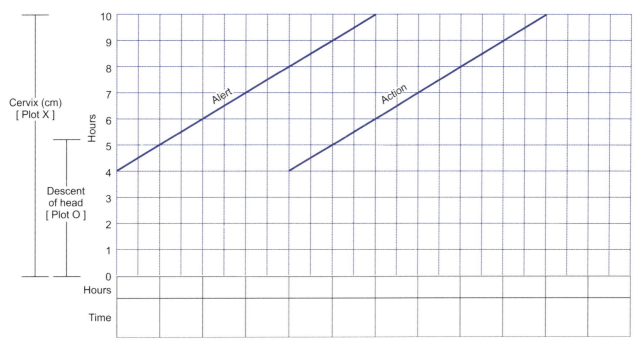

Fig. 9.1A: Modified WHO partograph

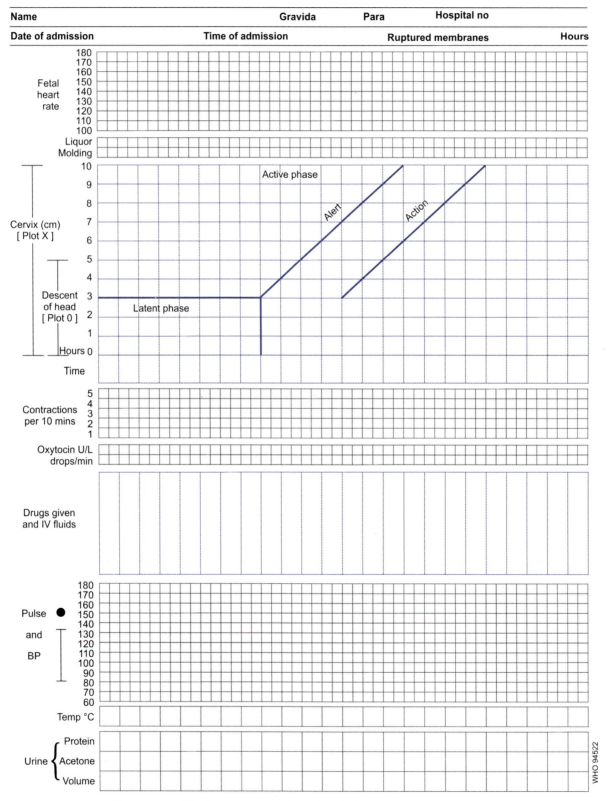

Fig. 9.1B: Modified WHO partograph is plotted after 4 cm of cervical dilatation

High-risk Pregnancy

Manorama Purwar, Ashish Zararia

1. Define high-risk pregnancy.

Pregnancy is defined as high-risk when the probability of an adverse outcome for the mother or neonate is increased over and above the baseline risk of that outcome among the general pregnant population by presence of one or more risk factors.

2. What do you mean by a risk in high-risk pregnancy and how do you calculate it?

Risk reflects the incidence of an adverse health outcome and it is calculated as odds ratio.

3. Why there is a need to focus on high-risk pregnancy?

At primary and secondary healthcare center, recognition of high-risk pregnancy and timely referral to higher healthcare center is essential. High-risk pregnancy needs vigilance and more care during antepartum, intrapartum and postpartum period to improve pregnancy outcome. For example, recognition of a case of pre-eclampsia can prevent its complications.

4. What is the role of preconception counseling in high-risk pregnancy?

By counseling, we can explain the magnitude of risk, discuss finances and special investigation may be carried out to improve obstetric outcome wherever possible.

5. How preconception care is helpful in diabetes and neural tube defect?

Normalization of blood glucose values in diabetic women and supplementation of folic acid may prevent neural tube defect.

6. What is the risk in pregnancy for following ethnic groups?

Ethnic group	Risk
A. Indian Subcontinent, Middle East	Thalassemia, sickle cell disease
B. Mediterranean, American Black	G6PD deficiency
C. Far East	Hepatitis B (chronic carrier)
D. Africa	HIV infection leading to MTCT (mother-to-child transmission).

7. What are the common health problems that make the pregnancy high-risk?

- Teenage pregnancy and age >35 years
- Lifestyle choices like smoking, alcohol and drug abuse
- Medical history, prior C-section, previous abortions, low birth weight or preterm birth, high-risk for genetic disease
- Underline conditions, such as diabetes, high blood pressure, epilepsy, anemia, infections, mental disorders
- Pregnancy complications, such as hyperemesis, threatened abortion, placental and amniotic fluid problems, Rh sensitization
- Multiple and postdate pregnancy.

8. What do you mean by teenage pregnancy?

Pregnancy in a girl aged between 13 and 19 years.

9. Define grand multipara and its complications.

Woman who had 4 or more viable births is a grand multipara.

Complications are:
- Antepartum hemorrhage
- Anemia
- Labor abnormalities
- Postpartum hemorrhage
- Abnormal presentation
- Macrosomia
- Precipitate labor.

10. Enumerate obstetric problems of elderly primi.

- Hypertension
- Gestational diabetes
- Prolonged labor
- Congenital abnormalities of newborn.

11. What are the maternal and fetal risks of smoking?

Maternal:
- Preterm delivery
- Placental complications like placental insufficiency and placental abruption
- Intrauterine growth retardation
- Premature rupture of membranes
- Ectopic pregnancy.

Fetal:
- Low birth weight babies (LBW)
- Neurobehavioral abnormality
- Sudden infant death syndrome
- Cleft lip/cleft palate.

12. How do you prevent it?

- Counseling and social support
- Stopping smoking by midpregnancy will improve outcome
- Reducing smoking is better for pregnancy if not possible to stop completely
- Specific targeted intervention program for high-risk group.

13. What is the daily requirement of folic acid during pregnancy?

400 µg/day (0.4 mg/day) periconceptionally (at least 4 weeks before and 8 weeks after conception).

14. How do you classify underweight and overweight woman during pregnancy?

Two ways:
1. Body mass index (BMI) calculated as (kg/m^2)
   Thin <20
   Normal 20–24
   Overweight 25–30
   Obese >30.
2. Prepregnancy body weight
   Underweight <45 kg
   Overweight >85 kg.

15. What are the obstetric problems of overweight woman?

- Pre-eclampsia
- Gestational diabetes
- Shoulder dystocia
- Postpartum hemorrhage
- Postoperative morbidity
- Thromboembolism (TEB).

16. What is the total weight gain by a healthy nulliparous pregnant woman during normal pregnancy?

- 12.5 kg
  - Upto 20 weeks: 4 kg
  - After 20 weeks: 8.5 kg.

17. Name few single gene disorders. To whom you will offer prenatal diagnosis for single gene disorder?

Single gene disorders are:
- Achondroplasia
- Sickle cell disease
- Thalassemia
- Cystic fibrosis
- Friedreich's ataxia
- Hemophilia.

Women will be offered prenatal diagnosis when there is:
- History of previously affected child
- Family history
- For recessive diseases carrier screening programs like sickle cell disease.

18. What are the options for prenatal genetic screening?

What it is?	When it is done?	What the results might tell you?	Follow-up
Noninvasive prenatal testing			
Blood test	As early as week 10 in high-risk groups	Risk of Down syndrome (trisomy 21) and certain other chromosomal conditions	Possible chorionic villus sampling or amniocentesis
First trimester screening			
Blood test and ultrasound	11–14 weeks	Risk of Down syndrome (trisomy 21) or Edward's syndrome (trisomy 18)	Possible chorionic villus sampling or amniocentesis
Quad screen			
Blood test	15–20 weeks	Risk of Down syndrome or spina bifida	Possible targeted ultrasound, chorionic villus sampling or amniocentesis

19. What must be the glycosylated Hb1c level in diabetes mellitus preconceptionally?

It should be <6.

20. What is Rh sensitization?

Rh negative mother giving birth to Rh positive child is Rh sensitization.

21. In which trimester chances of congenital syphilis are high?

Second trimester of pregnancy.

22. How TORCH group of infection affects a fetus?

Fetus may have:
- Hydrocephalus
- Chorioretinitis
- Convulsion
- Jaundice.

23. What is effect of epilepsy on pregnancy?
- Increased chances of convulsion
- Increased risk of congenital malformations because of effect of antiepileptic drug
- Increased risk of abruptio placentae.

24. What is the effect of antiepileptic drugs (AED) on pregnancy?
- Anthropometric changes—small for gestational age,
- Teratogenic effects, and
- Long-term cognitive effects.

25. How do you screen a high-risk woman through history?
- Age <20 or >29 years
- History of two or more abortions (spontaneous or induced)
- Stillbirth
- Previous congenital anomaly malformation
- Preterm birth
- Birth weight of previous baby >3.5 kg
- Grand multipara
- Previous lower segment cesarean section (LSCS) or uterine surgery
- Difficult forceps delivery
- Pre-eclampsia/eclampsia
- Antepartum hemorrhage
- Anemia
- Third stage complication
- Previous medical disease.

26. What investigations need to be done for evaluation of high-risk pregnancy preconceptionally?
- Hb, CBC
- ABO, Rh typing
- *Blood sugar:* Fasting and postmeal
- Screening for hemoglobinopathy
- VDRL
- TORCH infection
- HIV
- Hepatitis B, C
- Urine routine
- Cervical culture
- Cervical cytology
- Thyroid profile
- Hysteroscopy and laparoscopy for Müllerian duct anomaly
- Ultrasonography of pelvis
- Screening for sexually transmitted disease.

27. What is risk of Rh negative pregnancy? What is RAADP?
In a sensitized Rh negative woman, the maternal antibodies can cross placenta and result in hemolysis leading to hydrops fetalis in severe cases. All Rh negative woman with Rh positive husband should be screened for Rh alloimmunization. It is recommended that RAADP (routine antenatal anti-D prophylaxis) should be given to all nonsensitized woman at 28 weeks in dose of 300 mcg, which prevents sensitization due to repeated small fetomaternal hemorrhage during pregnancy.

28. What is significance of increased nuchal translucency (NT) at 11–13 weeks?
Increased NT is associated with chromosomal abnormalities and aneuploidy.

29. What steps need to be taken to promote healthy pregnancy if it is a high-risk one?
- Schedule a preconception appointment
- Be cautious when using assisted-reproductive technique (ART)
- Seek regular prenatal care
- Eat healthy diet, gain weight wisely
- Avoid smoking, alcohol and drug abuse.

30. How nutritional factor affects pregnancy?
- Folic acid deficiency causes neural tube defect
- Iron deficiency produces anemia and its complications
- Diet containing low proteins lead to hypoproteinemia and its complications; diet containing low proteins and low calories lead to intrauterine growth restriction
- Obesity has its own complications like gestational diabetes mellitus (GDM), pre-eclampsia, thromboembolism, etc.

31. What are the social factors, which makes pregnancy high-risk?
- Substance abuse
  - Drug abuse
  - Alcohol
  - Smoking
- Domestic violence
- Occupational hazard
- Improper housing
- Financial constraints.

32. How do you assess fetal well-being in high-risk pregnancy?
- Establish gestational age → Nuchal translucency-nasal bone (NT-NB) scan + Dual marker
- Monitor fetal growth
- Monitor fetal well-being by daily fetal movement count, nonstress test
- Biophysical profile, contraction stress test (CST), umbilical and uterine Doppler.

33. How do you evaluate a high-risk pregnancy?

These can be evaluated under 4 headings:

Social factors:
- Age <16 years, >35 years
- Parity primipara and grandmultipara
- Height >139 cm
- Weight <45 kg and >85 kg

Past pregnancy factors:
- History of infertility
- History of two or more abortions
- History of third stage complication
- History of child birth >9 lbs and <5 lbs
- History of difficult labor, history of LSCS
- History of pregnancy-induced hypertension (PIH).

Medical and surgical factors:
- Gestational diabetes
- Chronic renal disease
- Cardiac disease
- Other significant medical disorder.

Present pregnancy factors:
- Rh negative mother
- Anemia
- Malpresentation
- Hydramnios
- Intrauterine growth restriction (IUGR)
- Hypertension
- Postmaturity
- PROM
- Bleeding <20 weeks and >20 weeks.

MUST REMEMBER

- One of the important aims of antenatal care (ANC) is detection of high-risk pregnancy.
- All institutes should have a protocol mandatory for ANC.
- Preconception counceling plays a major role in detecting the high-risk factors before pregnancy.
- High-risk pregnancies are a small segment of obstetrical population that produces the majority of maternal and neonatal mortality and morbidity.
- The exhausting list of medical conditions and obstetric high-risk factors should be easily available in the ANC for ready reckoner.
- High-risk pregnancy management may need specialized clinics and hence early referral.
- The best time to confirm gestational age is USG at 14 weeks of pregnancy.

Prelabor Rupture of Membranes

Sadhana M Tayade, Chandan Gupta

1. What is prelabor rupture of membranes (PROM)?

Prelabor rupture of membranes is rupture of membranes beyond 37 weeks of pregnancy and one hour before the onset of labor.

2. What is PPROM/SPROM/prolonged ROM?

- *PPROM:* Preterm prelabor rupture of membranes before 37 weeks of gestation
- *SPROM:* Spontaneous prelabor rupture of membranes is ROM after or with onset of labor
- *Prolonged ROM:* Any ROM that persists for more than 24 hours and prior to the onset of labor.

3. What is the incidence of PROM and PPROM?

- Incidence of PROM is around 7–12%
- Incidence of PPROM is 2%.

4. What are the high-risk factors for PROM?

High-risk factors:
- History of PROM in previous pregnancy
- Low socioeconomic status
- Tobacco chewer
- Uterine over distention
- Polyhydramnios
- Multiple gestation pregnancy
- Cervical or vaginal infection
- Bacterial vaginosis
- Group B Streptococci
- *Mycoplasma*
- Ureaplasma
- *Neisseria gonococci*
- *Chlamydia.*

Infections:
- Cervical or vaginal infection
- Chorioamnionitis
- Bacterial vaginosis
- Group B *Streptococci*
- *Mycoplasma*
- Ureaplasma
- *Neisseria gonococci*
- *Chlamydia*
- Abnormal placentation
- Abnormal trophoblastic invasion of spiral arteries
- Repetitive stress
- Reduced tensile strength of membranes
- Multifetal gestation
- Polyhydramnios
- Cervical incompetence.

5. What will be the associated symptoms?

Patient will mainly have complaint of gushing of fluid from vagina. She may have complaint of fever and pain in abdomen, reduced/loss fetal movements.

6. What are the iatrogenic causes of PROM?

The PROM can be seen in following cases:
- Amniocentesis
- Cervical cerclage.

7. What will be the differential diagnosis according to the symptoms?

- Urinary incontinence
- Vaginal discharge/hydrorrhea gravidarum.

8. How will you confirm the diagnosis?

- *Methods to confirm rupture of membranes:*
    - Per speculum examination
    - Examination of collected fluid from posterior fornix
    - Nile blue sulphate test
    - USG
    - Intra-amniotic instillation of indigocarmine dye.
    - Fetal fibronectin—dectected by ELISA in endocervix/vagina in cases of PROM. This test is highly accurate and not affected by blood, but meconium may interfere.
    - Alpha-fetoprotein is present in high concentration in amniotic fluid but does not exist in vaginal secretion or urine.
    - Vaginal fluid ferning (result from drying out of salts contained in the amniotic fluid)
    - Vaginal fluid pH (nitrazine).
- *Other bedside evaluations:*
    - Visualize cervix with speculum to estimate dilation
    - DNA probe for Chlamydia and gonorrhea

- Group B *Streptococcus* culture from vagina and rectum
- Fetal monitoring for well-being.
- *Laboratory investigations of blood [complete blood count (CBC), C-reactive protein (CRP)]:*
  - Urine (routine and microscopy)
  - Vaginal swabs.
- *Advanced diagnostics to consider:*
  - *Consider ultrasound:*
    a. May help to confirm diagnosis (oligohydramnios)
    b. Determines fetal position and placental location
    c. Estimates fetal weight.
  - *Amniocentesis:*
    a. Evaluate fetal lung maturity
    b. Method to confirm ROM in uncertain cases
       i. Uses indigo carmine dye 1 mL in 9 mL sterile normal saline (NS)
       ii. Instilled into uterus via amniocentesis
       iii. Vaginal tampon turns blue within 30 minute in ROM.

9. What is the pathophysiology of PROM?

At term, programmed cell death and activation of catabolic enzyme, such as collagenases and mechanical forces result in ruptured membranes. PROM occurs probably due to the same mechanisms. It also appears to be linked to underlying pathological processes, most likely due to inflammation and infection of the membranes.

10. What is nitrazine paper test?

It is a diagnostic test that is around 90 percent sensitive. The normal vaginal pH is between 4.5 and 6.0, where amniotic fluid is more alkaline with a pH of 7.1–7.3. Nitrazine paper turns blue, if the patient has PROM as the pH of vaginal fluid will be more than 6.0.

11. What are the causes of false-positive nitrazine paper test?

- Bacterial vaginosis
- Blood/semen in vagina
- Alkaline antiseptics.

12. What is the significance of ferning pattern?

Ferning (arborization) under light microscope indicates PROM. A separate swab should be used to obtain fluid from posterior fornix or vaginal sidewalls. Contamination with vaginal blood may cause false-negative test and cervical mucus can result in false positive. Ferning is due to drying of salts contained in amniotic fluid.

13. What is high leak?

The patients with documented PROM show an intact sac at the time of delivery, these cases result from rupture of amnion with intact chorion. The patients have documented evidence of amniotic fluid losses who continue to leak fluid in small amounts for long duration, after initial episode and maintain adequate amount of fluid at all the times.

14. What are the types of swabs that should be taken?

- Posterior fornix
- Vaginal sidewalls
- Cervical swab for chlamydia, gonorrhea
- Perianal/anal swab for Group B *Streptococcus*.

15. What are the maternal complications?

- Chorioamnionitis—acute or subclinical
- Placental abruption
- Operative intervention
- Postpartum endometritis.

16. What are the fetal complications?

- Preterm birth
- Respiratory distress syndrome
- Fetal restriction deformities
- Pulmonary hypoplasia
- Increased neonatal morbidity and mortality
- Cerebral palsy.

17. How to diagnose chorioamnionitis?

Fever more than 37.8°C or 100.4°F and two or more of following criterias:
- Maternal pulse more than 100 bpm
- Fetal heart rate > 160 bpm
- Uterine tenderness
- Foul smelling vaginal discharge
- Leukocytosis >15,000/cmm
- CRP > 2.7 mg/dL
- No other site of infection.

18. When will you decide expectant line of management?

Expectant management of PROM includes a course of antibiotics with steroids. Expectant management and waiting for spontaneous labor may be considered in selected patients for first 12–24 hours, depending upon maternal and fetal condition.

19. What are the factors that determine outcome of PROM?

Outcome of PROM mainly depend upon maternal infection, duration of PROM and gestational age of pregnancy. Plan of management of PPROM remote from term should include the neonatal and maternal medical team. These patients should be delivered at places with the availability of neonatal intensive care unit (NICU).

20. What is the medical line PPROM of management?

Medical line of management includes antibiotics and steroids:

Corticosteroids: Decrease perinatal morbidity and mortality after preterm PROM. The most widely used and recommended regimens include intramuscular betamethasone (celestone) 12 mg every 24 hours for two days, or intramuscular dexamethasone 6 mg every 12 hours for four days.

Tocolytic therapy: This therapy may prolong the latent period for a short time but do not appear to improve neonatal outcome. A short course of tocolytic drugs can be administered to allow initiation of antibiotic, corticosteroid administration, and maternal transport.

21. How will you manage a case of PROM according to the gestation?

Management of a case of PROM according to the gestation is illustrated in Flow chart 11.1.

Flow chart 11.1: Managment of case of PROM according to the gestation

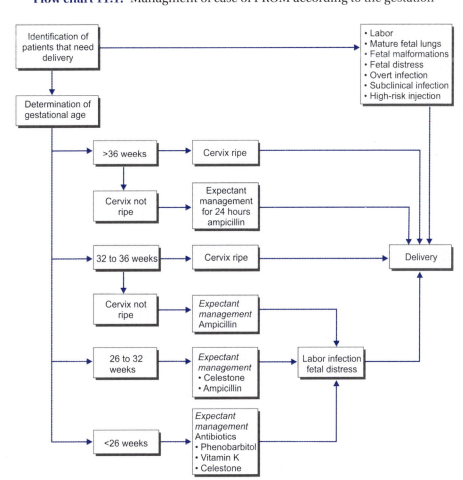

Antibiotics: Giving antibiotics to patients with preterm PROM can reduce neonatal infections and can be given according to the following regimen:

1. Erythromycin 250 mg
2. Co-amoxiclav 375 mg
3. Erythromycin and co-amoxiclav.

22. How you will manage term prelabor rupture of membranes (PROM)?

- *Induction of labor:*
  - Fetus of 36 weeks gestation
  - Weight >2500 g
  - Fetal lung maturity adequate.

- Methods for induction of labor
- *Consider oxytocin induction of labor:*
  - Spontaneous labor onset within 48 hours to 90%
  - Oxytocin decreases PROM infection rates
  - Oxytocin does not increase cesarean rates in PROM.
- *Consider cervical ripening, if unfavorable cervix:*
  - Decreases risk of chorioamnionitis in PROM
  - Does not increase cesarean rate in PROM.
- *Indications for GBS prophylaxis:*
  - Prolonged ruptured membranes anticipated >18 hours
  - Fever > 38°C.

23. When will you deliver the patient immediately?

- Impending labor
- Mature fetal lungs
- Fetal malformation
- Fetal distress
- Overt infection
- Subclinical—infection (as seen in repeated parainfluenzavirus (PIV)/diabetes mellitus (DM)/sickle cell/RhD, immunosuppressants).

MUST REMEMBER

- The clinical diagnosis of PROM is by evidence of clear fluid through vagina and can be confirmed through microscopic examination by nitrazine test, pH of the fluid and ferning pattern.
- All patients of PROM should be started with prophylactic antibiotics to prevent chorioamnionitis.
- Absent fetal breathing movement and nonreactive NST are first biophysical manifestations of impending infection.
- Chance of chorioamnionitis is inversely proportional to gestational age at time of ROM.
- Onset of labor after PROM is directly related to gestational age at time of rupture.
- Reduced amniotic fluid is best judged by ultrasound evaluation using amniotic fluid index (AFI) or maximum vertical pocket measurement.
- Incidence of hyaline membrane disease (HMD) is inversely related to gestational age at time of PROM.
- Administration of tocolysis is useful in selected patients with contractions at the time of admission, where time is required for action of steroids.
- Judicious use of tocolytic, antibiotics and steroids for better neonatal and maternal outcome is very important.

Prolonged Pregnancy

Vandana Nimbargi, Hemant Deshpande

INTRODUCTION

Prolonged pregnancy remains a challenge to the obstetrician and gynecologists.

The controversy that needs to be addressed is the issue of whether to use routine induction for all postdate patients or to selectively induce patients who have favorable cervices, nonreassuring antepartum test results, macrosomia, or other antepartum complications.

Evidence indicates that the use of routine induction in the postdate pregnancy leads to a significantly increased rate of cesarean section without improvement in outcome.

1. What is the definition of post-term?

Prolonged pregnancy is used to refer to those pregnancies advancing beyond the expected date of delivery (EDD).

Postdatism term can be used because she has crossed the dates, the gray zone between EDD and post-term period can be called postdated pregnancy.

Post-term is used to designate pregnancies that advance beyond 42 weeks or 294 days from the first day of last menstrual period.

2. What is the incidence of post-term?

Incidence: Average is 7–8 percent, although, it varies form 3–14 percent, using the definition of 294 days, the incidence of post-term pregnancy is 9–10 percent. When she is sure about her LMP, the incidence is about 7.5 percent when the first trimester ultrasound examination is considered it is 2.6 percent. The difference in incidence is on account of length of menstrual cycle. As far as possible the menstrual date and first trimester ultrasound scan should be considered.

3. What is the etiology of post-term pregnancy?

- Idiopathic—in most cases, the cause is unknown
- Anencephaly without hydramnios
- Placental sulfatase deficiency
- Adrenal hypoplasia in fetus
- Hereditary—in family and also in patient herself postdate, there is 3 times increased chance of recurrence
- Diabetes
- Hypothyroid gravida.

4. What is postmaturity/dysmaturity syndrome?

Only 20–40 percent cases of postdated pregnancy show features of postmaturity as follows:
- Loss of subcutaneous fat and muscle mass
- Long thin limbs
- Dry skin (dehydration) with wrinkling and desquamation of epidermis (scaling/peeling)
- Absence of vernix caseosa and lanugo hair
- Long nails and hair
- Meconium staining of skin, nails and amnion
- Attentive apprehensive look
- Sole-creases
- 25 percent of the remaining pregnancy show macrosomia (wt >4.5 kg) and 40–50 percent quite normal.

5. What is Clifford's classification of postdated infant?

- *Stage I (Mild):* Clear amniotic fluid
- *Stage II (Moderate):* Skin is discolored green
- *Stage III (Severe):* Skin yellowish-green.

6. Determination of gestational age?

Clinical: Excellent dates
Per vaginal (P/V) examination in 1st trimester
USG between 7 to 11 weeks.
Date of fruitful coitus (especially during ART):
- Quickening 18–20 weeks in primigravida, 16–18 weeks in multigravida
- USG between 16 weeks to 24 weeks.

7. What do you mean by excellent dates?

Known LMP with regular cycle, not using OC pills, during the last 3 months and the last period was normal in duration and amount of flow.
- USG between 7 to 11 weeks
- USG between 16 to 24 weeks.

Why we rely on USG, because:

Ultrasound biometry margins of error: Crown-rump length (CRL) till 12 weeks is 3–5 days, biparietal diameter (BPD) at 12–20 weeks is 1 week, BPD at 20–30 weeks is 2 weeks, and BPD after 30 weeks is 3 weeks.

8. What are the amniotic fluid changes associated with prolonged gestation?

Amniotic fluid volume decreases as following:
- 38 weeks 1,000 mL
- 40 weeks 800 mL
- 42 weeks 480 mL
- 43 weeks 250 mL
- 44 weeks 160 mL

Amniotic fluid <400 mL after 40 weeks of gestation is associated with fetal complications.

Oligohydramnios: It is a marker for fetal compromise and it puts the fetus at risk for cord accidents.

USG diagnosis of oligohydramnois: No vertical pocket >2 cm or amniotic fluid index (AFI) 5 cm or less. It is considered an indication for delivery.

9. What are the placental changes associated with prolonged gestation?

Placenta shows a decrease in diameter and fibrinoid deposition on chorionic villi with atherosclerotic changes in blood vessel in chorionic and decidual blood vessel. Appearance of hemorrhagic infarcts, foci for calcium deposition and formation of white infarcts seen. Infarcts are present in 60 and 80 percent of post-term placentas, and they are more common at the placental borders.

10. What are the maternal risks in post-term pregnancy?

As such per se, due to post-term, there is no risk to the mother except for secondary to induction and operative deliveries (forceps, LSCS).

11. What fetal problems are associated with prolongation of pregnancy?

- *Antepartum changes:* There is acute placental insufficiency, oligohydramnios leading to cord compression causing intrauterine death (IUD).
  Intrapartum: Due to intrauterine asphyxia → Meconium staining of liquor → intrapartum death. Intrapartum fetal distress—25 percent (umbilical cord compression and chronic placental insufficiency)
- Meconium aspiration syndrome (an eight-fold increase in meconium aspiration)
- Fetal trauma due to macrosomia (shoulder dystocia)
- Post-maturity syndrome.

Postpartum death:
- Hypoglycemia in newborn
- Hypovolemia
- Polycythemia
- Adrenocortical hypofunction
- Intracranial hemorrhage.
- Perinatal morbidity increases by 35 percent in post-term pregnancy.
- Mortality doubles in 43rd weeks and 5 times in 45th week.

12. What are the cord problems seen in post-term pregnancy?

- Cord compression due to oligohydramnios
- Wharton's jelly in cord decreases vulnerable to compression
- Percentage of fetal Hb decreases so oxygen saturation in umbilical vein decreases (from normal 60 to <30%)
- Hypoxia or vagal stimulation by cord compression leads to evacuation of meconium from large bowel to the amniotic fluid
- Thick particulate type.

13. What are the causes of oligohydramnios in post-term pregnancy?

- Oligohydramnios is due to less urine formation which may be:

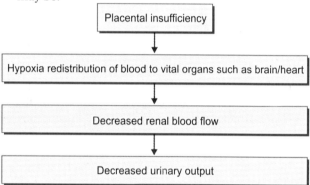

Oligohydramnios: It is a marker for fetal compromise and it puts the fetus at risk for cord accidents.

USG diagnosis: No vertical pocket >2 cm or amniotic fluid index (AFI) is 5 cm or less. It is considered an indication for delivery.

14. How will you assess fetal well-being in post-term pregnancy?

Clinical:
1. Clinical assessment of liquor
2. Daily fetal movement count (DFMC) chart.

Biophysical:
1. Nonstress test (NST): Acceleration of fetal heart rate with fetal movement in normal.
2. *Biophysical profile:* Introduced by Manning in 1980. It is done on USG
- *Modified BPP (Vintzileos et al. 1987):* Here NST (vibroacoustic stimulation test—VAST) + amniotic fluid index (AFI) are done
- *Doppler waveform studies:* Absence or reversal of blood flow during diastole in umbilical vessels indicate fetal jeopardy.

15. How often you will do the fetal well-being test?
- DFMC chart—daily
- NST twice (preferably thrice) a week, if necessary can be repeated (may be daily)
- AFI by USG twice or thrice a week
- Biophysical profile twice weekly.

16. How will you manage post-term?
If the fetal wellbeing test shows fetus is in good state, wait and watch till 41 weeks. After 41 weeks, pregnancy has to be terminated.

17. What is the labor management of post-term pregnancy?
Induction of labor is done, if pelvis is adequate, no cephalopelvic disproportion (CPD) and fetopelvic disproportion.

Bishop scoring is done:
- Cervix is ripe (score >5), induction is done by oxytocin drip or prostaglandins and ARM done as soon as feasible.
- Cervix is unripe/not favorable (score <5), cervical ripening prostaglandin (PGE_2 gel) and then oxytocin drip or prostaglandins and ARM.

18. What is the intrapartum management of prolonged pregnancy?
- Patient must be monitored by CTG and partogram.
- Left lateral position.
- ARM as soon as possible (it enhances the labor, detection of meconium-stained liquor, scalp pH testing/other tests as per availability such as fetal ECG).

With slightest abnormality during the course of labor, manage by operative intervention (LSCS/forceps/ventouse).

19. What do you mean by shoulder dystocia?
In vertex presentation when there is difficulty in delivery of the shoulders, due to macrosomia should dystocia is common in:

D Diabetes mellitus in pregnancy
O Obesity
P Postdatism
E Excessive weight gain of mother
A Anencephaly.

20. Describe the indications for cesarean section in postdate pregnancy.
- Detection of fetal compromise with fetal surveillance
- Fetal macrosomia
- Any other obstetrics indication (CPD/pelvic disproportion/fetal distress, etc.) (Flow chart 12.1)

Flow chart 12.1: Management of prolonged pregnancy

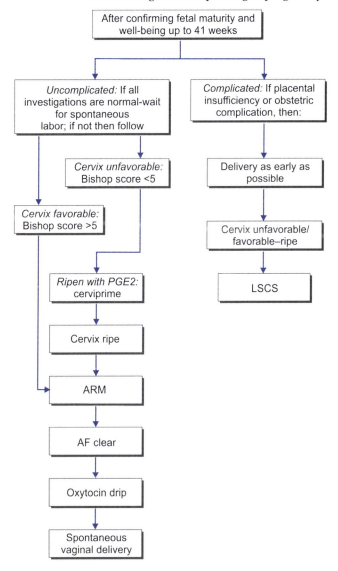

MUST REMEMBER
- Postdatism is better termed as prolonged pregnancy, which defines it as any pregnancy which crosses the EDD or goes beyond the dates.
- The placenta is an aging organ and hence functionally becomes less effective after 42 weeks of gestation called as postmaturity.
- The problems of prolonged pregnancy are macrosomia, intrapartum fetal distress due to oligohydramnios and cord compression leading to meconium aspiration.
- Low-risk pregnancy with prolonged dates should be induced at 41 completed weeks of gestation. High-risk pregnancy needs earlier induction of labor.
- Severe oligohydramnios should be managed with amnioinfusion during labor.
- Shoulder dystocia should always be kept in mind.

Previous Cesarean Section

Kanan Yelikar, Ashwini Yelikar

RECENT ADVANCES/UPDATE CHANGING TRENDS

Due to the advent of safety issues in LSCS, the spectrum of indications is widening. The main reasons are safe anesthesia, antimicrobials, blood transfusion, improved fetal monitoring equipment, neonatal ICU facilities due to which incidence is swinging between 10 and 40 percent.

HISTORY

Special Points Pertaining to LSCS

- Indication of LSCS (documented proof in the form of previous hospital records)
- Gestational age at the time of cesarean section
- Elective/emergency
- History of complications during previous LSCS.

Indications of Previous LSCS

- Contracted pelvis
- Cephalopelvic disproportion
- Malpresentations (breech/transverse lie/POP)
- Maternal diseases PIH/diabetes
- IUGR/PPROM
- Macrosomia.

Emergency

- Failure to progress
- Placenta previa (weak scar)
- Prolonged labor/obstructed labor (chances of sepsis are more).

Intraoperative History

- Duration of surgery
- Type of anesthesia
- History of blood transfusion
- Any complication during CS
- PPH
- Perinatal outcome
- Weight of the baby/cry at birth/NICU admission.

Postoperative

- Febrile illness/morbidity
- Hospital stay/removal of stitches
- History of wound infection.

Interval between present and past pregnancy. Previous vaginal delivery making the scar weak:
- Menstrual history
- Obstetric history
- General examination/systemic examination
- PV examination.

Diagnosis: Second gravida with previous LSCS at term (high-risk pregnancy).

1. How will you define LSCS?

This is defined as abdominal route of delivery by giving an incision over the abdomen and lower segment of uterus.

2. What are the types of cesarean section?

Cesarean sections are of two types, depending on the type of uterine incision:
i. *Classical cesarean section:* Incision is vertical and on the upper segment
ii. *Lower segment:* Incision is transcurvilinear on the lower uterine segment.

3. Define LUS.

LUS is defined as that portion, which develops from isthmus (portion between anatomical internal os and histological internal os). It is thin and passive during labor. The peritoneum is loosely attached. All incisions are taken on this segment of the uterus.

4. State advantages of lower segment cesarean section.

- Apposition is good
- Lower segment is inert during puerperium
- Scar is good. Rupture may occur only in labor in 1 to 2%.

5. State disadvantages of upper segment cesarean section.

- Healing of scar is poor
- Rupture occurs 5 to 10 times more (can occur during pregnancy also).

6. How do you classify CS depending on the time of CS?

- Elective CS done after 39 weeks of gestation
  - Patient not in labor
  - It is possible only in a booked patient, who attends the antenatal care (ANC) regularly
- Emergency CS when patient is already in labor.

7. What are the advantages/disadvantages of elective CS?

Advantages:
- Patient is well-prepared psychologically and surgically, for example, nil by mouth
- Relatives are available
- Senior surgeons/blood bank/anesthetists are available
- Patient is fit for anesthesia.

Disadvantages:
- LUS may not be well-formed
- If dates are not sure, possibility of prematurity cannot be ruled out (with USG this is becoming less).

8. What are the management options for previous LSCS?

Patient can be kept for VBAC/repeat LSCS.

Vaginal birth after cesarean section (VBAC) once a cesarean, always a cesarean (Craigin, 1916) is often misinterpreted and hence, many practitioners revert away from VBAC (from last 2 decades, VBAC is gaining more popularity since different studies, have proved that 60 to 80 percent of previous LSCS for nonrecurrent indication can deliver vaginally). A patient can be selected for VBAC after thorough counseling of the patient and her husband.

- Facility to carry out immediate LSCS must be present (within 10–15 minutes), i.e. fully equipped hospital set up
- Pelvis should be adequate. Rule out CPD single fetus/longitudinal lie/vertex presentation. Cervix should be favorable
- Placenta should not be low lying
- Strength of the scar as assessed by the history and local examination
- Contraindications for VBAC/indications for repeat LSCS elective repeat cesarean delivery (ERCD):
  - Previous 2 LSCS
  - Previous classical CS/hysterotomy/myomectomy
  - Previous CS with breech/placental previa/macrosomia/associated medical factors
  - History of previous perinatal death/long standing infertility/elderly patient.

9. What is the place of VBAC in modern obstetrics?

Vaginal birth after cesarean section (VBAC), once a cesarean always a cesarean (Craigin, 1916), is often misinterpreted and hence many practitioners revert away from VBAC (from last 2 decades, VBAC is gaining more popularity since different studies have proved that 60 to 80 percent of previous LSCS for nonrecurrent indication can deliver vaginally.

10. What is trial of labor and trial of scar?

All VBAC are trial of scar. Trial of labor is a terminology coined to define mode of delivery in a non-scarred uterus, where possibility of labor ending in a CS is kept in mind, e.g. primigravida with minor degree of CPD.

11. How will you conduct VBAC?

- All criteria for VBAC to be fulfilled
- Careful monitoring of labor
- Use of partogram to detect any abnormal labor pattern
- Slightest doubt about scar dehiscence—prepare the patient for CS.

12. What are the symptoms/signs for scar dehiscence?

Symptoms
- Suprapubic pain
- Vaginal bleeding
- Bladder tenesmus.

Signs
- Maternal tachycardia/hypotension
- Variable fetal heart rate pattern
- Tenderness over the uterine scar (palpated in a transverse direction)
  - Cessation of uterine contraction
  - Loss of station of presenting part.

13. What is scar dehiscence/rupture of uterus?

Scar dehiscence means whenever the scar tissue either partially or completely gives way. It is also called as rupture of the scar during labor. It could be complete when amniotic cavity and the peritoneal cavity communicate with each other, i.e. all the layers of uterine wall tear off. Incomplete scar rupture means the scar thickness partially tears off (both cavities do not communicate). Rupture of uterus is usually kept reserved for rupture during spontaneous labor in case of unscarred uterus.

14. How do you assess scar integrity?

Factors in History/Imaging Techniques

History:
- Technical skills of surgeon
- Previous indications for CS—placenta previa makes a scar healing weak. Obstructed labor associated with sepsis and hence weak scar
- Lateral extensions in incisions
- Short interval between previous and present pregnancy
- Previous VBAC makes a scar weak
- Present pregnancy factors like twins/hydramnios/placenta previa (anterior).

Imaging:
- USG for scar thickness.

15. Discuss indications to terminate VBAC.

- Fetal distress
- Scar dehiscence
- Unforeseen CPD.

16. Describe technique of LSCS.

Skin incisions—Vertical   Midline
                           Paramedian

- Transverse—Pfannenstiel
- Misgav Ladach—no sharp dissection/only stretching of tissue with figures
- Uterine incisions
  1. Upper segment
  2. Lower segment
     - Transcurvilinear
     - Inverted T
     - J-shaped
     - U-shaped

17. Write indications of classical CS/upper segment CS.

- Lower uterine segment is not accessible either due to adhesions or extreme vascularity as in major degree placenta previa
- When urgent delivery of the baby is must as in case of deteriorating maternal condition.

18. Discuss difficult situations in delivering the baby.

- Floating head: Which can be delivered with the help of forceps application
- Head is deep in pelvis as in obstructed labor. It can be delivered either by pushing the head from below or Patwardhan's method (where the shoulders are delivered first, followed by trunk, breech and then head)
- In major degree placenta previa—either go by the side of placenta or go through the placenta
- Dry labor where liqor is all drained out
- Transverse lie/hand prolapse.

19. Should you remove placenta manually during CS in all cases?

Temptation to remove placenta manually should be avoided. Since, it leads to more PPH and sometimes incomplete removal.

20. Define role of exteriorization of uterus.

It is bringing out the uterus through the abdominal incision for better visualization and proper suturing, is advantage under special situations. For example, uncontrolled PPH, where extension of incision is suspected, bleeder cannot be located. Exteriorization of the uterus is not recommended routinely because it is associated with more pain.

21. Discuss exploration of scar after VBAC.

Routine palpation/exploration of the scar is not required after every VBAC. It is indicated after:

- Instrumental delivery
- PPH
- Unexplained shock.

22. Discuss decision-induction—incision-delivery interval.

Delivery at emergency CS for maternal or fetal compromise should be accomplished as quickly as possible, taking into account that rapid delivery has the potential to do harm. A decision to delivery interval of less than 30 minutes is not in itself critical in influencing baby outcome, but has been accepted as an audit standard for response to emergencies within maternity services.

23. What is the plan of care in singleton uncomplicated pregnancy with previous scar?

- Antenatal booking as early as possible but before 16 weeks
- Around 20 weeks—anomaly scan and placental localization
- Around 32 weeks—reassessment of low lying placenta, if present
- Around 36 weeks—assess and decide mode of delivery
- Around 36-41 weeks—await for onset of spontaneous labor
- If for ERCS—do at 39 weeks
- If at 41 weeks, no onset of labor—assess and decide mode of delivery (consider chance of VBAC success, priority attached to vaginal birth and antepartum still-birth risk).

24. What are maternal and perinatal risks and benefits of VBAC compared to ERCS?

- Maternal benefits of VBAC—72-76% chance of successful VBAC which is associated with shorter hospital stay, increased likelihood that future pregnancies may be delivered vaginally.
- Maternal risks—0.5% risk of scar rupture associated with maternal and perinatal morbidity and mortality.
- Higher risk of blood transfusion (1.7%) and endometritis (2.9%).
- 24-28% chance of emergency LSCS.
- Infant benefits—1 percent risk of transient respiratory morbidity.
- Infant risks—0.1 percent prospective risk of antepartum stillbirth beyond 39 weeks while awaiting for spontaneous labor.
- 4% risk of delivery-related perinatal death.
- 8% risk of hypoxic ischemic encephalopathy.

25. What are the newer indications for CS?

Previous CS with breech, macrosomia, severe PIH with unripe cervix, multiple gestation, failure to progress, fetal distress. Since last 2 decades, the professionals are trying to reduce the incidence of primary cesarean section. Think 10 times before a patient. For primary cesarean section, do not think for 10 seconds to prepare a patient for previous LSCS.

26. How to reduce the incidence of primary LSCS?

Women with an uncomplicated pregnancy should be offered induction of labor beyond 41 weeks because this reduces the risk of perinatal mortality and the likelihood of CS.

A partogram with a 4-hour action line should be used to monitor progress of labor of women in spontaneous labor with an uncomplicated singleton pregnancy at term, because it reduces the likelihood of CS.

Consultant obstetricians should be involved in the decision-making for CS, because this reduces the likelihood of CS.

Electronic fetal monitoring is associated with an increased likelihood of CS. When CS is contemplated because of an abnormal fetal heart rate pattern, in cases of suspected fetal acidosis, fetal blood sampling should be offered if it is technically possible and there are no contraindications.

27. What are the minimum necessary investigations for LSCS?

Hb, urine routine, blood grouping and Rh typing, BT and CT.

MUST REMEMBER

- LSCS is commonly performed operative obstetric procedure.
- Optimum incidence is upto 10, however, in tertiary care center is upto 30%.
- Maternal and perinatal outcome is better in planned LSCS.
- Vaginal birth after cesarean section is gaining popularity. Upto 60–80% can deliver vaginally.
- VBAC should be conducted in well-equipped hospital.
- During VABC, scar dehiscence is a constant threat and rupture uterus is a life-threatening condition, as yet there is no standardized test to predict scar dehiscence.
- Common indication of previous LSCS:
  Fetal distress
  - Contracted pelvis
  - Cephalopelvic disproportion
  - Malpresentations (breech/transverse lie /POP)
  - Maternal diseases PIH/diabetes
  - IUGR/PPROM
  - Macrosomia
  - Failure to progress
  - Placenta previa (weak scar).
- Prolonged labor/obstructed labor (chances of sepsis are more).
- Contraindication to VBAC—previous 2 LSCS, previous classical cesarean section, previous uterine rupture, baby weight >4 kg.
- Contraception for 3 years after LSCS is advisable in the form of IUCD/progesterone containing contraception when she is exclusively breastfeeding.

Rh-Negative Mother

Kanan Yelikar, Sonali Deshpande

1. What is the incidence of Rh-ve women in India?

The incidence of Rh-ve women ranges from 5–10%.

2. What do you mean by isoimmunization?

Isoimmunization is defined as the production of immune antibodies in an individual, in response to an antigen derived from another individual of the same species, provided the first one lacks the antigen.

3. How is the pathogenesis of Rh disease in the fetus?

- Transplacental hemorrhage occurs in 75% of pregnancies, which is followed by primary immune response
- Primary immune response is slow (several weeks), weak and IgM antibodies which do not cross the placenta
- A secondary exposure to Rh+ve cells leads to a secondary immune response
- Secondary immune response is rapid (1 day), strong and predominantly IgG antibodies which cross the placenta
- After secondary immune response, IgG antibodies which are formed, cross the placental barrier and coat the fetal RBCs causing extravascular hemolysis. To overcome this situation, extramedullary erythropoiesis occurs in liver and spleen, and nucleated RBC precursors (erythroblasts) are released in peripheral circulation (Flow chart 14.1).

4. Why erythroblastosis fetalis term is used?

As a result of fetal anemia, extramedullary hemopoiesis occurs in the liver and spleen, and nucleated RBC precursors (erythroblasts) are released into the peripheral circulation, hence the name.

5. What are the manifestations of hemolytic disease of newborn?

- Congenital anemia of the newborn
- Icterus gravis neonatorum
- Hydrops fetalis.

6. What are the characteristic features of hydrops fetalis?

Hydrops fetalis is characterized by ascites, pericardial and pleural effusion, skin edema, cardiac failure leading to fetal loss.

7. What is the incidence and extent of Rh isoimmunization?

- Risk of immunization increases with the amount of fetomaternal hemorrhage.

RBCs Risk of Rh-isoimmunization

- First trimester in 0.03 mL 3%
- Third trimester in 0.25 mL 45%

8. How will you quantify fetomaternal hemorrhage?

Fetomaternal hemorrhage (FMH) will be quantified either by technique of immunofluorescence flow cytometry (IFC) compared with traditional Betke Kleihauer testing. IFC detects approximately twice the number of fetal RBCs as compared to Kleihauer.

9. What is Kleihauer count?

Approximate volume of fetal blood entering into the maternal circulation is estimated by Kleihauer count, using acid elution technique to note the number of fetal RBCs per 50 low power fields (LPF).

Flow chart 14.1: Pathogenesis of Rh disease in fetus

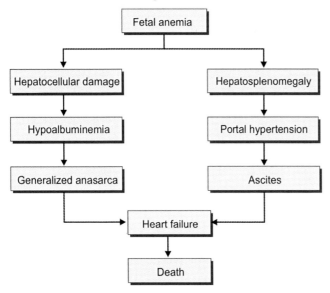

If there are 80 fetal erythrocytes in 50 LPF in maternal peripheral blood films, it represents a FMH to the extent of 4 mL of fetal blood.

10. What are the indications for anti-D prophylaxis?
- Antepartum at 28 weeks in unsensitized women
- After spontaneous/induced abortion/ectopic pregnancy
- Postpartum, if fetus is Rh +ve
- After CVS, amnio and cordocentesis
- After bleeding episodes during pregnancy.

11. What is the rational for giving antepartum prophylaxis?
Fifteen percent of Rh sensitizations are caused by small FMH that occurs between 20-40 weeks. Before 20 weeks, the chances of FMH are very less.

12. What is the recommended dose of anti-D?
Recommended dose of anti-D:
- First trimester abortion: 50 μg
- First trimester ectopic: 50 μg
- Second trimester abortion: 300 μg
- Second trimester ectopic: 300 μg
- Prophylaxis at/about 28 weeks: 300 μg
- Third trimester amniocentesis: 300 μg
- FMH (as estimated by different test); depending on quantum of hemorrhage.

13. What is Rh immunoglobulin?
It is a biological product derived from human placenta. It is efficacious, safe, stable, free from other blood group antigens or antibodies and free from HIV, Hepatitis B, C and other viral diseases like mumps and measles.

14. Choice of prophylaxis—monoclonal/polyclonal.
Polyclonal:
- Proven technology
- Covers all 30 epitopes of Rh antigen
- Approved by US FDA
- Dependent on plasma donor.

Monoclonal:
- Unproven technology
- Covers only 1 epitope of Rh antigen
- Not approved by US FDA
- Independent plasma donor.

15. How to minimize FMH?
- Precautions during lower segment cesarian section:
  - Prevent blood spillage in the peritoneal cavity
  - Manual removal of placenta (MRP) should be avoided.
- Avoid administration of ergometrine for active management of III stage of labor
- Amniocentesis should be done by USG, guided so as to avoid injury to the placenta
- Early clamping of the cord
- Forcible attempt to perform external cephalic version (ECV) under anesthesia should be avoided
- MRP should be done gently
- To refrain from abdominal palpation as far as possible in abruptio placentae
- Avoid Rh +ve blood to Rh –ve female
- Prevent active immunization by giving anti-D. Do not allow pregnancy to overrun the dates.

16. Up to how many days, anti-D can be administered?
Up to 4 weeks of delivery. Ideal is within 72 hours.

17. What is the critical value of serum bilirubin to develop kernicterus?
The neonate with severe hyperbilirubinemia is at risk of developing kernicterus, if bilirubin levels are in excess of 25 mg/dL at term or even 12 mg/dL in preterm neonates.

18. What are the indications of intrauterine blood transfusion?
Indicators of fetal anemia:
- Edema
- Hydrops
- Fetal hematocrit <30% in nonhydropic fetus.
- Increased middle cerebral artery (MCA) peak systolic velocity Doppler.

19. How is intrauterine transfusion given?
- Intraperitoneal: Transplacental
- Intravascular: Transperitoneal
- Intracardiac
- Amount of blood to be transfused is calculated by Bowman's formula (Weeks of gestation –20) × 10 mL
- Packed O Rh –ve blood is used.

20. What are the complications of intrauterine therapy?
- Cord constriction
- Umbilical cord hematoma
- Fetal bradycardia
- Fetal exsanguination
- Preterm labor
- Increase in maternal antibody level.

21. What are the investigations to be done in cord blood?
- Five millilitres of blood should be taken
- Plain bulb: Blood group Rh typing, direct Coombs test, serum bilirubin
- Oxalated bulb: Hb percent, blood smear for the presence of immature RBCs.

22. How will you manage the affected newborn?

- Phototherapy at 420–480 nm—Degrades the bilirubin by photooxidation and excreted out. Fiberoptic delivery system
- Phenobarbitone: Increases the activity of glucoronyl transferase. Dose—2 mg/kg, thrice a day
- Intravenous immunoglobulin
- Hemoxygenase inhibitor
- Double volume exchange transfusion
- Erythropoietin.

23. What are the indications of exchange transfusion in a newborn?

- Cord blood Hb <15%
- Previous definite history of an affected baby due to homolytic disease
- Birth weight <2.5 kg
- Rapidly developing jaundice with unconjugated bilirubin rises more than 5 mg percent
- When there is progressive rise of bilirubin >1 mg/dL/hr inspite of phototherapy
- Rate of bilirubin rise > 0.5 mg/dL despite phototherapy when Hb 11–13 g
- To improve anemia and CCF of neonate
- Progressive anemia of neonate.

24. What are the different antibodies formed as a result of Rh-isoimmunization?

Two types of antibodies are formed:
- *Saline antibodies (IgM):* These are in the maternal circulation and these are larger molecules, they cannot pass through placenta and are not harmful to the fetus.
- *Albumin antibodies (IgG):* These type of antibodies appears in the maternal circulation as a result of secondary immune response. These are small molecules and can pass through the placenta and cause damage to the fetus.

25. When does the icterus becomes evident? Why?

In Rh-sensitized baby, within 24 hours, hemolysis starts in utero.

26. Discuses the management of Rh –ve mother

i. Nonimmunized mother blood grouping and Rh typing of the husband (Flow chart 14.2).
ii. *Immunized mother:*
- USG should be done frequently, depending on the severity of the cause to assess fetal health.

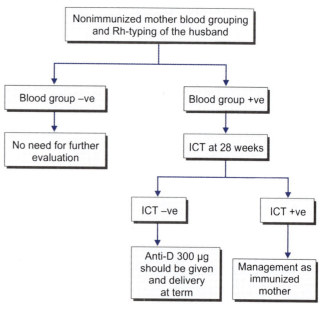

Flow chart 14.2: Management of Rh-negative mother

Abbreviation: ICI, indirect Coombs test

- Doppler velocimetry—increase MCA peak systolic velocity.
- Nonstress test (NST) is done from 28 weeks onward. Sinusoidal and deceleration patterns correlate with severe fetal anemia (Flow chart 14.3).

27. Is anti-D immunoglobulin indicated in sensitized pregnancy?

No benefits to patients.

28. Should anti-D be given in molar pregnancy, IUFD, postdated pregnancy, threatened abortion?

In molar pregnancy, threatened abortion and IUFD, anti-D should be given. In case of postdated pregnancy, a patient who received anti-D at 28 weeks of gestation, repeat anti-D after an interval of 12 weeks.

29. How long the effect of anti-D immunoglobulin lasts?

The half-life of anti-D is 24 days. If delivery occurs within 3 weeks of standard antenatal dose, the postnatal dose may be withheld in absence of significant fetomaternal hemorrhage.

30. What are the newer modalities used in the management of sensitized pregnancy?

In Doppler findings, peak systolic velocity of middle cerebral artery corresponds with fetal Hb concentration.

Flow chart 14.3: Management of immunized mother

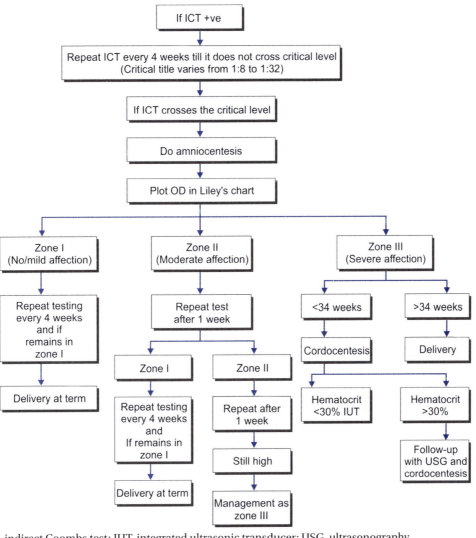

Abbreviations: ICI, indirect Coombs test; IUT, integrated ultrasonic transducer; USG, ultrasonography

MUST REMEMBER
- RhD-negative women who are not RhD alloimmunized should receive anti-D immunoglobulin.
- Anti-D prophylaxis also should be administered after pregnancy loss, invasive procedure like amniocentesis, after any antenatal bleeding episodes and after ECV.
- Consider administration of agumented dose of anti-D based on FMH assessment after any operative delivery like LSCS, MRP.
- RhD-negative women who are nonsensitized should receive anti-D immunoglobulin.
- All pregnant women with husband RhD positive should receive anti-D prophylaxis at 28 weeks of gestation.
- Anti-D prophylaxis should be advocated after pregnancy loss, invasive procedures like amniocentesis, CVS and after ECV.
- For first trimester, the recommended dose of anti-D is 50 µg IM.
- For ectopic pregnancy, amniocentesis, second trimester MTP, ECV, antenatal and postdelivery prophylaxis, the recommended dose of anti-D is 300 µg IM.

Preterm Labor

Jyoti Bindal, Ashwini Yelikar

1. What is preterm labor?

Frank uterine contraction with or without pain with progressive cervical dilatation and effacement from 20 weeks (developed countries) and 28 weeks (developing countries like India) to 37 weeks of gestation, (onset of labor with intact membrane before 37 weeks) (labor and delivery before 20 weeks of gestation is called as miscarriage).

2. What causes preterm labor?

General maternal problems/behavioral problem:
- Smoking, alcoholism, cocaine abuse
- Malnutrition
  - Stress
  - Coitus

Pregnancy complications:
- PIH, thyrotoxicosis and SLE syndrome
- Hydramnios
- Multiple pregnancy
- APH
- Previous history of abortion and preterm birth
- Chronic diseases (anemia, liver disease, renal disease and cardiac).

Uterine causes:
- Bicornuate/unicornuate/septate uterus
- Submucous fibroid
- Cervical incompetence
- Uterine hypersensitivity.

Infections:
- PROM
- Chorioamnionitis
- Asymptomatic bacteriuria
- Bacterial vaginosis
- Intrauterine infections (*Chlamydia*, group B *Streptococci*).

Fetal causes: Chromosomal and structural anomalies.

Iatrogenic:
- Induction of labor
- External version
- Amniocentesis
- Cordocentesis.

Etiology:
- 1/3rd are idiopathic
- 1/3rd are associated with PROM
- 1/3rd associated with complications
  - Uterine anomaly
  - Infection
  - Iatrogenic

3. Define risk factors for preterm labor.
- Poor socioeconomic status
- Maternal smoking
- Low pre-pregnant weight
- Maternal age <18 years or >40 years
- Prolonged standing
- Longer hours of work
- Coitus after 30 weeks
- Lack of weight gain or weight loss during pregnancy
- Low birth weight of previous infant.

4. Discuss pathophysiology of preterm labor.

Pathophysiology of preterm labor is illustrated in Flow chart 15.1.

5. Write warning signs of preterm labor.
- Menstrual like cramps
- Low, dull backache
- Pressure (feels like baby is pushing down)
- Increase or change in vaginal discharge
- Fluid leak from vagina
- Uterine contraction with or without pain, 10 minutes apart or closer.

6. Discuss management of patient at-risk of preterm labor.
- Regular antenatal visits
- Education about preterm labor
- Aggressive treatment of cervical and vaginal discharge
- Serial pelvic examination
- Serial USG examination
- Coital abstinence
- Limitation of physical activity
- Change in working condition
- For patients with history of second trimester loss or spontaneous preterm birth, close monitoring during antenatal case (ANC).

7. Write predictors of preterm labor.
- *Risk markers:* As described earlier.
- *Home uterine activity monitoring (HUAM):* Involves telemetric recording of uterine contraction and its transmission to a monitoring center and daily feedback from the healthcare practitioner to offer patient's support and advice. Not recommended nowadays.

Flow chart 15.1 Pathophysiology of preterm labor

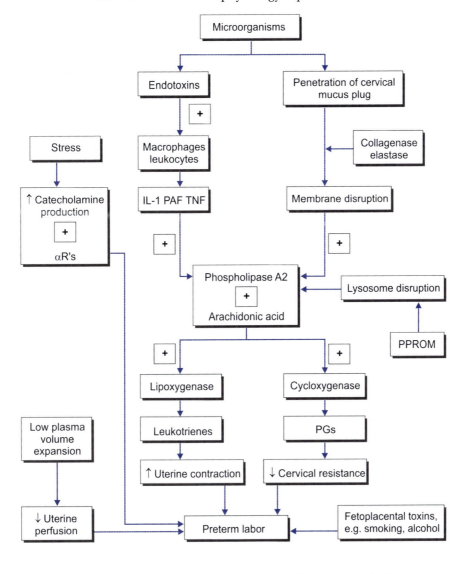

- *Biochemical markers:*
  a. *Salivary estriol:*
     - >18 ng/mL before 34 weeks indicate preterm labor
     - Poor sensitivity and specificity.
  b. *Serum collagenase:*
     - Increases in preterm labor
     - Detected by ELISA.
  c. *Relaxin hormone:* Increases in preterm labor.
  d. *Fetal fibronectin.*
- Most important predictor of preterm labor.
- Its presence in cervicovaginal secretion >50 ng/mL during 20–37 weeks indicated preterm labor
- *USG can reveal:*
  - Fetal malformation
  - Hydramnios, multiple pregnancy
  - Fetal age
  - BPP, breathing pattern
  - Cervical length and extent of dilatation
  - Risk factors for preterm labor
  - Funneling of cervix with internal os dilatation >20 mm and shortening of cervix (cervical length <25 mm) between 24–28 weeks may increase the relative risk of preterm labor
  - Normal fetal breathing stops 24–48 hours before the onset of labor, this finding is specific in presence of intact membrane and in absence of APH.
  - *USG:* 65–70% predictive for preterm labor.
- Screening for lower genital tract infection including bacterial vaginosis.

8. What is bacterial vaginosis?

Normal *Lactobacillus* predominant vaginal flora, is replaced by anerobic bacteria, i.e. *Gardnerella vaginalis* and *Mycoplasma hominis.*

9. How do you diagnose bacterial vaginosis?

- Vaginal pH >4.5
- Amine (fishy) odor with KOH
- Presence of clue cells (vaginal epithelial cells glued with dead bacilli)
- Few WBC with mixed flora.

10. Discuss investigations/laboratory studies in preterm labor.

- Complete hemogram—including CBC, differential count
- Urine analysis and culture
- Serum C reactive protein (>0.8 = chances of preterm labor)
- *Electrolytes and serum glucose:* In cases requiring B_2 agonist tocolytics
- USG examination
- *Amniocentesis:*
  - For fetal lung maturity
  - Bacteriological study
- *Cervicovaginal fluid:* Microscopic with Gram staining
  - Culture and sensitivity
  - Fetal fibronectin levels.

11. Define role of amniocentesis to detect infection.

Infection indicated by:
- Increased leukocyte count
- Decreased glucose
- Increased IL-6 (most sensitive test for detection of amniotic fluid containing bacteria)
- Positive Gram staining
- Positive culture.

12. Discuss diagnosis of preterm labor.

- More subjective than objective
- Require serial examination (preferably by same examiner)

Criteria (proposed by AICOG in 1997)
- Four contraction in 2 minutes or 8 in 60 minutes plus progressive change in the cervix
- Cervical dilatation >1 cm
- Cervical effacement > 80%.

13. What is the management of preterm labor?

It varies according to the condition of the patient:
Group A: Patient who are at risk
Management as described earlier.

Group B: Patient with warning signs of threatened preterm labor
- Limitation of physical activity
- Referral to tertiary care center
- Antibiotics—Ampicillin/ampicillin + Sulbactam (commonly used)
- Tocolytics—Beta-adrenergics, calcium channel blockers, magnesium salts, etc.

Group C: Management of patient with established preterm labor.

a. *Patients who need to be delivered immediately:*
   - *Maternal diseases:* PIH, hypertension, chronic renal disease, cardiac disease, SLE, acute or chronic infection
   - Advanced labor—5 cm dilatation or >80% effacement with membrane bulging
   - PPROM
   - Congenital and chromosomal anomalies in fetus
   - IUGR
   - Chorioamnionitis
   - If adequate, fetal lung maturity is present.

b. *Patients who do not require immediate delivery:*
   Drugs given
   - *Tocolytics*: After ruling out their contraindications, IV route is effective than oral
     Antibiotics: It is only helpful when preterm is associated with chorioamnionitis or PPROM or any condition predisposing to maternal infection, e.g. immunosuppressive drugs.
   - *Glucocorticoids:*
     - Rule out contraindications (e.g. diabetes mellitus, as steroids aggravate the hyperglycemia)
     - Used where maturity is within 34 weeks with immature fetal lung and there is definite interval of >24 hours between delivery and drug administration with maximum limit within 7 days of last dose.

     Agents used are:
     Betamethasone—12 mg—24 hours—apart
     Dexamethasone—6 mg—12 hourly—4 doses
   - *Phenobarbitone*:
     - Dose 10 mg/kg maximum upto 500–700 mg IV in 30 minutes
     - It may prevent intraventricular bleeding in newborn
     - Role is controversial.
   - *Vitamin K_1:*
     - Dose 10 mg IM followed by 20 mg orally or injection to be repeated every week before 32 weeks
     - It may prevent intraventricular bleeding in newborn
     - Role is controversial.

14. What steps should be taken during delivery of preterm infant?

Ist stage of labor
- *Epidural anesthesia:* Alleviates labor pain
  Improves oxygenation.
- Avoid strong sedatives—suppress the fetal respiratory center.

IInd stage of labor
- Premature bearing down should be discouraged otherwise fetus may suffer ICH
- Intrapartum fetal monitoring
  Avoid fetal scalp monitoring—may cause scalp hemorrhage
- *Liberal episiotomy:*
  - To shorten the 2nd stage
  - To reduce the force compressing the soft fetal skull
- Outlet forceps superior to ventouse extraction—less likely to cause ICH
- Elective cesarean delivery does not confer much benefit to the baby and should be done only after weighing the benefit to the neonate against the maternal morbidity of operative delivery
- The possibility of a PPH should be borne in mind, if the woman was administered tocolytic drugs before delivery and preventive measures should be taken.

15. What steps should be taken for the neonate immediately after birth?

- Cut and clamp umbilical cord immediately to prevent overloading of blood circulation
- For immediate resuscitation by pediatrician
- Establish breathing fast and avoid prolonged anoxia, but remember that prolonged oxygen therapy is also harmful and can lead to bronchopulmonary dysplasia and retrolental fibroplasia
- Avoid infection by proper antibiotics
- Vitamin K and phenobarbitone—not recommended nowadays
- Intratracheal surfactant, if available
- Maintain euthermia
- IV nutrition preferred to oral feed for first few days. Breastfeeding is started once the suckling reflex is established.

16. What are the consequences of preterm labor?

Prematurity is the major consequence, resulting in risk of neonatal morbidity and mortality. This mostly occurs due to:

- Birth asphyxia
- Respiratory distress syndrome
- Jaundice
- Hemorrhage
- Hypocalcemia
- Hypoglycemia
- Sepsis
- Feeding difficulties
- Necrotizing enterocolitis
- PDA
- IVH
- Sensorineural deafness
- Developmental delay
- Iatrogenic complications, e.g. retrolental fibroplasia
- Reduced growth potential
- Recurrent respiratory infection
- Learning difficulties
- Social enforced separation of mother and baby
- Sudden infant death syndrome (SIDS)
- Blindness.

17. What are tocolytic drugs? Why they are used in preterm labor?

Drugs that inhibit uterine contraction are called as tocolytic drugs.

Tocolytic are useful in preterm labor for:
- Adding few days to fetal maturity. To provide time for completing corticosteroid therapy and utero transfer.
- Pulmonary maturity will reduce the risk of respiratory distress syndrome (RDS) in the newborn.

18. What are the contraindications of tocolytic therapy?

The conditions are the following:
- Severe hemorrhage
- Abruptio placentae
- Pregnancy-induced hypertension
- Intrauterine fetal death
- Chorioamnionitis
- Pulmonary hypertension
- Known intolerance to tocolytics
- Fetal maturity (after 34 weeks of pregnancy)
- Lethal fetal anomaly
- Severe intrauterine growth retardation
- Uncontrolled insulin-dependent diabetes
- Asthmatic patient (tachyphylaxis)
- Patient on monoamine oxidase (MAO) inhibitor.

19. What are the different tocolytic agents and how are they used?

	Drugs	Class of drugs	Dose IV	Dose oral
1.	Isoxsuprine (Duvadilan)	β-mimetic	30–60 mg in 500 mL dextrose (0.1–1 mg/min)	5–10 mg
2.	Ritodrine	β-mimetic	150 mg in 500 mL (4–12 mg/hour)	10 mg 2 hourly (1st dose 30 min before stopping IV drip) to maximum 120 mg in 24 hours
3.	Terbutaline	β-mimetic	5 mg/min maintenance dose 2–5 mg/min max 30 mg	5 mg 6–8 hourly subcutaneous 2–5 mg, 3–4 hourly
4.	Salbutamol	β-mimetic	20–50 mg/min maintenance dose 2–5 mg/min	—
5.	Indomethacin	Anti-prostaglandin	50 mg initially reduced to 25 mg 4 hourly × 24 hours	Same as IV dose loading 50–100 mg followed by 24
6.	Sulindac	Prostaglandin synthetase inhibitor	—	200 mg 12 hourly for 48 hours
7.	Magnesium salt		$MgSO_4$—4 g in 10% dextrose over 20 min followed by 2% maintenance infusion at 2 g/hour	Oral salts—Magnesium gluconate 1 g BD, magnesium oxide—200 mg TDS, magnesium chloride—535 mg QID
8.	Nifedipine	Calcium-channel blockers		30 mg followed by 20 mg TDS Sublingual—10 mg every 15–20 min in the 1st hour thereafter 60–160 mg/day
9.	Atosiban or Antocin or Tractocile	Oxytocin antagonist	7.5 mg bolus, then 7.5 mg in doses of 300 mg/min for 3 hours (18 mg/hour), then 100 mg/min upto 48 hours (6 mg/hour) total dose should not exceed 330 mg over 48 hours	—
10.	Nitroglycerine	No donors	Used as transdermal patch—10 mg patch approximately to lateral aspect of thigh and is repeated after 2 hours, if contraction do not stop. Not more than 2 patches are used in 24 hours. Can be kept for 48 hours	
11.	L-arginine	No donor	Under trial	
12.	Na nitroprusside	No donor		

20. What are the adverse effects of commonly used tocolytic agents?

	Drugs	Maternal effect	Fetal effect
1.	β-mimetic	Tachycardia, hypotension, hyperglycemia, hyperinsulinemia, hypokalemia, hypocalcemia, hyperlipidemia, tremor, cardiac arrythmia, myocardial infarction, pulmonary edema and fluid retention headache, chest pain, liver damage. Contraindication in cardiac disease diabetes, hyperthyroidism, pregnancy induced hypertension, intrauterine growth retardation, fetal death, antepartum hemorrhage	Fetal hypoglycemia, hypocalcemia, hypotension, ileus
2.	Indomethacin	Hepatitis, renal failure, gastrointestinal bleeding	Premature closure of ductus arteriosus and pulmonary hypertension, intracranial hemorrhage, necrotizing enterocolitis, renal dysfunction
3.	Nifedipine	Hypotension, tachycardia, headache, dizziness, nausea	Acidosis and fetal asphyxia, jaundice
4.	Magnesium sulfate	Hypotension, MS paralysis, drowsiness, cardiac arrest, pulmonary edema, respiratory depression, tetany	Fetal hyperglycemia, neonatal drowsiness, lethargy, respiratory depression
5.	Atosiban	Nausea, vomiting, headache	

21. What is the mode of action of various tocolytics?

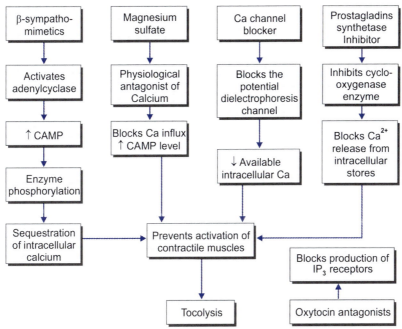

22. What is the role of corticosteroids in preterm labor?

Antenatal corticosteroid therapy reduces the risk of respiratory distress syndrome (by 50%), necrotizing enterocolitis and intraventricular hemorrhage in the preterm newborn.

- *Effective between 30 and 34 weeks of gestation:*
  (<30 weeks—type II pneumocytes scanty—drug not effective)
  (>34 weeks—cells produce adequate surfactant—no use of drug)
- Betamethasone 12 mg 24 hourly × 2 doses
  Dexamethasone 4 mg 6 hourly × 4 doses
- These drugs have negligible immunosuppressive effect and are safe even in presence of infection, pregnancy-induced hypertension and tuberculosis also in diabetes with caution
- The drug effect appears 24 hours after the infusion and persists for 7 days
- Multiple weekly doses of corticosteroids is not recommended nowadays
- Betamethasone is better than dexamethasone
- Dexamethasone causes intraventricular and periventricular leukomalacia leading to cerebral palsy.

23. Discuss ineffective treatment for preterm labor.

Bed rest (expectant management)
- Strict bed rest for >3 days increases risk of developing blood clots in the legs or lungs (1 in 1000 to 16 in 1000)
- There is no evidence that long-term bed rest lowers the risk of preterm labor.

Cervical encirclage
Cervical encirclage is the surgical closure of an incompetent cervix:
- A recent study has shown that cerclage used to close a shortened cervix (identified using TVS) is ineffective for preventing preterm labor and delivery
- It also carries a risk of infection and pregnancy loss. It is also associated with increased medical intervention and doubling of the risk of puerperal pyrexia
- So it should not be done in cases other than proved cervical incompetence.

Home uterine activity monitoring (HUAM)
Research has shown that HUAM is expensive and has no proven effect on delaying early birth.

24. Some important and vital statistical data.

Impact of preterm labor
- Incidence in developed countries   6–7%
- Incidence in India   10%
- Responsible for 75% of all neonatal mortality
- Responsible for 50% of long-term neurological impairment in children

Relative risk of preterm labor
- Low socioeconomic status   2 times
- Black race   2 times
- Recent cocaine use   4 times

- Prolonged periods of standing during pregnancy — 1.3 times
- Weight gain <0.27 kg/week during pregnancy — 2.54 times
- Patient with asymptomatic bacteriuria — 2 times
- Group B streptococci in vaginal culture — 18.7%
- Increased incidence of preterm labor is found among women delivering male infants (odds ratio 1:2)
- Low magnesium and high relaxin level are also associated with increased incidence of preterm labor.

Risk in subsequent pregnancy
- One preterm birth = 14.3%
- Two preterm birth = 28%
- Bacterial vaginosis has been suggested as the causative agent in upto 50% cases of idiopathic preterm labor.

Relation between fetal weight and survival
- 1000–1500 g >90% survival
- <1000 g—survival decreases 10–15% for each decrement of 100 g
- <500 g—survival is rare.

According to gestational age survival rate
- 72% at 28 weeks
- While it is 50–60% at 26 weeks and increases 0.9–3% per day from 25–30 weeks
- 50% neonatal deaths occur in 24 hours and another 15% in 48 hours of birth.

25. Recent predictor of preterm labor.

Fetal Fibronectin
- Glycoprotein present in high concentration in maternal blood and in amniotic fluid
- Plays role in intercellular adhesion during implantation and in maintenance of placental adhesion to decidua
- Detectable in cervix vaginal secretion until 16–20 weeks of gestation thereafter disappears until near term unless premature rupture of membrane occurs
- >50 ng/mL during 20–37 weeks indicates preterm labor
- Positive test at 24 weeks—60 fold increase in risk of preterm labor within 4 weeks of sampling
- 20 times risk of clinical chorioamnionitis
- Negative predictive value—90–95%.

26. What are the indications of iatrogenic preterm labor?
- Maternal—severe PIH, eclampsia, APH
- Fetal—fetal distress, severe IUGR, noncompatible fetus.

27. What is risk scoring system?
Risk scoring system aims to identify those at high-risk of preterm labor by using primary predictors such as previous obstetrics history, sociodemographic factors.

MUST REMEMBER
- Incidence of preterm labor—5–10%.
- Sociodemographic factors, previous history of preterm labor, multiple gestations, vaginal infections, cervical incompetence, congenital anomaly are important contributing factors for preterm labor.
- Correction of anemia, improvement of nutrition, elimination of septic foci, limited drug and substance abuse and regular antenatal check up reduce the incidence of preterm labor.
- Threatened preterm labor is characterized by regular and frequent uterine contractions, but cervical dilatation less than 1 cm.
- The subclinical chorioamnionitis is one of the important etiological factors.
- Tocolysis should be given only till cervix is less than 3 cm. Later on, labor should be allowed.
- The role of antibiotics in prevention of preterm labor is controversial.
- Management of preterm labor consists of detecting which patients can be conserved with tocolysis and glucocorticoid treatment and which patients need to be delivered.

HIV Infection during Pregnancy

Deepti Dongaonkar, Sachin Khedkar

It is essential for every MBBS graduate to know about diagnosis and principles of managing HIV infection. HIV infection during pregnancy needs special attention.

HISTORY

When was first HIV case reported in the world?
When was the first case reported in India and which city?
When was the word HIV coined?
When and where the organism for HIV was discovered?
What is window period?
What is the natural history of HIV? (Stages of the disease)

- Universal precautions to be taken by care providers
- Postexposure prophylaxis and drug given for the same
- HIV controlling organization at center and state levels.

TYPES OF HIV VIRUSES

- HIV type 1—serology A, B, C, D...................L, M, N
- HIV type II (seen in North India)
- (HIV I type E is common in India).

PREVALENCE AND INCIDENCE (NACO 2004–2005)

- Cumulative—Total 5.3 million in India (Dec 2005) affected
- Male to female ratio: 60:40
- New infection per year—16,000 per year (20,000 in 2005)
- General population less than 1%
- Pregnant women in South India (including Maharashtra) more than 1%
- Commercial sex worker—40-60%
- In STD clinics—20-30%.

Modes of transmission:

- *Horizontal transmission:*
  - Sexual—homosexual, heterosexual, bisexual
  - Intravenous drug abuse
  - Infected blood transfusion
- *Vertical transmission:*
  - Mother to child during pregnancy and childbirth
- *Minor route of transmission:*
  - Postmortem examination
  - Ear prick or tattooing needles
  - Wet kissing with oral ulcer in one partner
  - Intramuscular/subcutaneous injection
  - Washing and cleaning surgical instrument/linen
  - Washing/wiping blood splash with cuts on finger
  - Surgery procedure/open wound dressing
  - Blood collection/tooth bite.

Indications for HIV testing:

- Screening during every pregnancy
- Recurrent pelvic infection, vaginal ulcers or discharge
- Chronic ill health, 10% weight loss in 6 months, unexplained fever, loose motions since 1 month.
- Screening each tuberculosis patient
- Person who received multiple blood transfusion
- Suspected opportunistic infection
- Second marriage following death of a partner in young age
- Person with drug abuse/chronic alcoholism
- Malignancy before 40 years of age (for prognosis).

Screening during pregnancy:

Under PPTCT (Prevention of parent-to-child transmission) program. All pregnant women, irrespective of gestational age are offered voluntary testing. "Opt out".

During ANC, a patient goes through:

- Pretest counseling, written consent, distribution of reports, post-test counseling
- Nevirapine prophylaxis: HAART Prophylaxis.

TYPES OF TESTS FOR HIV DIAGNOSIS

Adult:

- Antibodies detection tests—ELISA test, rapid test, ImmunoComb test
- Antigen detection tests—Western blot, immunoblot
- Viral detection—bDNA PCR, RT PCR (RNA PCR), NASBA.

Neonates:

- Up to 2 months—p24 antigen (western blot)
- Up to 18 months—RT-PCR, DNA PCR

- After 18 months—ELISA based like adults
- HIV risk associated per exposure with high-risk behavior (UNAIDS/NACO)
- Blood transfusion—95%
- Vertical transmission—25-40%
- IV drug abuse—0.67%
- Homosexual—0.04%
- Heterosexual—0.1-0.3%
- Needle injury to HCW—0.4%
  (heterosexual is common mode of transmission in India due to frency of exposure).

Prevalent Mode of HIV Spread (Differ in Northern and Southern States) NACO

- Sexual—80-90% (in southern states)
- Among women 80-90% are housewives (from promiscuous husband)
- Blood transfusion—2-5%
- IVDU—15-20% (in southern states)—70-80% (in Manipur and Nagaland).

Determinant of mother-to-child transmission of HIV

Prenatal factors	Intrapartum factors	Postpartum factors
Nutrition	ART	Breast versus formula feed
CD4	Duration of rupture of membranes	Breastfeed duration
CD8		Mixed feed
Viral load	Vagina douche*	Mastitis/nipple infection
STI	Vaginal vs cesarean	ART to baby
ART	Duration of labor	Maternal ART with BF

*Savlon or 1% betadine is good for vaginal douches

ASSOCIATION OF HIV AND TUBERCULOSIS

- 25-30% of Tuberculosis patients may be HIV positive 60% of HIV patient may suffer from TB in lifetime
- Extrapulmonary TB is common among HIV infected person
- TB is common cause of death among Indians with HIV (adult and children)
- Presence of TB during pregnancy increases risk of transmission
- Risk reactivation of old healed TB lesion is known occurrence of TB hastens the progression of the disease.

Antiretroviral drugs available

Nucleoside analogue (NRTI)	Non-nucleoside analogue (NNRTI)	Protease inhibitor (PI)	Fusion inhibitors (FI) (under trial)
Zidovudine	Nevirapine	Indinavir	
Lamivudine	Delavirdine	Ritonavir	
Didanosine	Efavirenz	Saquinavir	
Stavudine	Nelfinavir	Amprenavir	
Abacavir			
Zalcitabine			
Adefovir			
Tenofovir			

ART in red are commonly used in pregnancy

Indications for starting ART:
- Symptomatic HIV disease
- CD4 cell count fewer than 350 copies/cmm
- Viral load more than
- 10,000 copies/mL by branched DNA PCR
- 20,000 copies/mL by RNA PCR
- Acute retroviral syndrome within 6 months of documented seroconversion
- Prevention of mother-to-child transmission
- Postexposure prophylaxis.

Contraindications for ART

Maternal factors	Fetal factors
Hb less than 8.0 g%	Fetal demise
Thrombocytopenia (<100,000/cmm)	Fetal anomaly
Total WBC <1,000/cmm	Fetal hydrops or ascitis
Radiotherapy or chemotherapy	Fetal severe anemia
Anti-HIV vaccine	Oligo- or polyhydramnios
S creatinine more than 1.5 mg% (130 µmol/L) Creatinine clearance >70 mL/min	

Preferred ART combinations

- For PPTCT—single NRTI or 2 NRTIs or 2 NRTIs + 1 NNRTI
- PEP—2 NRTI or 2 NRT + 1 NNRTI or 2 NRTI + 1 PI
- Other patient—2 NRTI + 1 NNRTI or 2NRTI + 1 PI (Consult expert before stating therapy to avoid drug interaction and toxicity).

Monitoring patient on ART—Every three to four monthly

Specific	Nonspecific	Extra, if required
CD4 count	Hb, CBC, total	Urine or stool culture
CD8 count	Lymphocyte count	ART drug sensitivity
Viral load	LFT, RFT	X-ray chest for chronic cough
Specific fungi	X-ray chest, if known	USG for liver, kidney, pelvis
Virus culture	Tuberculosis	Bone marrow aspiration, MRI

Side-effects and toxicity known with long-term use of ART

Hematological	Metabolic	Systemic	Bones
Anemia	Lipodystrophy	Hepatotoxicity	Avascular necrosis of femur neck
Pancytopenia	Insulin resistance	Nephrotoxicity	
Thrombocytopenia	Lactic acidemia	Polyneuropathy	Osteopenia
	Hypertriglyceridemia	Hypersensitivity	Osteoporosis
		GIT disturbances	

Drugs	Side-effects
Zidovudine	Anemia
Efavirenz	Neural tube defects
Indinavir/Ritonavir	Nephrolithiasis/Lipodystrophy
Stavudine	Pancreatitis

Indications for discontinuation of ART

Toxicity-related	Disease progression related
Hb fall below 8.0 g%, pancytopenia	No fall in viral load with 3-4 months ART
Lactic acidemia	Development of malignancy
Hepatic dysfunction with HBV/HCV infection	Try change of ART combination or do drug resistance test
Drug intolerance/drug sensitivity	

Always change drug with known toxicity or stop all drugs at a time to avoid development of drug resistance. Consult expert.

1. Should HIV testing be mandatory or voluntary during pregnancy?

Voluntary: Mandatory testing may cause program failure in long-term. Voluntary testing with pretest counseling gives an opportunity for health education and for HIV awareness drive. It also encourages for behavioral change.

2. What is HIV transmission rate from Mother-to-child in India?

- Without drug (ART) it 25-40% (36% author study in 1998).
- With drug (ART) intervention 2-12% (differ with combination and duration).

3. When does MTCT occur?

- It can occur any time during pregnancy.
- It is more (15-20%) in late months of pregnancy and maximum (70%) during labor. Breastfeeding can risk 7-15% children fed for more than 5 months.

4. What care should be taken during pregnancy in HIV infected mother?

Routine ANC visit pattern followed. Avoid any maternal infection, which may reduce immunity. Promote health with good hygiene and nutrition. Screen for TB, genital infections. Prevent anemia, hypoproteinemia. Encourage hospital delivery and early arrival to hospital in labor. Encourage ART.

5. What care should be taken during labor in HIV infected women?

Should arrive early in labor. Vaginal douche should be given to minimize neonatal infection. Avoid prolong labor and rupture of membranes (ROM). ROM (ARM) may be done in indicated cases. Avoid instrumental delivery and CS. Cesarean section should be done for obstetrics indications only. Continue ART. Avoid milking of card. Encourage early clamping. Healthcare provider should observe universal precaution for self-protection.

6. What ART should be given?

Zidovudine, lamivudine and nevirapine are standard drugs used during pregnancy and labor. Selection of drugs (ART) depends on viral load, CD4 and CD8 count.

7. What are different ART regimen given in prenatal period for pregnancy with HIV?

A. ACTG 076 (NY 1992)—ZDV 100 mg five times a day, 14-38 weeks
B. Thai (1995)—ZDV 300 mg twice a day from 36 to 40 weeks
C. PETRA regimen (S. Africa, Tanzania, 1998)
D. PACT 185 regimen (USA 1998)
E. Uganda regimen—Nevirapin 200 mg stat single dose.

Grand Multipara

Pushpa S Junghare, Kanan Yelikar, Kalpana Kalyankar

HISTORY

- Obstetric history should be asked in details, including:
  - Duration of marriage
  - *Gravidity:* No. of times she was pregnant
  - *Parity:* No. of times she delivered.
  - Details regarding her previous pregnancies and deliveries.
- Socioeconomic history
- Educational history
- Awareness regarding contraception
- History pertaining to presence of anemia, diabetes hypertension.

1. Define grand multipara.

A woman who has delivered 4 or more viable babies, and is pregnant for the fifth time.

2. Is it very commonly encountered condition?

As family size is decreasing a case with grand multiparity is less commonly encountered.

3. What are the risks of grand multiparity?

Anemia, PIH, pregnancy aggravated hypertension are more common. The hemorrhage of all varieties, i.e. before, during and after delivery is doubled, uterine rupture tripled. The incidence of cesarean section rate is also increased.

4. Are there any other associated risk factors?

Patient is older in age, her cardiovascular system is less resilient, obesity might have set in. Majority of these patients may be poor, overworked and tired, unregistered or not having antenatal care. Prolonged lactation can deplete them of calcium.

5. What obstetrical complications are encountered in a grand multipara?

- Twin pregnancy
- Placenta previa
- Abruptio placentae
- Malpresentations
- Preterm labor.

6. What are complications during labor?

- Malpresentation—due to pendulous abdomen together with the high angle of pelvic inclination—breech presentation, transverse and oblique lie are more common
- Delayed engagement of head can give rise to PROM and cord complications
- Cephalopelvic disproportion may occur. The babies tend to get larger with successive pregnancies. Moreover, the pelvic inclination is increased and forward subluxation of sacrum upon the sacroiliac joints reduces the true conjugate
- Incidence of cesarean section is thereby increased
- Precipitate labor might occur
- Obstructed labor
- Rupture of uterus.

7. What are third or postpartum problems?

With every pregnancy and delivery, the uterus undergoes increase in fibrous tissue and decrease in elastic tissue. This affects the contractility. Third stage bleeding and postpartum bleeding is more common. Operative interference may add to traumatic PPH.

Patient is asked to attend regular antenatal OPD as a high-risk patient. Her anemia should be prevented or corrected with appropriate iron therapy. Patient reporting late in pregnancy may need blood transfusion for the same. One should be vigilant regarding hypertension or presence of diabetes mellitus.

8. What about obstetric management for grand multipara?

After ruling out malpresentation and cephalopelvic disproportion, patient can be given trial of vaginal delivery. It should be a hospital delivery.

Labor should be more meticulously monitored so as to detect cord complications, malpresentation like brow presentation or obstructed labor. Timely intervention will be helpful. Patient should be electively taken for LSCS, if there is transverse lie at term or cephalopelvic disproportion.

9. How to manage third stage?

As this patient is at high-risk for third stage bleeding and PPH, prophylactic measures against this complication should be taken. IV line should have been set up during labor, blood should be kept ready and uterotonic drugs can be used to prevent postpartum hemorrhage.

10. Give details about management of third stage.

IV methargin 0.4 mg can be given to mother immediately after delivery or 10 units of pitocin can be given IM or combined methergine and oxytocin can be given IM injection—carboprost 125 mg IM can also be given.

11. Write any newer alternatives for management of third stage?

If it is not possible to give injectables and drugs which require cold storage, tablet misoprostol 200–1000 mcg can be given orally, sublingually or kept in rectum for prevention of PPH.

12. What if patient does not respond to all methods and develops PPH?

After trying all conservative methods to treat atonic PPH and after ruling out traumatic PPH, patient can be treated more vigorously. Laparotomy should be performed to expedite hysterectomy rapidly. Blood transfusion should be given as required. Delay in treatment might land the patient in irreversible shock, Sheehan's syndrome, DIC, etc.

13. What about obstructed labor and rupture uterus?

These are preventable complications and good antenatal and intrapartum supervision should take care of this. Still unbooked patient may come with these problems. After resuscitation, irrespective of fetal outcome, patient should be operated. After doing cesarean section for obstructed labor, bilateral tubectomy should be ideally carried out. After rupture of uterus, patient can be salvaged by laparotomy and repair of uterus followed by tubectomy. If the trauma is irreparable, one should go ahead with hysterectomy.

14. What advise you will give after delivery?

If patient delivers vaginally with no complications, she should be advised tubectomy operation before discharge.

15. Are complications of grand multiparity preventable?

One should discourage grand multiparity. Every patient coming for antenatal care and delivery should be counseled regarding small family size and family planning methods. A grand multi coming in first-half of pregnancy should be given the option for MTP followed by some contraception.

16. How to tackle malpresentation?

Transverse, oblique or unstable lie is more common in grand multipara simply because of pendulous abdomen, baby size may be average and pelvis might be adequate. In such cases, external cephalic version during last few weeks of pregnancy or early labor may be attempted. If this fails, stabilized induction should be done. If this also fails, patient should posted for LSCS.

17. How to minimize morbidity and prevent mortality in mother and child?

One should be necessarily very alert when a grand multipara patient is admitted with any compliant anticipate the complications and she should be treated as a dire emergency. A transverse lie may end up as neglected shoulder presentation, cord prolapse, obstructed labor or even rupture uterus. A senior obstetrician should be informed early when ever such patient is admitted, so that the patient is properly managed.

MUST REMEMBER

- Multipara is composed of two Latin words: "Multi" meaning "much" and "para" from "pario," meaning "to bring forth".
- Incidence of anemia, hypertensive diseases, uterine rupture and primary cesarean section rate increases in grand multipara.
- Grand multipara is a major hindrance to safe motherhood
- Grand multipara shows poor acceptance of family planning methods.
- Twin pregnancy is 3 times more common in grand multipara
- During labor following guidelines are prescribed: (1) Pelvic assessment should be done as routine. (2) Presentation and position are to be checked. (3) Undue delay in progress should be viewed with caution.
- Atonic PPH is common in grand multipara.
- Rupture of uterus is most common cause of maternal death in grand multipara.
- Most common cause of fetal death in grand multipara is prematurity.

Occipitoposterior Position

Ashwini Yelikar, Chandan Gupta, Kanan Yelikar

1. How will you define presentation?
It is defined as that part of the fetus, which occupies the lower pole of the uterus, e.g. cephalic and podalic.

2. Define lie, position, attitude, and presenting part.
Lie: It is the relation of the long-axis of the fetus to the long-axis of uterus or maternal spine, e.g. longitudinal lie, oblique lie, and transverse lie.

Position: This is the relation of the denominator on the presenting part, with the four quadrants of the pelvis, e.g. LOA, left occipitoanterior means, the presentation is vertex, denominator is occiput, position is left anterior, and lie is of course longitudinal.

Attitude: It is the relation of different parts of the fetus with each other, e.g. the universal attitude is that of flexion.

Presenting part: It is that part of the fetus, which is at the cervix or which is first felt on doing a pelvic examination.

3. What are the incidences of different presentation?
- Cephalic 96%
- Vertex 95.5%
- Face 0.4%
- Brow 0.1%
- Podalic 4%
- Breach 3.5%
- Transverse 0.5%.

4. Define occipitoposterior position.
In vertex presentation, when the occiput lies in one of the posterior quadrants or lies over sacroiliac joints or on the sacrum directly.

5. What are varieties of OP?
- Oblique
- Direct OP or occipitosacral.

6. Which position is more common?
Right occipitoposterior (ROP) is more common, because right oblique diameter of the pelvis is slightly more than the left oblique and presence of rectosigmoid on left side.

7. What are the etiological factors for OP?
- Anthropoid shape of the pelvis
- Deflexed head
- Poor uterine action
- Cephalopelvic disproportion.

8. How to confirm the diagnosis?
- On inspection, abdomen looks flat below umbilicus
- Fetal limbs are easily felt near the midline
- Head is not engaged
- FHS are difficult to locate, but in direct occipitoposterior position, fetal heart is distinctly felt in midline
- Elongated bag of membranes that rupture early
- Sagittal suture in oblique diameter
- Anterior fontanelle is easily felt due to deflexion of the head
- In late labor after formation of caput, unfolded pinna points towards occiput.

9. How will you manage OP?
Watchful expectancy 80–90% of OP rotate anteriorly and deliver vaginally.

10. What are the unfavorable mechanisms?
POP persistents occipitoposterior position, if the head fails to rotate, in spite of good uterine contractions, till the end of second stage of labor.

11. How will you manage POP?
- Cesarean section in modern obstetrics
- Manual rotation
- Forceps rotation and extraction (Keilland's forceps)

- Ventouse
- Craniotomy, if baby is dead.

12. How can deep transverse arrest occur in case of oblique OP position? What is oblique posterior arrest?

In cases of incomplete forward rotation, the occiput rotates through 1/8th of circle so that the sagittal sutures come to lie in bispinous diameter. Nonrotation of head in moderate degree of deflexion leads to oblique posterior arrest of labor.

13. What is mechanism of 'face to pubis' delivery?

It is more common in anthropoid type of pelvis. Further descent of head occurs till root of nose hinges under pubic symphysis. First brow occiput and vertex deliver by flexion, and face is born by extension. Restitution and external rotation occur.

MUST REMEMBER
- Occipitoposterior is malposition for 3rd or 4th position of vertex.
- It is not abnormal presentation.
- Dextrorotation of uterus and sigmoid colon on the left favor ROP position.
- OP is commonly associated with anthropoid or android pelvis.
- In direct occipitoposterior position, small sinciput may be confused with breech.
- Engagement of head is delayed due to deflexion.
- Long rotation by 3/8th of circle in 80% cases leads to favorable outcome.
- Nonrotation or incomplete rotation may complicate course of labor.
- Face to pubis delivery can occur and head is born by flexion.

Breech Presentation

Sonali Deshpande

1. What is the incidence of breech presentation?

The incidence of breech presentation is 20% at 28 weeks and drops to 5% at 34 weeks and 3% at term.

2. What are the etiological factors for breech presentation?

The etiological factors are:
a. Prematurity
b. Maternal factors—multiparity, polyhydramnios, contracted pelvis, uterine anomalies, fibroid uterus
c. Placental—cornual-fundal attachment of placenta, placenta previa
d. Fetal—multiple pregnancy, hydrocephalus, anencephaly, IUFD.

3. What are the different varieties of breech presentation?

There are four varieties:
a. Complete (20%)—flexion at thighs and knees
b. Frank (60–80%)—flexion at thighs and extension at knees
c. Footling (10%)—single or double, with extension at thighs and knees
d. Knee—single or double, with extension at thighs and flexion at knees.

4. What do you mean by recurrent or habitual breech?

When the breech presentation occurs in 3 or more consecutive pregnancies, it is called as habitual or recurrent breech. The causes are congenital malformation of uterus and repeated cornu-fundal attachment of placenta.

5. How will you diagnose breech presentation clinically?
- P/A hard globular ballotable fetal head is found to occupy fundus
- Lateral grips indicate back on one side and small fetal parts on other
- On Pawlik's grip, ballotable breech, if not engaged and after engagement the fourth maneuver shows the firm breech to be beneath the symphysis. Fetal heart sounds are above the level of umbilicus
- On PV examination, both ischial tuberosities, the sacrum, the anus, and sometimes the external genitalia. Sometimes the finger may be meconium-stained.

6. What do you mean by complicated breech?

When the breech presentation is associated with obstetric conditions which adversely influence the prognosis such as prematurity, placenta previa and contracted pelvis.

7. What is the importance of meconium in breech presentation?

Presence of meconium before the fetus is in pelvis is abnormal and should be considered as a possible sign of fetal distress.

8. What is the role of USG in breech presentation at term?

USG should be done to know the type of breech, placental localization, estimated fetal weight (EFW), fetal anomalies, amniotic fluid index and to know the flexion of head.

9. What is difference between spontaneous, assisted breech and total breech extraction?
- In spontaneous breech delivery, the entire fetus is expelled by natural forces of mother, with no assistance other than support of baby as it is being born.
- *Assisted breech:* The fetus is delivered by the natural forces as far as the umbilicus. The remainder of the baby is extracted by the attendant (assistance is required above the level of umbilicus).
- *Total breech extraction:* The entire body of the fetus is extracted by the attendant (assistance is required below the level of umbilicus).

10. How will you select the mode of delivery in breech presentation?

The choice of abdominal/vaginal route depends upon the history of previous breech delivery, type of breech, flexion of fetal head, fetal size, estimated fetal weight, quality of uterine contractions, size of maternal pelvis and other obstetric complications.

11. What is ECV? How is it performed?

External cephalic version (ECV) is the procedure of converting breech of a longitudinal lie or transverse lie into cephalic presentation.

One or two operators are necessary for the procedure. The procedure should be performed in a setting where fetus can be monitored and LSCS can be performed immediately. NST should be done before and after the procedure. USG to confirm breech presentation and to assess the AFI. Administration of tocolytics may be beneficial.

The patient should be tilted laterally to prevent supine hypotension. First the fetal breech is elevated out of the maternal pelvis. The version is attempted by turning the fetus in forward roll (move the fetus in the direction of the fetal nose). If attempts at inducing a forward roll motion are unsuccessful, the opposite direction may be attempted. The amount of force exerted is gauged by the patient's pain tolerance.

After versions, fetus should be monitored for 30 minutes. Rh-immunoglobulin should be administered to Rh-negative mothers.

12. What are the contraindications for ECV?

Absolute contraindications: III trimester bleeding, ruptured membranes, severe fetal anomalies, uterine anomalies, multiple pregnancy, pre-eclampsia.

Relative contraindications: Uterine scar, maternal obesity, oligohydramnios, IUGR.

13. What are the complications of ECV?

Fetal heart rate deceleration, fetomaternal hemorrhage, PROM, abruption placenta, fetal brachial plexus injury and rarely amniotic fluid embolization.

14. What are the advantages of ECV?

The success rate is 70–80%. The benefits of ECV include the increased probability that the fetus will be in the cephalic presentation when labor sets in and to achieve uncomplicated vaginal delivery. It also decreases the LSCS rates.

15. Why to perform ECV at 36 completed weeks?

- If spontaneous version was to occur, it would have happened spontaneously
- Risk of spontaneous reversion is decreased after a successful version at term
- Should complication arise during attempted version, it is possible to accomplish an emergency delivery at term.

16. What are the factors associated with successful version?

Multiparity, less gestational age frank breech are associated with successful version. Lower success rates with nullipara, advanced cervical dilatation, anterior placenta, low station of breech, EFW <2.5 kg and >3.5 kg.

17. What are the principles of breech delivery?

- Progress of labor should be left undisturbed until the presenting part starts descending the perineum and then give liberal episiotomy
- Avoid undue haste. Gentle suprapubic pressure to maintain the flexion of fetal head by the assistant
- Keep the back anteriorly. Never pull from below, let it get pushed from above.

18. What is Zatuchni and Andros scoring system?

For making the decision of abdominal/vaginal route in breech presentation, this system is used (Table 19.1).

Table 19.1: Zatuchni–Andros Breech scoring

	Add 0 point	Add 1 point	Add 2 points
Parity	0	1	2
Gestational age, week	39+	38	<37
EFW, lb	8	7–8	<7
Previous breech	0	1	2
Dilation	2	3	4
Station	–3	–2	–1

If the score is 0–4, cesarean delivery is recommended.

19. What are the fetal dangers in breech delivery?

- Intracranial hemorrhage
- *Asphyxia:* Cord compression, cord prolapse, prolonged labor, and aspiration of amniotic fluid and vaginal contents caused by active breathing before the head has been born.
- *Injuries:* Hematomas-brain, testicles, sternomastoid and thigh.
  - *Fractures:* Femur, humerus, clavicle and skull.
  - *Viscera:* Liver, adrenals, kidneys and lungs.
  - *Nerves:* Brachial plexus and spinal cord.

20. Why the perinatal mortality is more in breech delivery?

Prematurity, congenital anomalies, birth asphyxia, fetal injury and cord prolapse.

21. What is the incidence of cord prolapse with different varieties of breech?

- For footling—15%
- Complete breech—5%
- Frank breech—0.5%.

22. What is hyperextension of fetal head?

When the angle of extension of fetal neck is more than 90 degrees, it is called hyperextension or the star gazing breech. It is diagnosed on ultrasound by viewing the upper region of spine and fetal head in sagittal plain.

23. What is your opinion about induction/augmentation of labor in breech delivery?

Selective oxytocin augmentation should be considered when the clinician is confident that the cause of failed progress is inefficient uterine contractions and not the fetopelvic disproportion. Induction of labor should not be entertained if the cervix is unfavorable.

24. What is the overall incidence of LSCS for breech presentation?

The overall incidence is 15–50%, out of which 80% are elective.

25. How will you manage breech presentation at and beyond 36 weeks?

- Breech presentation without contraindication for vaginal birth → perform ECV.

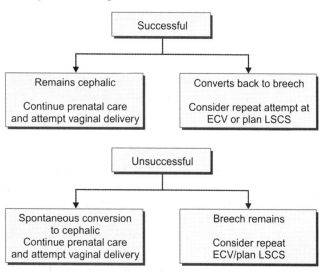

26. Why the risk of vaginal delivery is more in preterm breech?

In addition to the complications of prematurity, the preterm breech is at risk of entrapment of fetal head in an incompletely dilated cervix, cord prolapse, hypoxia and intraventricular hemorrhage.

27. Is LSCS justified for preterm breech?

LSCS will probably reduce the trauma but unlikely to eliminate the complications of prematurity. Cochrane database study does not justify a policy of elective LSCS for preterm breech.

28. What are the indications for elective LSCS in breech?

Elective LSCS is generally planned for patients with complicated breech presentations. The high-risk factors may include previous LSCS, contracted pelvis, BOH, history of infertility, placenta previa, IUGR, footling presentation, hyperextension and fetopelvic disproportion.

29. What is the timing and what are the advantages of episiotomy in breech delivery?

After the climbing of breech at perineum, liberal episiotomy is given. The advantages of episiotomy are:
- It helps in vaginal manipulations
- Facilitates easy delivery
- For unmolded aftercoming head, it avoids compression and decompression.

30. Write RCOG guidelines for the management of breech presentation. Reducing the incidence of breech presentation by ECV.

- There is no evidence to support routine recommendation of the knee-chest position
- All women with an uncomplicated breech pregnancy at term (37–42 weeks) should be offered ECV
- Tocolysis is effective, both when used routinely and when used selectively
- ECV should be done near to facilities for emergency delivery. A cardiotocograph is necessary. Ultrasound is helpful
- There is insufficient evidence to support the use of regional anesthesia to facilitate ECV
- The best method of delivering a term frank or complete breech singleton is by planned cesarean section
- A trial of labor should be precluded in the presence of medical or obstetric complications that are likely to be associated with mechanical difficulties at delivery.

Intrapartum management

There is no evidence that epidural analgesia is essential and, in selected cases, induction or augmentation may be justified. Fetal blood sampling from the buttocks provides an accurate assessment of the acid-base status, when the fetal heart rate trace is suspect.

Management of the preterm breech and twin breech:
- ECV before term has not been shown to offer any benefits
- There is insufficient evidence to support routine cesarean section for the delivery of preterm breech
- There is insufficient evidence to support cesarean section for the delivery of the first or second twin
- It is essential that all details of care are clearly documented, including the identity of all those involved in the procedures.

31. Do you know any postural management of breech presentation?
- Knee-chest position
- Supine position with pelvis elevated with a wedge-shaped cushion.

32. What are the indications of breech extraction?
Acute fetal distress in fully dilated cervix and to deliver second twin.

33. What are the causes of arrest of aftercoming head?
- Arrest at brim, deflexed head, contracted pelvis, hydrocephalus
- Arrest in the cavity deflexed head and contracted pelvis
- Arrest at outlet deflexed head and rigid perineum.

34. What are the causes of arrest of breech at different levels?
- Arrest at brim—Fetopelvic disproportion, extended breech, uterine inertia
- Arrest at outlet—Fetopelvic disproportion, rigid perineum, uterine inertia, hydrocephalus.

35. What will you do if the delivery of head occurs through an incompletely dilated cervix?
The cervix is to be pushed up while traction of the fetal trunk is made by jaw flexion and shoulder traction method. If necessary, Duhrssen's incision at 2 and 10 O'clock position of the cervix.

36. Which forceps are applied for the delivery of aftercoming head?
The Piper's forceps: These are specialized forceps with pelvic noncephalic application which maintains head in flexed position.

37. How will you differentiate between breech and face presentation?

Breech	Face
1. Anal opening and two ischial tuberosities in one line	1. Mouth and 2 malar prominences make a triangle
2. Suckling absent	2. Suckling present
3. Fingers stained with meconium	3. Not stained
4. External genitalia diagnostic	4. Eyes and nose diagnostic

38. How will you differentiate between foot and hand?

Foot	Hand
1. Toes are of equal length	1. Fingers are of unequal length
2. Toes are shorter	2. Fingers are longer
3. Great toe has lesser mobility	3. Thumb can be abducted easily
4. Firm heel can be felt	4. No equivalent hard thing

39. What is Pinard's maneuver?
The Pinard's maneuver may be needed with a frank breech to facilitate delivery of the leg, only after the fetal umbilicus has reached. Flexion of the fetal knee by giving pressure in the popliteal fossa associated with abduction of the thigh. This is done under general anesthesia. Procedure is obsolete in modern obstetrics.

40. What is Løvset's maneuver?
This is used where arrest of labor is due to extended arms. Løvset's maneuver is used widely for bringing down an arm in breech presentation. In this, the baby is grasped using both the hands by femuropelvic grip keeping the thumbs parallel to the vertebral column. It includes rotation of the trunk, lowering the trunk, and delivery of the arm.

41. What is Burns–Marshall technique?
This technique is used for delivering the aftercoming head. The baby is allowed to hang by its own weight. The assistant is asked to give suprapubic pressure.

When the nape of neck is visible, baby is rotated towards maternal abdomen by holding the ankles forming a wide arc.

42. What is Mauriceau–Smellie–Veit maneuver?
This is jaw flexion and shoulder traction method used to deliver aftercoming head. The assistant is asked to give suprapubic pressure. The baby is placed on the left supinated forearm. The middle and the index finger of the left hand are placed on the malar bones on either sides to maintain the flexion of the head. The index finger of the right hand is kept on left shoulder, middle finger is on suboccipital region and the ring and the little finger on the right shoulder. Traction is given in downward and backward direction till the nape of neck is visible and then fetus is rotated towards maternal abdomen.

43. What is Prague maneuver?
This maneuver is used in occipitoposterior position of aftercoming head. Back remains posterior. Two fingers of

one hand grasping the shoulder from the back draw fetus from below while the other hand draws the feet up over the abdomen of the mother.

44. What is term breech trial?

Term breech trial by Hannah, et al was published in 2000 in the Lancet. This was a planned RCT between planned vaginal verses planned cesarean study. This study was discontinued since April 2001, because it confirmed vaginal delivery more hazardous when compared to C section. PNM was reduced by 75% following elective C section (RR 0.23, 95% CI 0.07-0.81).

MUST REMEMBER
- Breech is the most common malpresentation.
- Prematurity is the most common cause.
- Fetal heart rate auscultated at or above umbilicus.
- *Inherent risks of breech presentation:* Prolonged labor, manipulative trauma, increased perinatal morbidity and mortality.
- The goal of ECV is to increase the proportion of vertex presentation amongst fetuses that were formerly in breech position.
- It was advantageous to deliver term breech patients by C section to improve the ultimate perinatal outcome.

Transverse Lie/Shoulder Presentation

Kanan Yelikar, Ashwini Yelikar

1. What is transverse lie and its incidence?
When the long axis of the fetus lies perpendicular to the maternal spine or centralized uterine axis, the lie is called transverse lie. Transverse lie accounts for 0.3–0.5% of singleton births and occurs in 5–10% of multiple births.

2. What are the etiological factors?
- Prematurity (most common factor)
- High parity
- Placenta previa
- Contracted pelvis
- Uterine anomalies—arcuate or subseptate uterus
- Pelvic tumors
- Polyhydromnios
- Fetal anomaly
- Multiple pregnancy
- Intrauterine fetal demise.

3. Why there is increased risk of maternal and perinatal morbidity in transverse lie?
Placenta previa, prolapse of the umbilical cord, fetal trauma during delivery and uterine rupture from prolonged labor increase the risk of maternal and perinatal morbidity.

4. What is the internal podalic version (IPV)?
It is type of version, which is done through vaginal approach and podalic end is drawn inside vagina to make presentation breech and lie longitudinal, following version fetus is delivered by breech extraction.

Indications of IPV
The only indication of IPV in modern obstetrics is second of twin baby with transverse lie.

Pre-requisites for IPV
- Cervix should be fully dilated
- Uterus should be well-relaxed
- IPV is done under general anesthesia
- Adequate liquor, membrane intact
- Fetus should be alive
- Experienced obstetrician must do the procedure.

Contraindications
- Absence of liquor
- Postcesarean pregnancy
- Neglected shoulder presentation.

Complications
- Rupture uterus
- Fetal trauma
- Fetal asphyxia
- Fetal mortality.

5. What is neglected shoulder presentation?
It comprises series of complications that may arise in a patient of transverse lie/shoulder presentation when the labor is left uncared.

Complications are impacted shoulder—obstructed labor—rupture uterus with clinical shock and sepsis, examination of dehydration and ketoacidosis.

MUST REMEMBER
- Most common position in transverse lie is dorsoanterior.
- In dorsoposterior position, chance of fetal extension is common with increased risk of arm prolapse.
- Transverse lie in twin pregnancy is found in 40% cases.
- USG is confirmatory in transverse lie.
- FHS are best heard on one side of umbilicus towards the fetal head.
- Cesarean is the best and the safest method of management in nearly all the cases of persistent transverse lie, even if baby is dead.

Obstructed Labor

Kanan Yelikar, Ashwini Yelikar

1. Define obstructed labor.

When the labor comes to a standstill, in spite of good uterine contractions due to fault in the passage or passenger.

2. What are the common causes of obstructed labor?

Fault in passage:
- Contracted pelvis
- Soft tissue obstruction due to tumors.

Fault in passenger:
- Malpresentation
- Malposition
- Congenital anomalies
- Big baby
- Locked twins.

3. Write about clinical features of obstructed labor.
- History of prolonged labor
- Maternal exhaustion
- Dehydration
- Metabolic acidosis
- Genital sepsis
- Per abdomen Bandl's ring
- Colonic distention
- Advanced and edematous bladder
- Hematuria.

4. What is Bandl's ring?

It is a pathological retraction ring at the junction of active upper segment and distended lower segment. Bandl's ring is the effect of obstructed labor. Constriction ring is the cause of obstructed labor.

5. Write about complications of obstructed labor.

Immediate signs
- Dehydration, exhaustion
- Metabolic acidosis
- Sepsis
- PPH and shock
- Rupture uterus
- Death due to rupture of uterus shock and sepsis
- Urinary complications.

Remote complications
- Genitourinary fistula
- Rectovaginal fistula (RVF)
- Variable degree of vaginal atresia
- Sheehan syndrome.

6. Write the effects of obstructed labor on fetus.
- Asphyxia
- Acidosis
- Intracranial hemorrhage
- Infection
- Perinatal loss.

7. State difference between constriction ring and retraction ring.

Constriction ring	Bandl's rings
• It is manifestation of localized, incoordinate uterine contractions around the narrow part of the fetus, i.e. neck. The uterine contractions usually occur around presenting part during 1st stage of labor due to prolonged labor. • *2nd stage of labor*: Prolonged second stage, no obvious cause. • *3rd stage*: Retained placenta or diagnosed during MRP. • Treated by deep plane of anesthesia.	• It rises towards umbilicus as labor advances. Tenderness over the abdomen present. Round ligaments are taut and tender.

8. What is the treatment of obstructed labor?

Correction of dehydration, antibiotics and lower segment cesarean section (LSCS).

9. What are the difficulties during LSCS?
- Overstretched LUS
- Sings of threatened rupture
- Bladder is edematous and overstretched.

MUST REMEMBER
- Obstructed labor should not occur with good antenatal care.
- Intelligent use of partogram by medical and paramedical staff helps to monitor the progress of labor and early pick-up of prolonged and obstructed labor.
- If obstructed labor remains undetected, can end up with life-threatening conditions such as ruptured uterus, septicemia, and death.

Third Stage Complications

Kalpana Mahadik

POSTPARTUM HEMORRHAGE (PPH)

Definition: Apparent blood loss more than 500 mL after delivery of fetus.

Clinical Definition

Any amount of bleeding from or into the genital tract following birth of the baby up to the end of the puerperium which adversely affects the general condition of the patient evidenced by rising pulse rate and falling blood pressure.

Quick Clinical Review

Think of predisposing causes like:
- Over-distended uterus
- Hypotonic uterus (twins, hydramnios, inertia in first stage)
- Instrumental delivery
- Grand multipara
- Placenta previa
- History of PPH in previous pregnancy.

All these etiological causes are to be thought before occurrence of the complication. A rule has to be followed that delivery of such patient should be personally attended by the treating gynecologist.

Some do's and don'ts to be followed are:

Do's

Keep a oxytocin drip going to such patients even after the fetus and placenta is out. Convert the physiological oxytocin drip to high concentration oxytocin drip.
- Keep the uterotonic drugs like oxytocin, prostaglandin, misoprostol ready in labor room when such patient is in labor
- Keep the bladder empty
- Watchful cat's eye, i.e. after delivery of placenta assessing the women every 15 minutes for expression of clots.

Don'ts

- Not omitting the IV drip after the delivery of placenta
- Not leaving the women alone after placental delivery
- No hurry to shift the patient to bed. Patient must be observed for minimum period of two hours and shifted to bed from labor room after passing urine.

Frequently Asked Questions (FAQs)

1. What are types of PPH?
- Primary (occurring within 24 hours)
- Secondary (after 24 hours but up to puerperium).

2. What are the causes of PPH?
- *Atonic uterus 80%:* Overdistended uterus, grand multipara, malnutrition, anemia, APH, prolonged labor, anesthetics (ether, halothane, cyclopropane) labors-induced by oxytocin, mismanaged third stage (retained clots), constriction ring, precipitate labor
- *Traumatic 20%:* Episiotomy, vaginal and cervical tears, paraurethral tears, colporrhexis.
- Combined.
- *Coagulation disorder:* Diminished procoagulants (washout phenomenon) or increased fibrinolytic activity like in DIC, abruptio placentae, jaundice in pregnancy, thrombocytopenic purpura, HELLP syndrome, intrauterine death of fetus.
- Retained placenta, placental bits or membranes.

3. What is prognosis in PPH?

Depends on—In how big center the patient is:
- If blood bank is available
- How smart is team around
- How much you anticipate the PPH.

4. What is important—prevention or treatment?

Both are equally important.

5. What are preventable causes and how do you act in such situation?
- Anemia treatment, use of parenteral iron sucrose, autologous blood transfusion
- High-risk patients to be recognized like twins, hydramnios, grand multipara, APH, history of previous 3rd stage complication

- Anticipation of blood grouping and Rh-typing with probability of blood transfusion arrangement
- Slow delivery of trunk
- Preference to local anesthesia than general anesthesia
- Active management of third stage of labor
- No fiddling or kneading of the uterus
- Complete examination of the placenta
- Continue oxytocin even after delivery of placenta
- PNC observation for 2 hours post delivery.

6. Write management of 3rd stage bleeding in brief.

Principles
- Replacement of blood loss by fluid and blood
- Keep uterus empty
- Never forget traumatic PPH.

Management started simultaneously on all fronts
- IV drip with 5-10 units oxytocin in half liter fluid
- IM carboprost 250 µg or rectal suppository of misoprostol 800 µg
- Fundal massage and recognizing sign of lost fundus, i.e. inversion
- Catheterize patient
- Controlled cord traction to deliver placenta
- Decision of manual removal of placenta is to be reserved for half an hour with watchful expectancy
- Anticipation, diagnosis and enthusiastic treatment of traumatic bleeding.

7. Write management of atonic PPH.
- General management as discussed above
- High concentration (10–20 units) oxytocin drip or IM carboprost or misoprostol suppository
- Organize your team, nurses, resident, registrar, laboratory, blood bank people and operation theater staff, immediately as soon as you see slightest indication of bleeding
- Massage uterus, expel clots
- Bimanual compression
- Exploration of uterus under general anesthesia
- Bilateral internal iliac artery ligation
- Uterine tamponade—uterine packing by Sengstakens Blakemore tube
- Uterine artery embolization
- B-Lynch stitch, compression sutures
- Shivkar's pack
- Hysterectomy.

8. What are the causes of secondary PPH and how do you manage it?
- It occurs commonly between 8th and 14th day of delivery.

Causes:
- Retained bits of placenta
- Infection of vaginal/cervical lacerations/episiotomy wound
- Subinvolution—low grade infection
- LSCS—10th to 14th day, infection of uterine wound
- Patient who is on estrogen therapy for suppression of lactation, may exhibit withdrawal bleeding
- Chorionepithelioma
- Placental polyp
- Infected fibroid
- Fibroid polyp
- Subacute inversion of uterus.

RETAINED PLACENTA

Definition: Placenta is said to be retained when it is not expelled after 30 minutes of birth of baby. According to WHO, it is 15 minutes.

Four Clinical Types
1. Placenta completely separated but retained
2. Simple adherent placenta in uterine atony
3. Placenta incarcerated in uterine cavity (constriction ring)
4. Morbidly adherent placenta.

Frequently Asked Questions (FAQs)

1. What is risk involved in placental retention
- Hemorrhage
- Shock due to blood loss, unrelated to blood loss when period is more than 1 hour
- Sepsis
- Risk of recurrence in next pregnancy.

2. What is the management of retained placenta?

Manual removal of placenta (MRP) is to be done under general anesthesia, if separated, only removal, if adherent it has to be separated from uterine wall and removed followed by a high concentration oxytocin drip.

3. What are associated complications of retained placenta?
- Retained placenta with shock but no hemorrhage, treated by treatment of shock first, then MRP
- Retained placenta with hemorrhage same as in third stage hemorrhage
- Retained placenta with sepsis. Mostly separated and septic. Treatment is removal and broad spectrum antibiotics—use of parenteral imipenem and metronidazole.

4. What is placenta accreta, its signs and management?

This is rare condition in which placenta directly anchored to myometrium usually with low lying placenta. In this, decidual layer is absent. Diagnosis by failure to find line of cleavage between placenta and uterine wall. General treatment is acute normovolemic hemodilution on OT table. 500–1000 mL of whole blood is collected through central line from the patient and replaced with colloid and crystalloid (3:1) to maintain blood pressure. The previously collected blood is retransfused as soon as surgical bleeding is controlled. Preoperative bilateral common iliac artery balloon catheterization immediately after delivery of the fetus is a newer modality. Selective embolization of uterine vessels using polyvinyl alcohol, gel, foam or coils is also tried. Treatment is hysterectomy. In young women, placenta is left for being autolyzed, so that conservation of reproductive function is achieved and subsequent treatment with methotrexate.

INVERSION OF UTERUS

Definition: When uterus is turned inside out partially or completely. It is acute, following normal delivery, rarely chronic.

Frequently Asked Questions (FAQs)

1. What are causes of inversion of uterus?

- Uterine atony
- Placenta accreta
- Short cord
- Pulling of cord
- Crede's expression
- Faulty technique in MRP, i.e. rapid withdrawal of hand.

2. What are complications of inversion?

- Shock—neurogenic
- Associated hemorrhage
- Infection
- Associated pulmonary embolism.

3. How inversion is diagnosed?

Cupping of fundus or absent fundus, presence of pear-shaped mass, reddish purple in color per vaginum.

4. What is the prognosis of inversion of uterus?

If not treated timely, death due to shock, hemorrhage or embolism.

5. What is the management of inverted uterus?

Treatment of shock, antibiotics, and reposition under general anesthesia as early as possible.

POSTPARTUM SHOCK

Causes

- Amniotic fluid embolism
- Intractable postpartum hemorrhage
- Pulmonary thromboembolism
- Unexplained sudden postpartum collapse.

Frequently Asked Questions (FAQs)

1. What is the modern concept of fluid replacement in massive hemorrhage?

- Use of FFP, platelets and packed red cells in proportion of 1:1:1
- Do not give crystalloids in unlimited volumes
- Permissive hypotension to maintain BP between 80 and 100 is considered till packed cells are arranged.

2. What is hemostatic resuscitation?

Till the blood transfusion is arranged, huge quantity of crystalloids should not be given.

3. What is dilutional coagulopathy?

Use of crystalloids will lead to dilution of coagulation factors. If platelet count <50,000/cumm, fibrinogen <100 mg/dL, prothrombin time or activated partial thromboplastin time (aPTT >1.5 × normal), there is indication for use of FFP.

4. What is abdominal compartment syndrome?

Use of crystalloids and colloids will lead to third spacing of fluids resulting in bowel edema and ascites. An associated ileus put together increases intra-abdominal pressure to a point where compression of abdominal and retroperitoneal vessels will compromise preload to the heart, leading to drop in cardiac output and hypotension. Also associated with oliguria, cephalad displacement of diaphragm, leading to bilateral basal atelectasis, with right to left shunt and consequent hypoxemia.

5. How do we manage abdominal compartment syndrome?

Surgical decompression with vacuum-assisted closure.

MUST REMEMBER
- Third stage of labor starts from delivery of the baby and ends with complete expulsion of the products of conception.
- Complications can occur even before and after expulsion of placenta. The complications after expulsion of placenta are atonic or traumatic PPH or retained products of conception.
- Atonic PPH is the commonest cause of PPH.
- Always explore the genital tract in all cases of PPH to confirm atonic or traumatic PPH.
- Active management of the third stage should be routinely done for every high-risk pregnancy.
- Oxytocin should be continued for at least one hour after delivery in all cases induced or accelerated by oxytocin.
- During cesarean section, spontaneous separation and delivery of the placenta reduce blood loss.
- Fiddling or kneading with the uterus or pulling of cord should be avoided.
- Every patient should be observed for at least two hours before shifting them to postnatal ward.
- High-risk cases should be managed at the tertiary care where facilities for blood, anesthetist, expert obstetrician are available.

Multiple Pregnancy

Kanan Yelikar, Varsha Deshmukh

When more than one fetus simultaneously develops in the uterus, it is called multiple pregnancy. They may be dizygotic twins (80%) or monozygotic twins (20%). Depending upon division of blastodermic vesicle, they are further divided into:

- Diamniotic dichorionic or D/D—30%, division takes place within 72 hours after fertilization
- Diamniotic monochorionic twins—division takes place between 4 and 8 days
- Monoamniotic-monochorionic twin—division takes place after 8th day
- Conjoined twin <1%—division takes place after 2 weeks of development of embryonic disc. Four types of fusion may occur: (i) Thoracopagus (commonest) (ii) Pyopagus (posterior fusion) (iii) Craniopagus (cephalic) (iv) Ischiopagus (caudal).

Incidence of multiple pregnancy is increasing due to ART procedures.

DIAGNOSIS

Overdistension of the abdomen, palpation of multiple fetal parts (two heads or three fetal poles) are the findings suggestive of twins. Auscultation of two fetal hearts simultaneously by two different personnel, with a difference of 10 beats per minute.

Maternal Risk Associated with Twins

- I Trimester abortions, congenital malformations and hyperemesis
- II Trimester anemia, PIH, polyhydramnios, preterm labor
- III Trimester APH (placenta previa and abruption placentae), malpresentations, PROM, labor—malpresentations, PROM, cord prolapse, increased operative interference, PPH
- Puerperium-failing lactation, subinvolution.

Fetal Risk Associated with Twins

- Preterm labor—50% deliver before 37 weeks
- IUGR—10–25%
- Increased perinatal morbidity—5 times of singleton pregnancy
- Abortions—2 times of singleton pregnancy
- Malformations—2 times of singleton pregnancy.

Precautions to be Taken in Labor

- Anticipate and recognize the increase potential for complication of labor and delivery in twins
- Establish IV access
- Strict FHR monitoring
- Trained obstetrician available
- Immediate availability of anesthetist
- Availability of trained neonatologist.

Generally, vertex-vertex are delivered vaginally. Sets in which twin A is non-vertex is delivered by lower segment cesarean section (LSCS).

Precautions to be Taken after Delivery of First Baby

- Do not give ergometrine
- Set up oxytocin drip so that the contractions start and presenting part is fixed
- Then do ARM so that the chances of cord prolapse are minimized.

The second baby has a higher chance of fetal distress secondary to cord prolapse and abruption placentae.

1. What is Hellin's law?

- Hellin's law expresses the incidence of multiple pregnancy
- Twins—1:89
- Triplets—$1:(89)^2$
- Quadriplets—$1:(89)^3$.

2. What are the characteristic features of development of twins?

Characteristic Features of the Twins

- Somewhat lighter and smaller than a singleton
- Sometimes the two are unequal in size
- Sometimes one grows normally and the other perishes
- Malformations are common
- Monsters, e.g. thoracopagus are rarely seen.

3. What is the arrangement of placenta and membranes in twins?

In binovular twins, the placentae are either separate or fused. Although fused, there is no vascular connection. In uniovular twins, the placenta is single and there is sharing of fetal circulation. There is single chorion and two amnions.

4. Clinically, when do you suspect multiple pregnancy?

The following conditions should alert you of multiple pregnancy:
- Positive family history of twins
- Hyperemesis
- Unexplained excessive weight gain
- Early onset PIH
- Unexplained severe anemia
- Abnormally elevated serum alpha proteins in second trimester
- History of excessive fetal movements
- Height of uterus more than the period of gestation
- Polyhydramnios.

5. How do you confirm the diagnosis of twins?

Ultrasonography shows two sacs and two fetal poles by 5 weeks of gestation.

6. What is the antenatal care in twins?

Frequent visits are recommended in twins, i.e. every two weekly after 26–30 weeks. Patient is advised to increase the calorie intake by 300 kcal/day, take extra bed rest, and to report immediately, if backache starts. The obstetrician should be vigilant about early diagnosis of preterm labor, PIH and IUGR. Proper advice is given to the patient.

7. Why PPH occurs more commonly in twins?

The causes of PPH are uterine overdistention leading to atonicity, more incidence of placenta previa, larger placenta taking more time to separate leading to more blood loss and more sinuses are opened up which again lead to blood loss.

8. What information is obtained from first trimester USG?

- Two sacs with fetal poles
- Determination of chronicity
- Determination of gestational age.

9. What information is obtained from second trimester USG?

Second trimester USG gives an idea about chronicity, gestational age, placental localization, AFI, congenital anomaly, cervical status and conjoined twins.

10. What weight gain is recommended in twin pregnancy?

25–35 lb or 12.5–15 kg.

11. What dose of iron is recommended in twin pregnancy?

Ferrous sulfate is given in the dose of 60–120 mg till Hb becomes normal, then it is given as 60 mg/day.

12. What dose of calcium is recommended in twin pregnancy?

1800 mg/day of calcium is recommended in twin pregnancy.

13. When is the cervical evaluation done in twin pregnancy?

The cervical evaluation is done in twin pregnancy if there is a probability of impending preterm labor or as early as 16–20 weeks of gestation. The features of impending preterm labor are evidence short cervix, history of bleeding per vaginum (P/V), dilatation of the cervix or descent of the presenting part.

14. What are the features of twin pregnancy in labor?

The characteristic features of twin pregnancy in labor are short latent phase, common in multigravidae, birth weight less than 2.5 kg and associated with malpresentations.

15. How fetal presentation affects delivery in twins?

On admission, the fetal presentation is established. If there is any doubt, USG help can be taken. Generally vertex-vertex are delivered vaginally. Sets in which twin A is nonvertex is delivered by LSCS. Management of vertex-nonvertex set is controversial.

16. Of the two babies, which one is at a higher risk?

The second baby has a higher chance of fetal distress secondary to cord prolapse and abruptio placentae.

17. What are the management options, if the second baby is by breech?

The management options if the second baby is by breech are either to do ECV or deliver by breech.

18. What are the management options, if the second baby is by transverse lie?

The management options if the second baby is by transverse lie are to do ECV or LSCS. If the obstetrician is experienced, IPV is also an option if the baby weight ≤2 kg.

19. What are the indications of LSCS in twins?

- Malpresentations
- Placenta previa
- Cord prolapse
- Conjoint twins
- Monochorionic twin.

20. What is fetus papyraceous?

Of the two fetuses, one perishes *in utero*. The fluid in the dead amnion is absorbed. The body of the dead fetus is compressed in between the live fetus and the uterine wall. This results in a curiously flattened mummified fetus known as fetus papyraceous.

21. What is vanishing twin syndrome?

Very early pregnancy begins as twins. But of the two fetuses, one is absorbed. This is known as vanishing twin syndrome.

22. What is the definitive evidence of uniovular twins?

The definitive evidence of uniovular twins is the acceptance of tissue graft.

23. What is superfecundation?

Two ova from the same cycle may be fertilized by the sperms from different acts of coitus within a short period, it is known as superfecundation.

24. What is superfetation?

It is the fertilization of two ova from different cycles, separated by weeks or even months. There is no evidence of this phenomenon in human beings.

25. What is twin-to-twin transfusion syndrome?

When there is intercommunication of blood vessels in the placentae, it results in twin-to-twin transfusion syndrome. When one placenta is fed by an artery from the first twin and drained by a vein that leads to the II twin, it leads to the shifting of blood from the donor twin to the recipient twin, this is known as twin-to-twin transfusion syndrome.

26. What are locked twins?

It is a rare phenomenon. When the first baby is by breech and the second baby is by vertex, the babies may get locked with each other. This occurs more commonly with monoamniotic twins.

27. What is the role of selective reduction in multiple pregnancy?

With ART, high order gestations occur frequently. Both the fetal and maternal outcomes are compromised in the high order gestations. These outcomes are believed to improve if the pregnancy is reduced to a lower gestation number in late first trimester. In selective reduction in multiple pregnancy injectable KCl is injected in the fetus who is to be reduced.

28. Do twins differ from singleton pregnancy in pulmonary maturity?

Overall, pulmonary maturity is attended at a earlier gestation (3-4 weeks) in twins than singleton pregnancy.

29. What difficulty is seen in the treatment of preterm labor in twins?

In twins, the plasma volume is increased up to 50-60%, whereas it increases by 45% in singleton pregnancy. Therefore, the cardiac load increases. This poses a special risk for pulmonary edema after giving tocolytics. Hence, tocolytics should be used cautiously.

30. What is the incidence of twins in India?

The incidence of monozygotic twins is almost the same throughout the world. The incidence of dizygotic twins, however, changes from place to place. In India, it is about 6-8/1000 live births.
Mumbai 6.8/1000
Bengaluru 7.3/1000
Kolkata 8.1/1000.

MUST REMEMBER

When more than one fetus is present *in utero,* it is known as multiple pregnancy. They may be dizygous (75%) or monozygous (25%). Ultrasonography showing two sacs and two fetal poles by 5 weeks of gestation is diagnostic of twins. Antenatally frequent visits are recommended in twins, i.e. every two weekly after 26-30 weeks. Patient is advised to increase the calorie intake by 300 kcal/day, take extra bed rest, and to report immediately if backache starts. Various maternal risks associated with multiple pregnancy are:
- I trimester-abortions, congenital malformations and hyperemesis.
- II trimester anemia, PIH, polyhydramnios, preterm labor.
- III trimester APH (placenta previa and abruptio placentae), malpresentations, PROM, labor—malpresentations, PROM, cord prolapse, increased operative interference, PPH.
- Puerperium—failing lactation, subinvolution. The causes of PPH are uterine overdistention leading to atonicity, more incidence of placenta previa, larger placenta taking more time to separate leading to more blood loss and more sinuses are opened up which again lead to blood loss. Weight gain is recommended in twin pregnancy which is 25-35 lb or 12.5-15 kg. Ferrous sulfate is given in the dose of 60-120 mg till Hb becomes normal, then it is given as 60 mg/day, 1800 mg/day of calcium is recommended in twin pregnancy. Fetal complications in multiple pregnancy are preterm labor, IUGR, increased perinatal morbidity, abortions and malformations. The second baby has a higher chance of fetal distress, secondary to cord prolapse and abruption placentae.

Drugs in Obstetrics and Gynecology

24

Shrinivas Gadappa, Kanan Yelikar, Sonali Deshpande

MAGNESIUM SULFATE

Class—Anticonvulsant and sedative.

Category A

Mechanism of action:
- Reduces end plate sensitivity to acetyl choline
- Reduces acetyl choline release
- Blocks Ca^{++} channels
- Direct depressant action on uterine muscle
- Tocolysis
- Neural stabilization.

Uses:
- Local—anti-inflammatory
- Parenteral—drug of choice in prevention and treatment of seizure in pre-eclampsia and eclampsia, tocolytic in preterm labor.

Contraindications: Myasthenia gravis, impaired renal function.

Side effects:
- *Maternal:* Respiratory depression, muscular paresis, flushing, perspiration, headache, rarely pulmonary edema
- *Fetal:* Lethargy, hypotonic, rarely respiratory depression.

Anti-dote: Injectable calcium gluconate 10%, 10 mL IV.

Monitoring

The maintenance dose of magnesium sulfate is given only after assuring that:
- Patellar reflex is present
- Respiration not depressed (RR >16/minute)
- Urine output during previous 4 hours exceeded 100 mL (25 mL/hour).

LABETALOL

Class—Antihypertensive.

Category C

Mechanism of action: $\beta_1 + \beta_2 + \alpha_1$ adrenergic blocker with weak β2 agonist (5 times more capable of locking β than α).

Uses: Hypertension in pregnancy, hypertensive crisis.

Contraindications: Hepatic disorders, asthma and CCF.

Side effects: Rash and liver damage and fetal hypoglycemia. $T_{½}$ = 4–6 hours.

Regimen

- Orally 100 mg tds upto 800 mg daily
- Intravenous starting with 20 mg IV bolus, if no response in 10 minutes 40 mg IV bolus, then 80 mg every 10 minutes with total dose of 220 mg per episode.

Table 24.1 Alternative regimens for magnesium sulfate

Regimen	Loading dose	Maintenance dose	Total dose
Pritchard	4 g IV over 3–5 minutes followed by 10 g IM deep	5 g IM 4 hourly in alternate buttock	30 g in pre-eclampsia, continued upto 24 hours after last convulsion or delivery whichever is later
Zuspan	4 g IV over 15–20 minutes	1–2 g/hour IV infusion	
Low dose regimen	4 g IV over period of 3–5 minutes	2 g IM/diluted IV 3 hourly	
IV/IM MgSO$_4$			
<ul><li>No evidence from the collaborative trial of any difference between the intramuscular and intravenous regimens.</li><li>However, intramuscular injections are painful and are complicated by local abscess formation in 0.5% of cases.</li><li>MAGPIE trial (magnesium sulfate for prevention of eclampsia</li><li>Therapeutic level 4–7 mEq/L</li><li>Toxicity appears after 8 mEq/L</li></ul>		<ul><li>When magnesium sulfate is admin IV, the onset of action is immediate and the duration of action is about 30 minutes.</li><li>Following IM admin of the drug, the onset of action occurs in about 1 hour and the duration of action is 3–4 hour.</li><li>Onset—IV > IM</li><li>Duration of action—IV < IM</li><li>Orally, it acts as an antacid, IV as an anticonvulsant, IM as neural stabilizing agent.</li><li>First sign of toxicity is loss of reflexes.</li></ul>	

NIFEDEPINE

Class: Dihydropyridine calcium channel blocker.

Category C

Mechanism of action: Voltage-gated calcium channel blockage in cardiac muscle and blood vessels (vasodilatation).

Uses: Hypertension, angina pectoris, prevention of preterm labor.
Precaution: Use with $MgSO_4$ can be hazardous
Side effects: Flushing, hypotension, headache, tachycardia and inhibition of labor.
$T_{1/2}$ = 2 to 5 hours.

Regimen
- 5–20 mg bd/tds maximum dose 200 mg
- Prevention of preterm labor—20–30 mg stat and 10–20 mg every 6 hourly.

ALPHA-METHYLDOPA

Class—Antihypertensive.

Category B

Mechanism of action:
- Stimulates α-receptors and decreases sympathetic outflow from CNS
- Decreases peripheral vascular resistance.

Uses: Pregnancy-induced hypertension.

Maximum effect in 4 hours, total duration of action is 8 hours.

Contraindications: Hepatic disorders, psychiatric disorders CCF.
Side effects: Postural hypotension, sedation, lethargy, reduced mental capacity, dryness of mouth, rebound hypertension and Coombs positive.

Regimen
250 mg tds maximum dose 2 g.

OXYTOCIN

Invented by Vincent du Vigneaud in 1953 and received noble prize in chemistry in 1955.
Class—uterine stimulant.

Category C

Mechanism of action:
- Acts through receptors and voltage-mediated Ca^{++} channels
- Stimulates amniotic and decidual PG production.

Uses:
- Induction and augmentation of labor
- Uterine inertia
- Prevention and treatment PPH
- Breast engorgement
- Oxytocin challenge test.

Contraindications:

Pregnancy	Labor	Anytime
Grand multipara	As in pregnancy	Hypovolemic state
Contracted pelvis	Obstructed labor	Cardiac disease
History of cesarean section or hysterotomy	Incoordinate uterine contraction	
Malpresentation	Fetal distress	

Side effects:
- *Maternal:* Uterine hyperstimulation, uterine rupture, water intoxication and hypotension.
- *Fetal:* Fetal distress.

Plasma half-life: 3–4 minutes, duration of action 20 minutes.

Regimen

High dose (4–6 mIU/minutes), low dose (1–4 mIU/minutes). Oxytocin escalating doses (Anderson's logarithmic method of titration) start in a dose of 4 U in 500 mL of RL and double the dose with every pint, i.e. 8-16-32 and so on up to maximum of 100 U.

Oxytocin Regimen

Oxytocin 2.5 U in 500 mL NS started at 10 drops/minute (2- 2.5 mU/min), dose is raised every 30 minutes till 4 contractions per 10 minutes each lasting for >40 seconds are obtained.

Set 1 mL = 20 drops	Set 1 mL = 15 drops
10 drops/min = 2.5 mu/min	10 drops/min = 3.4 mu/min
20 drops/min = 5 mu/min	20 drops/min = 6.6 mu/min
30 drops/min = 7.5 mu/min	30 drops/min = 9.9 mu/min
40 drops/min = 10 mu/min	40 drops/min = 13.2 mu/min
50 drops/min = 12.5 mu/min	

METHYLERGOMETRINE

Class—Uterine stimulant.

Category C

Mechanism of action:
- Blood vessel constrictor and smooth muscle agonist
- Acts directly on the smooth muscle of the uterus and increases the tone, rate, and amplitude of rhythmic contractions
- 4 week interval is necessary for the secondary immune response
- *Onset of action:* Oral—10 minutes, IM—4–7 minutes, IV—40 seconds.

Uses:
- Routine management after delivery of the placenta, PPH
- Subinvolution
- Most commonly used to prevent or control excessive bleeding
- Uterine contractions to aid in expulsion of retained products of conception
- Incomplete abortion:

Side effects: Cholinergic effects such as nausea, vomiting, and diarrhea, cramping, dizziness, pulmonary hypertension, coronary artery vasoconstriction, severe systemic hypertension (especially in patients with preeclampsia) and convulsions.

Contraindications: Hypertension, toxemia of pregnancy, and hypersensitivity, before second twin is born, heart disease, Rh-negative status, vascular disease.

Half-life = 1–2 hours.

Regimen

- *Parenteral:* 1 mL (0.2 mg) after delivery of the anterior shoulder, after delivery of the placenta, or during the puerperium. May be repeated as required, at intervals of 2–4 hours.
- *Oral:* One tablet, 0.2 mg, 3 or 4 times daily in the puerperium for a maximum of 1 week.

MISOPROSTOL (PGE$_1$)

Class—Uterine stimulant.

Category X

Mechanism of action:
- Binds to myometrial cells to cause strong myometrial contractions
- Cervical ripening with softening and dilatation of cervix
- Increase water content of cervix and lysis of glycoaminoglycogens.

Uses: Abortion, induction and augmentation of labor, prevention of PPH, cervical priming before gynecological procedures like D & C and hysteroscopy [vaginal route-action is slow and sustained, oral-action is rapid and short duration]. Medical termination of pregnancy, peptic ulcers, patent ductus arteriosus to maintain patency.

Complications

- Uterine hyperstimulation
- Uterine rupture
- Fetal heart rate abnormalities
- Amniotic fluid embolism
- Retained placenta
- Tachysystole, meconium passage
- Meconium aspiration syndrome.

$T_{1/2}$ = 1–2 minutes

Antidote—0.25 mg terbutaline SC.

Clinical situations and dose:
- For MTP use:
  Ist trimester—400 mcg every 4 hourly (maximum 1600 mcg)
  IInd trimester—400 mcg every 4 hourly
- For preinduction
  Cx ripening use: 25–50 mcg 4–6 hourly.
  (max dose 150 mcg)
- For IUD 13–24 weeks 200 mcg/4 hourly,
  late—100 mcg/6–12 hours
- *For viable pregnancy:* 25 mcg intravaginal, 4 hourly maximum doses 150 mcg
- *For PPH:* Prophylaxis 600 mcg/rectal
  Treatment 1000 mcg/rectal.

DINOPROSTONE PGE2

Class—Prostaglandin

Mechanism of action:
- Binds to myometrial cells to cause strong myometrial contractions
- Cervical ripening with softening and dilatation of cervix.

Uses: Induction of labor.

Contraindications:
- For induction of labor in women with:
  – Scarred uterus (pre-LSCS or uterine surgery)
  – Grand multiparae.
- Hypersensitivity
- Asthma.

Side effects: Nausea, vomiting, diarrhea, vaginal irritation and hyperstimulation syndrome.

$T_{1/2}$—contraction starts within 1 hour and peaks at 4 hour.

Regimen

0.5 mg (3 mL) over 6 hours with 3 doses in 24 hours.
Antidote—0.25 mg terbutaline SC.

CARBOPROST 15-METHYL-PGF2-ALPHA

Class—Prostaglandin.

Mechanism of action:
- Binds to myometrial cells to cause strong myometrial contractions

- Cervical ripening with softening and dilatation of cervix.

Uses:
- Prophylaxis and treatment of PPH
- IInd trimester MTP
- Ist trimester MTP for softening of cervix.

Contraindications:
- For induction of labor in women with:
  - Scarred uterus (pre LSCS or uterine surgery)
  - Grand multiparae.
- Hypersensitivity
- Asthma.

Side effects: Nausea, vomiting, diarrhea, vaginal irritation and rupture of uterus.

Regimen

250 mcg IM every 20 minutes till bleeding stops or maximum 8 ampoules.

MIFEPRISTONE RU-486 (RUSSELL UNIT)

Class—Antiprogestine.
Mechanism of action (Competetive antiprogestational and antiglucocorticoid):
- Attenuate midcycle Gn (gonadotropin) surge
- Prevents secretory change by progesterone
- Stimulates uterine contractions
- Blocks decidualization.

Uses:
- Termination of pregnancy up to 7 weeks
- Cervical ripening
- Postcoital contraceptive and once a month contraceptive
- Induction of labor.
- Treatment of Cushing's disease
- Medical management of fibroid.

Contraindications
Side effects: Nausea, vomiting, diarrhea, headache, dizziness, chills or hot flushes, shivering, fatigue
$T_{1/2}$ = 20–36 hours.

Regimen

200 g single dose.

ETHACRIDINE LACTATE

Class—Uterine stimulant.
Mechanism of action: Stripping of membranes with liberation of PGs.

Uses:
- Antiseptic in solutions of 0.1%
- Second trimester abortion. Up to 150 mL of a 0.1% solution is instilled extraamniotically using a Foleys catheter.

Contraindications: Hypersensitivity.
Side effects: Anaphylactic reaction, hypersensitivity, prolonged use delays wound healing.

Regimen

10 mL/gestational week of 0.1% solution (max 200 mL).

ORAL IRON

Ferrous sulfate, ferrous gluconate, ferrous fumarate, ferrous ascorbate, sodium feredetate, iron hydroxide polymaltose, ferric ammonium citrate, carbonyl iron.
Class—Hematinics.

Uses: Iron deficiency, anemia prophylaxis and treatment, megaloblastic anemia.

Contraindications:
Side effects: Epigastric pain, nausea, vomiting, staining of teeth, metallic taste, bloating, constipation.

Regimen

200 mg (60 mg elemental iron) tds.

FOLIC ACID

Class—Hematinics.

Category A

Uses: Megaloblastic anemia treatment and prophylaxis, in methotrexate toxicity, phenytoin toxicity, prevention of abruption, prevention of neural tube defects.

Side effects: Nontoxic.

Folinic acid—Used for prevention and treatment of methotrexate toxicity within 3 hours of administration, treatment of hyperhomocysteinemia.

Regimen

- Therapeutic—2–5 mg/day
- Prophylactic—0.5 mg/day.

TERBUTALINE

Class—Tocolytic.

Category B

Mechanism of action: β_2 adrenergic stimulant (↓ intracellular Ca^{++} → inhibits MLCK → inhibits interaction of actin and myosin → smooth muscle relaxation).

Uses:
- Prevention of preterm labor for at least 48 hours for action of corticosteroids
- Antidote for prostaglandin-induced uterine hyperstimulation.

Side effects:
Maternal: Headache, palpitation, tachycardia, pulmonary edema, hypotension.
Fetal: Tachycardia, heart failure and IUFD.

Regimen
0.25 mg SC every 3-4 hourly.

RITODRINE

Beta 2 agonist

Class—Tocolytic.
Mechanism of action: β₂ adrenergic stimulant (↓ intracellular Ca⁺⁺ → inhibits MLCK → inhibits interaction of actin and myosin → smooth muscle relaxation)

Uses:
- Prevention of preterm labor
- External cephalic version.

Side effects:
Maternal: Tachycardia, hypotension, palpitation, hyperglycemia, hypokalemia, pulmonary edema.
Fetal: Hyperkalemia, hypoglycemia, hypotension, respiratory distress syndrome.

Regimen
Tablet 10 mg, 10 mg/mL, 0.05-0.35 mg/minute for 12 hours increased by 50 mcg/min every 10 minutes, orals started ½ hour before discontinuation of IV drip. Then tablet 2 hourly for first day and then 4-6 hourly on subsequent days.

ISOXSUPRINE

Class—Tocolytic.
Mechanism of action: β₂ adrenergic stimulant (↓ intracellular Ca⁺⁺ → inhibits MLCK → inhibits interaction of actin and myosin → smooth muscle relaxation)

Uses:
- Prevention of preterm labor
- External cephalic version

Contraindications:
Chronic cardiac disease, hyperdynamic circulation, chorioamnionitis, fetal demise, fetal malformation.

Side effects:
Maternal: Tachycardia, hypotension, palpitation, hyperglycemia, hypokalemia, pulmonary edema.

Fetal: Hyperkalemia, hypoglycemia, hypotension, respiratory distress syndrome.
Plasma half life: 1.5-3 hours.

Regimen
2 cc IM every 8 hourly
10 mg bd/tds.

MATERNAL CORTICOSTEROIDS

Betamethasone and Dexamethasone

- Betamethasone 2 doses 12 mg IM 24 hours apart
- Dexamethasone 6 mg IM every 6 hours total 4 doses
- Repeat or booster doses are not needed
- *Relative contraindications:*
  - May be used with caution in severe preeclampsia
  - Impaired GTT (glucose tolerance test)
  - Severe adrenal insufficiency between 28 and 34 weeks
- Dexamethasone also used in HELLP syndrome.

CORTICOSTEROIDS

- Indicated between 28 and 34 weeks
- *Contraindications:*
  - Diabetic mother
  - Chorioamnionitis.

CEFOTAXIME

Class—Cephalosporin (third generation—parenteral)

Category B

Mechanism of action: Inhibits bacterial cell wall synthesis.

Uses:
- Respiratory, urinary and soft tissue infection
- Surgical prophylaxis
- Infections such as meningitis, typhoid, gonorrhea, hospital acquired infections.

Side effects: Thrombophlebitis, diarrhea, hypersensitivity.
$T_{½}$ = 1 hour but longer for deacetylated metabolite.

Regimen
1-2 grams IV 8-12 hourly.

METRONIDAZOLE

Class—Tissue amebicide (nitroimidazole).

Category B

Mechanism of action: Nitro group disrupts pyruvate pathway energy metabolism in anerobes.

Uses: Amebiasis, giardiasis, *trichomonas vaginalis*, anerobic bacterial infection.

Contraindications: In neurological diseases, blood dyscrasias, Ist trimester pregnancy, chronic alcoholism.

Side effects: Anorexia, nausea, vomiting, metallic taste, abdominal cramps.

$T_{1/2}$ = 8 hours.

Regimen
- Orally 400 mg tds
- Parenterally 500 mg/100 mL IV suspension tds.

CIPROFLOXACIN

Class—Fluoroquinolones.

Category C

Mechanism of action: Damages bacterial DNA→ damaged DNA digested by endonuclease → cell lysis.

Uses: UTI, gynecological and wound infection, gonorrhea, bacterial gastroenteritis, typhoid, MDR-TB.

Contraindications: Pregnancy and lactation.

Side effects: Nausea, vomiting, bad taste, headache, anxiety and skin hypersensitivity.

$T_{1/2}$ = 3–5 hours.

Regimen
Oral: 500 mg bd.
IV: 200 mg bd.

CLOTRIMAZOLE

Class—Anti-fungal (azole).

Category B

Mechanism of action: Inhibits cytochrome P450 → cascade of membrane instability.

Side effects: Local irritation.

Uses: Vaginal candidiasis.

Regimen
1% lotion/cream
100 mg vaginal tablet.

CLINDAMYCIN

Class—Lincosamide antibiotic.

Category B

Mechanism of action: Inhibits protein synthesis.
Uses: Anerobic and mixed infection (abdominal/lung/pelvic abscess), bacterial vaginosis.

Contraindications:

Side effects: Urticaria, abdominal pain, diarrhea and pseudomembranous enterocolitis.

Regimen
150–300 mg qid orally or
200–600 mg IV 8 hourly.

FLUCONAZOLE

Class—Triazole antifungal.

Category C

Mechanism of action: Inhibits cytochrome P450 → cascade of membrane instability.

Uses: Cryptococcal meningitis, systemic/local candidiasis, recurrent candidiasis.

Side effects: Nausea, vomiting, abdominal pain, rash.

$T_{1/2}$ = 25–30 hours.

Regimen
150 mg single dose for vaginal candidiasis.

NEVIRAPINE

Class—Antiretroviral [non-nucleoside reverse transcriptase inhibitor (NNRTI)].

Category C

Mechanism of action: Inhibits non-nucleoside reverse transcriptase, an essential viral enzyme which transcribes viral RNA into DNA. Active only against HIV 1 infection.

Uses:
- Triple combination therapy has been shown to suppress viral load effectively in HIV-AIDS
- Prevention of vertical transmission—single dose of nevirapine given to both mother and child reduces the rate of HIV transmission by almost 50%.

Contraindications:

Side effects:
- Mild or moderate rash, Stevens-Johnson syndrome, toxic epidermal necrolysis and hypersensitivity, hepatotoxicity
- Severe or life-threatening liver toxicity.

Dosing of Nevirapine

Adult

Immediate-release (IR) tablet or oral suspension: 200 mg QD for 14 days, then 200 mg BID.

Extended-release (XR) Tablet

- *400 mg QD if initiating treatment with nevirapine:* Start with IR tablet, 200 mg QD for 14 days then change to XR tablet, 400 mg QD if switching from nevirapine IR formulation (200 mg BID) to XR formulation; start XR tablet, 400 mg QD (without lead-in dosage adjustment)
- Pediatric age 15 days—adolescence 150 mg/m^2 QD for the first 14 days, then 150 mg/m^2 BID; maximum total daily dose 400 mg
- Prevention of mother-to-child transmission, single dose 200 mg in active labor.

METHOTREXATE

Class—antimetabolite.

Category X

Mechanism of action: Inhibits dihydrofolate reductase → blocks DNA synthesis.

Uses: Invasive mole, choriocarcinoma, leukemias, rheumatoid arthritis, psoriasis, conservative management of ectopic pregnancy, embryo reduction.

Side effects: Ulcerative stomatitis, low white blood cell count and thus predisposition to infection, nausea, abdominal pain, fatigue, fever, dizziness and rarely pulmonary fibrosis teratogenic, bone marrow depression, renal tubular necrosis.

Regimen

One mg/kg, 100 mg/m^2 body surface area.

METFORMIN

Class—Oral hypoglycemic (Biguanides).

Category B

Mechanism of action:
- Suppress hepatic gluconeogenesis and glucose output from liver
- Enhances insulin-mediated glucose disposal in muscle and fat
- Retards glucose absorption in GIT
- Enhances peripheral glucose utilization.

Contraindications: Hypersensitivity, hypotension, CVS, RS, hepatic and renal disturbance.

Side effects: Abdominal pain, anorexia, metallic taste, tiredness, lactic acidosis.

Regimen

0.5–2.5 g, 2–3 doses.

CABERGOLINE

Class—D$_2$ agonist.

Category B

Mechanism of action: Long-acting dopamine D$_2$-receptor agonist (decreases prolactin secretion by activating dopaminergic receptors).

Uses:
- Prevention of lactation
- Hyperprolactinemia
- *Contraindications:*
  - Hypersensitivity
  - Severely impaired liver function or cholestasis
  - *Cautions:* Severe cardiovascular disease, Raynaud's disease, gastroduodenal ulcers, active gastrointestinal bleeding, hypotension.

Side effects: Nausea, vomiting, stomach upset, constipation, dizziness, lightheadedness or tiredness.

Regimen

2.5 mg stat for breast suppression.

TETANUS VACCINE

Class—toxoids.

Category C

Uses:
- Routine immunization of children and mothers
- After injury that might lead to introduction of tetanus bacilli.
- 4 weeks interval is necessary for secondary immune response.

Contraindications: Hypersensitivity.

Side effects: Local pain, erythema, induration, fever chills, malaise.

Regimen

0.5 mL single dose IM.

ANTI-Rc IMMUNOGLOBULIN

Class—vaccine.

Category C

Mechanism of action: Masks Rh-antigen on fetal RBCs after fetomaternal bleed hence prevents maternal sensitization.

Uses: Prevention and prophylaxis of postdelivery or postdelivery Rh-isoimmunization.

Contraindications: Hypersensitivity, should be given within 72 hours of delivery.

$T_{1/2}$ = 22–28 days but action lasts till 42 days.

Regimen

300 mcg post delivery

150 mcg post abortion

(10 mcg/mL of whole blood or 20 mcg/mL of PRC feto-maternal bleed).

TRANEXAMIC ACID

Class—Antifibrinolytic.

Category B

Mechanism of action: Binds to lysine binding site on plasminogen and prevents its combination with fibrin.

Uses:
- Dysfunctional uterine bleeding (DUB)
- Cu-T menorrhagia.

Side effects: Nausea, diarrhea, headache, giddiness, thrombophlebitis.

Contraindications: Severe renal insufficiency, hematuria.

Regimen

10–15 mg/kg, 2–3 times a day.

HORMONES IN GYNECOLOGY

Estrogen

Female sexual hormone and growth hormone for Müllerian system.

Synthesis of Estrogen

Steroidal hormone derived from lipid precursor cholesterol in graafian follicle, corpus luteum and placenta.

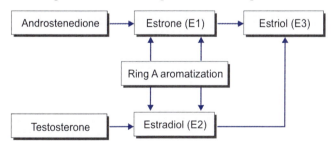

Natural Estrogens

- Estradiol (17β-Estradiol/E2) is the major estrogen secreted by ovary
- Estrone (E1)
- Estriol (E3)

- Principle estrogen before menopause—estradiol, after menopause—estrone.

Synthetic Estrogens

- Natural estrogens are inactive orally and have shorter duration of action due to rapid metabolism in liver
- To overcome these shortcomings, synthetic estrogens have been introduced
- However, currently introduced micronized estradiol preparations are orally active.

Conjugated Steroidal Estrogens

Estrone sulfate, estradiol valerate, estradiol benzoate, estradiol succinate or hemisuccinate.

Nonconjugated Synthetic Estrogens

17α-ethinylestradiol, mestranol.

Nonsteroidal

Diethylstilbestrol (oral), hexoestrol, dienestrol (topical).

Estrogen Analogos

Clomiphene, tamoxifen, raloxifene, ormeloxifene, chlorotrianisene.

Mechanism of action
- 2 types of receptors ERα and ERβ
- Most tissues express both subtypes but ERα predominates in uterus, vagina, breast, hypothalamous and blood vessels while ERβ predominates in prostate gland
- Binding of agonist to receptor causes dimerization of receptor and its interaction with 'estrogen responsive elements' (EREs) of target genes
- Gene transcription is promoted through certain coactivator proteins
- In case of antagonist binding, the receptor assumes a different conformation and interacts with corepressor proteins inhibiting gene transcription.

Physiological actions
- Stimulates development of vagina, uterus and breasts
- Development of secondary sexual characters
- Redistribution of fat to hips and breasts
- Responsible for accelerated growth phase and epiphyseal closure of long bones at puberty
- Maintenance of normal structure of skin and blood vessels
- Stimulates hepatic synthesis of many proteins like transcortin, thyroxine binding globulin, sex hormone binding protein, transferrin, renin substrate, fibrinogen causing increased circulating levels of thyroxin, estrogen, testosterone, iron and copper.

- Decrease in resorption of bone by antagonising effects of PTH
- Increased coagulability of blood by increasing concentrations of factors II, VII, IX, X and increased plasminogen and decreased platelet adhesiveness
- Increased HDL cholesterol and triglycerides and decreased total and LDL cholesterol
- Facilitate movement of fluid from the plasma to the extravascular space.

Uses

HRT:
- Estradiol is the safest estrogen
- If osteoporosis is a risk, it is best treated with tibolone
  - Estradiol, if necessary, may be considered in doses 1 mg/day
- If cardiovascular risk is predominant, tibolone is most suited
  - Estradiol, if necessary, may be considered in doses 1 mg/day
- For those with risk of breast and endometrial cancer tibolone is best, estradiol is better avoided
- Those with vasomotor symptoms and neuroendocrine deficits, estradiol is best
- Those at risk of venous thromboembolism and hot flushes should avoid raloxifene
- Oophorectomized subjects should be on estradiol from immediate postoperative period and may be shifted to tibolone after few months.

Oral contraceptive pills:
- Estrogen of choice is 17α ethinyl estradiol
- Usual dose ranges from 50 mg to 10 mcg
- Dose of 20–30 mcg has been found to be most optimal in combination with progestin.

Senile vaginitis:

Effective in both preventing and treating atrophic vaginitis, topical preparations are commonly used
- Delayed puberty in girls
- It can also be used in acne, hirsutism, palliative treatment of carcinoma prostate
- Tamoxiphene is the first choice hormonal therapy in breast cancer in both pre- and postmenopausal women.

Adverse Effects
- Increased risk of endometrial carcinoma
- Increased incidence of breast carcinoma
- Increased incidence of gallstones and benign hepatomas
- Increased risk of thromboembolic phenomenon
- Stilbesterol given to pregnant women causes increased incidence of vaginal and cervical carcinoma in the female offspring
- Migraine and endometriosis may be worsened.

PROGESTINS
- Progestin = favoring pregnancy
- Steroidal hormone derived from cholesterol, secreted by corpus luteum in early pregnancy and later by placenta
- Progesterone is a 21 carbon compound, natural progestin
- Progesterone means only good things to women and does not cause any harm
- Unfortunately, clinical usefulness is limited by poor absorption from oral route
- Orally active progestins in clinical practice are micronized progesterone, esters of progesterone and 19-norsteroid progestins.

Classification

Progesterone Derivatives
- *Derived from pregnane ring:*
  - *Micronized progesterone:* Oral, transdermal, IM, vaginal and rectal applications (prometrium, utrogestan, crinone)
  - *Derivatives of progesterone:* Retroprogesterone dydrogesterone–oral application (Duphaston)
  - *Esters of progesterone:* Pregnane steroids (21 carbon compounds)
  - *Hydroxyprogesterone derivatives:* Medroxyprogesterone acetate oral and parenteral application (Provera, Farlutal) 17α hydroxyprogesterone 17-n-caproate (Proluton injectable)
- *Progestins derived from androsten ring (19 carbon compounds):*
  - *Androstene steroids:* Testosterone derivatives, Ethisterone, dimethisterone, danazol—oral application
  - Progestins derived from estrane ring
  - *Estrane steroids* (18 carbon compounds) 19 nor testosterone derivatives: Norethisterone, norethisterone acetate, allyestrenol application (Orgametril, pregmate, lyndiol, gestin)
- Progestins derived from gonane ring
  - *Gonane steroids (19 carbon compounds):* Structural modification of estrane and ethyl group at position 13
  - Norgestrel (primovular)

- *Newer gonane steroids (19 carbon compounds):* Structural modification of gonane and methylene group at position 11
- Desogestrel, gestodene, norgestimate (novelon, femilon).

Mechanism of action
- Unlike other steroid receptors, progesterone receptors (PR) have limited distribution in body mostly confined to female genital tract, breasts, pituitary and CNS
- PR exists as two isoforms PR (A and B)
- After binding to progesterone, it undergoes dimerization, attaches to progesterone responsive element and regulates transcription through coactivators
- Natural progesteron is inactive orally, most of the synthetic progestins are active orally.

Physiological actions
- Brings about secretory changes in estrogen primed endometrium
- Brings about decidual changes in endometrium
- Converts watery cervical secretions into viscid scanty secretion
- Acting along with estrogen prepares mammary gland for lactation
- Weak inhibitor of Gn secretion from pituitary
- Causes rise in basal body temperature by 0.5 degree centigrade
- It also has respiratory stimulant and CNS depressant effect.

Uses:

Progestin	Indication
19 norsteroids (norgestrel, desogestrel, norgestimate)	Contraception
19 norsteroids (norethisterone, norethisterone acetate)	Hemostatic progestins (DUB)
Dydrogesterone (short acting progesterone like)	LPD, PMS, DUB, endometrial protection, menopause
Esters of progesterone (medroxyprogesterone)	Long-term contraception, endometrial protection
Micronized progesterone	LPD, PMS, DUB, endometrial protection, menopause
19 norsteroids (tibolone)	Menopausal support bone and CVS protection

MUST REMEMBER
- Breast engorgement, headache, rise in body temperature, esophageal reflux, acne, mood swings.
- Irregular bleeding and amenorrhea.
- 19 nortestosterone derivatives lower HDL levels and may promote atherogenesis.
- Blood sugar levels may rise and diabetis may be precipitated by long-term use of agents like levonorgestrel.
- If given in early pregnancy may cause masculanization of female fetus.
- Intramuscular injections are painful.

Induction of Labor

Kanan Yelikar, Varsha Deshmukh

INTRODUCTION

Induction of labor (IOL) is the artificial initiation of labor before its spontaneous onset for the purpose of delivery of the fetoplacental unit. The rate of induction varies by location and institution and appears to be increasing.

Induction of labor is a common procedure and about 20% pregnant women have labor induced for a variety of reasons.

The prevalence of induced labor is 18% in England and Wales (2001, RCOG), 20% in the USA (1999, Ventura) and 19% in Canada.

In India, however, no large scale studies on the prevalence of induction of labor have been made.

Induction of labor in women with recognized risk factors should take place in a well-equipped place with facilities for monitoring and emergency C-section.

ASSESSMENT BEFORE INDUCTION

- Indication for induction/contraindication
- Gestational age determination
- Cervical favorability
- Assessment of pelvis and fetal size
- Membrane status
- Fetal well-being/FHR monitoring
- Informed consent.

1. What do you mean by induction of labor?

Induction of labor (IOL) is defined as an intervention intended to artificially initiate uterine contractions resulting in the progressive dilatation and effacement of cervix with descent of the presenting part progressing to vaginal delivery.

2. What are the different indications for induction of labor?

- Prolonged pregnancy
- IUGR
- Pre-eclampsia
- IUD
- Antepartum hemorrhage (APH)
- PROM/chorioamnionitis.

3. What do you mean by stabilizing induction?

Stabilizing induction describes induction where the presenting part is not within the pelvis. If the delivery cannot be delayed, then an infusion of oxytocin should be commenced prior to amniotomy to ensure that contractions have commenced and head is over the brim.

4. What is Bishop's score?

Cervix		*Score*		
	0	1	2	3
Position	Posterior	Midposition	Anterior	-
Consistency	Firm	Medium	Soft	-
Effacement	0-30%	40-50%	60-70%	>80%
Dilation	Closed	1-2 cm	3-4 cm	>5 cm
Baby's station	-3	-2	-1	+1, +2

Favorable = 6–13
Unfavorable = 0–5.

5. What is modified Bishop's score?

Bishop score = ... (total)		*Date of Bishop score ..../..../....*		
Score	0	1	2	3
Dilation	Closed	1-2	3-4	5
Length (cm)	>4	3-4	1-2	0
Consistency	Firm	Medium	Soft	—
Position	Posterior	Midline	Anterior	—
Head station	-3	-2	-1, 0	+1, +2

Total = 13
Favorable > 6, Unfavorable < 6

6. What are the contraindications of inductions of labor?

- Contracted pelvis
- CPD
- *Malpresentation:* Like transverse lie, placenta previa
- Grand multipara
- Heart disease
- Pre 2 LSCS or previous classical LSCS
- Pregnancy following VVF repair
- Presence of pelvic tumor/carcinoma cervix
- Active genital herpes.

7. What are the different methods of induction?
- Medical
- Surgical
- Mechanical.

8. What are nonmedical methods of induction of labor?
Castor-oil, bath, enemas breast stimulation, acupuncture, sexual intercourse are suggested to be effective methods of inducing labor. But their benefits are not proved.

9. What is sweeping of membranes?
Sweeping or stripping of the membranes involves the digital separation of the membranes from the lower uterine segment which causes an increase in the level of PGF2-alpha.

10. What are the different mechanical methods of induction of labor?
Mechanical methods in the form of hygroscopic tents such as natural laminaria or synthetic sponges impregnated with $MgSO_4$ (lamicela), inflation of balloon of a urinary catheter within the cervical canal.

11. What is ARM?
Artificial rupture of membranes/amniotomy is frequently used as a method of induction. This is one of the surgical methods. Rupture of membranes leads to endogenous release of prostaglandins.

12. What do you mean by failure to respond?
It is defined as failure to enter the active phase of labor after 9 hours of regular uterine contraction. Failure of induction is defined as failure to deliver vaginally at the end of 24 hours and patient ends in lower segment cesarean section (LSCS) for indication other than fetal distress.

13. What happens to the cervix during ripening?
During ripening, a gradual dissociation and collagenolytic activity of the collagenase and protease enzyme on collagen bundles and a change in the type of proteoglycans in the ground substance, brings about the ripening effect.

14. Which drugs are used for cervical ripening?
Prostaglandins, oxytocin, estradiol, relaxin, mifepristone.

15. Which prostaglandin is used for cervical ripening?
PGE2 gel is used for cervical ripening. It is instilled in the cervical canal in a dose of 0.5 mg and can be repeated after 6 hours. A maximum 3 doses can be applied. Misoprostol 25 micrograms is highly effective for induction of labor especially in cases with intrauterine fetal demise (IUFD) and premature rupture of membranes (PROM) preterm premature rupture of membranes (PPROM), but there is slight risk of hyperstimulation. It can be used by sublingual or vaginal route every 4 hourly.

16. What are the complications of IOL?
Maternal—cervical tear, rupture uterus, operative delivery, accidental hemorrhage, infection, fetal distress, sepsis and neonatal jaundice.

17. What are the contraindications to prostaglandins?
Bronchial asthma, heart disease are the absolute contraindication to PGE2 and PGF2-alpha.

18. What is the antidote for hyperstimulation after PGE2 gel?
Terbutaline is used as an antidote.

19. What is the dose of oral PGE2 tablets for induction of labor?
- 0.5 mg tablet every hour, such 4 tablets in 4 hours.
- After 4 hours, 2 tablets every hour for 6 tablets.
- Maximum 10 tablets.

Side effects—nausea, vomiting, diarrhea.

20. What is the initial dose of oxytocin? What are the drug increments?
- Oxytocin 2.5 U in 500 cc of normal saline cardiotocography for 20 minutes to check the fetal condition and frequency of contraction.
- Escalation every 30 minutes infusion pump until 4–5 contraction/10 minutes.

Giving set	1 cc = 20 drops	1 cc = 15 drops
2.5 units oxytocin in 500 mL of N saline		
Drops/minute	mU/minute	mU/minute
10	2.5	3.3
20	5	6.6
30	7.5	9.9
40	10	13.2
50	12.5	16.5

21. State the types of induction of labor.
Elective and indicated. Elective induction is done for the convenience of the patient and the doctor. Indicated induction is done for maternal or fetal indications, e.g. PROM, postdated, pre-eclampsia, congenital malformation of the fetus.

22. What are the pre-requisites of IOL?
When possibility of vaginal delivery is fully anticipated.
- Confirmation of gestational age
- Fetal presentation, position
- Estimated fetal size
- Cervical favor ability
- Pelvic adequacy.

23. What is induction of labor in special situation?

IUFD, pre-LSCS, intrauterine growth restriction (IUGR), twins, preterm, PROM.

Pre-LSCS induction should be considered very carefully. However, the incidence of scar dehiscence is not different than in a spontaneous labor.

Multiple pregnancies, no definitive merits of an active policy of induction of labor.

PROM induction of labor is advantageous to reduce the infective sequelae in mother and baby.

IUGR carefully done since incidence of intrapartum fetal hypoxia is common.

24. What is the basic difference in the efficacy of oxytocic agents: PG and pitocin?

Prostaglandins are effective in preterm induction/in unfavorable cervix/ IUFD/preterm PROM.

25. What are the complications of induction of labor?

- Infections, accidental hemorrhage/dry labor/rupture uterus, amniotic fluid embolism/fluid retention with pitocin/uterine hypertonus
- *Fetal complications:* Prematurity/fetal distress/neonatal hyperbilirubinemia (more common with oxytocin).

26. Describe different complications of uterine contractions.

- *A hypertonus:* Single contraction lasting for >2 minutes
- *Tachysystole:* >5 uterine contractions in 10 minutes time
- *Hyperstimulation:* Hypertonus or tachysystole when associated with abnormal fetal heart pattern.

27. Define augmentation of labor.

Augmentation is the process of stimulation of uterine contraction (both in frequency and intensity) that are already present, but found to be inadequate.

28. Which are exclusive indications of ARM and oxytocin?

ARM: 1. APH
      2. Acute hydramnios
      3. Severe pre-eclampsia, eclampsia.
Oxytocin: IUD.

29. What are the hazards of ARM?

- Chances of umbilical cord prolapse
- Amnionitis
- It is a permanent procedure
- Accidental injury to fetal parts, placenta and cervix uterus
- Liquor amnii embolism (rare).

30. When do you call a women in active labor?

When the cervix is dilated at 3 cm with at least 3 contractions each lasting for 20 seconds over 10 minues.

MUST REMEMBER

- IOL is defined as an intervention intended to artificially initiate uterine contractions resulting in the progressive dilatation and effacement of cervix with descent of the presenting part.
- Common indications include wherever the continuation of pregnancy is detrimental for the health of the mother or the baby.
- With availability of better monitoring methods of high-risk pregnancies such as USG/color Doppler, the indications of induction of labor are increasing.
- The efficacy and safety of drugs such as oral and vaginal route of prostaglandins has been proved by different studies.
- Misoprostol is promising drug and helpful in cases with poor Bishop's score.
- Intrapartum electronic fetal monitoring during IOL is recommended.
- Failed IOL defined as when patient fails to deliver vaginally within 24 hours consideration of LSCS is done in this situation.
- For successful induction, cervix should be favorable, i.e. Bishop's score more than 7.
- Maternal complications include infections, accidental hemorrhage/dry labor/rupture uterus, amniotic fluid embolism/fluid retention with pitocin/uterine hypertonus.
- When induction of labor is to be done in women with recognized risk factors, should take place in a well-equipped place with facilities for monitoring and emergency C-section.

Instrumental Vaginal Delivery: Forceps and Ventouse

26

Shaila Sapre, Vidya Thobbi, Suguna

1. What is assisted vaginal delivery?

In some vaginal deliveries, additional assistance is employed to assist delivery by giving episiotomy, using forceps or vacuum extraction, or by manual maneuvers in cases of breech presentation (Figs 26.1A and B).

2. Who invented forceps and when?

- Peter Chamberlen of England invented forceps in the later part of 16th century or the beginning of 17th century. However, it was not generally known until the early part of the 18th century. The invention was preserved as a family secret through four generations. Even Sanskrit writing from approximately 1500 BC contains evidence of single and paired instruments.
- Chamberlen forceps—Iron blades which had only cephalic curve and handle.
- Leveret of Paris [1747]—Added the pelvic curve in 1747 and French lock with butterfly screw.
- Smellie of England—Added the English lock or double slot lock.
- Shank [1751]—Increased the length of the instrument and used it in breech presentation.
- Tarnier [1877]—Introduced axis-traction.
- Barton and Kjeillands introduced specialized forceps.

3. What are the types of forceps?

Classical instruments: It was designed by James Young Simpson, Wrigley and George L Elliot Jr in mid-19th century. It was commonly used for outlet and low pelvic rotational delivery (Fig. 26.2A).

Modified classical instruments: Overlapping solid blades with extended shanks like Tucker-Mclane forceps, elliot type, commonly used as mid-pelvic rotators or outlet blades.

Specialized instruments: Designed for specific indications like:
- Barton's for transverse arrest in platypelloid pelvis
- Keilland's for mid-pelvic rotation and correction of asynclitism (Fig. 26.2B)
- Piper's for delivery of aftercoming head in breech.

Divergent or parallel blades instrument:
Designed to limit fetal cranial compression; for example, Laufe, Shute and Hay.

Axis traction instruments:
- As a separate handle attached to any standard forceps
- Axis traction as an integral part of the forceps like Howk-Dennon's and de Wee's forceps.

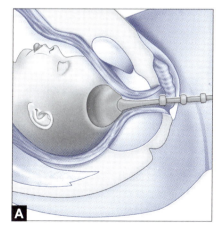 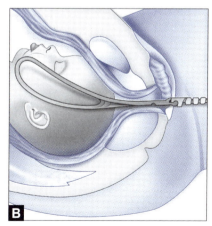

Figs 26.1A and B: Assisted vaginal delivery: (A) Vacuum-assisted birth; (B) Forceps-assisted birth

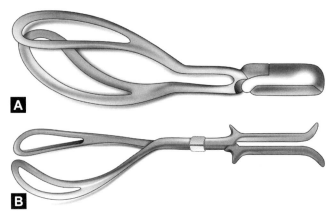

Figs 26.2A and B: Forceps: (A) Wrigley's outlet forceps; (B) Keilland's forceps

4. What is the classification of forceps application?

Classical (old) classification:
- Low/outlet forceps—forceps applied when the fetal head/skull has reached the pelvic floor, sagittal suture has reached the AP diameter of pelvis, and scalp is visible without separating the vulva
- Mid forceps—forceps applied when head is engaged but criteria for low forceps not reached
- High forceps—forceps applied when head is not engaged.

Newer classification as per ACOG (Revised in 1991):
- Outlet forceps
- Low forceps
- Mid forceps
- High forceps.

Outlet:
- Fetal scalp visible without separating the labia
- Fetal skull has reached the pelvic floor
- Sagittal suture is in the anteroposterior diameter or right or left occiput anterior or posterior position (rotation does not exceed 45º)
- Fetal head is at or on the perineum.

Low:
- Leading point of the skull (not caput) is at station plus 2 or more and not on the pelvic floor
- Two subdivisions:
  - Rotation of 45º or less from the occipitoanterior position
  - Rotation of more than 45º, including the occipitoposterior position.

Mid:
- Fetal head is no more than 1/5th palpable per abdomen
- Leading point of the skull is above station plus 2 but not above the ischial spines.
  - Two subdivisions:
  - Rotation of 45º or less from the occipitoanterior position
  - Rotation of more than 45º, including the occipitoposterior position.

High:
Not included in the classification as operative vaginal delivery is not recommended in this situation where the head is 2/5th or more palpable abdominally and the presenting part is above the level of the ischial spines.

5. How do you name forceps?
- *Long curved forceps:* High and mid cavity
- *Short curved forceps:* Outlet forceps.

6. What are the functions of forceps?
- To apply traction on the fetal head
- Compression effect which facilitates and aids in easy delivery
- It brings about rotation of head of the fetus
- It acts as a protective cage preventing any injury to the fetal head during delivery
- *As a vectis:* By applying one blade to deliver the head in cesarean section.

7. What are the indications for forceps delivery?

I. Maternal
- Maternal exhaustion
- Maternal conditions requiring cutting short of the second stage of labor where bearing down is contraindicated like in cardiac and pulmonary diseases and anemia
- *Delay in second stage occurs:*
  - Due to uterine inertia
  - Failure of progress of labor—fetal head is on the perineum for more than 20–30 minutes
- In patients with eclampsia
- Vaginal birth after cesarean section.

II. Fetal indications
- Fetal distress
- Nonreassuring fetal heart rate
- In cases of after coming head in breech deliveries
- Cord prolapse in second stage
- Low birth weight babies.

8. What are the prerequisites for forceps application?
- Suitable presentation and position
- Vertex or face presentation or for aftercoming head in breech deliveries
- Head must be engaged. Station should be at +2
- Cervix must be fully dilated and effaced and it should be completely taken up
- Membranes must be ruptured
- Uterus should be acting
- Bladder must be empty
- Appropriate anesthesia and a liberal mediolateral episiotomy should be given

- Consent and proper documentation should be maintained.

It can be remembered as the pneumonic FORCEPS
F: Full dilatation
O: Occipitoanterior
R: Rupture of membranes
C: Contractions—uterine, good, catheterization
E: Engagement—empty bowel
P: Position—pelvis adequate
S: Station of the presenting part.

9. What are the different parts of the forceps?
- Handles
- Locks—English, French, Sliding
- Shank
- Blades.

10. How will you decide the side of the blade?
The right or left blade is decided depending on the side of the maternal pelvis to which they are applied.

11. What do you mean by trial forceps?
It is a tentative attempt of forceps delivery in a case of suspected mid pelvic contraction with a predetermined decision of abandoning it in favor of LSCS, if moderate traction fails to overcome the resistance. This should preferably be performed in operation theater so that patient can be immediately taken up for LSCS.

12. What do you mean by failed forceps?
When an attempt in vaginal delivery with forceps has failed to extract the baby, it is called as failed forceps. The causes are poor clinical judgment of disproportion CPD, malposition and application before full dilatation of cervix or very early application of forceps before the head is low.

According to WHO [2003], forceps is labeled as failed forceps when fetus is undelivered after 3 pulls with no descent or after 30 minutes which should be managed by cesarean section.

13. What is elective or prophylactic forceps delivery? Who coined this term?
- The term was proposed by De Lee [1920].
- When interference with forceps is elective for the purpose of preventing maternal and fetal complications in cases where it is not really indicated or necessary, is known as elective or prophylactic forceps delivery like in cases of eclampsia, heart disease and previous cesarean section and anemia.

14. Why the forceps have different curves?
The forceps have two curves (Fig. 26.3):
- *Cephalic curve*: Fits the shape of the baby's head and reduces the danger of compression.

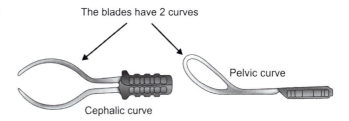

Fig. 26.3: Curves of blade

- *Pelvic curve*: Follows the direction of the birth canal and makes application and extraction easier and also decreases the damage to the maternal tissues.

15. What are the type of forceps application?
Cephalic application: Blades are applied along the sides of the head and the biparietal diameter is grasped in between the widest part of the blades. The long-axis of the blades correspond to the occipitomental plane (Figs 26.4A and B).

Pelvic application: Blades are applied on the lateral pelvic wall ignoring the position of the head, if the head is not

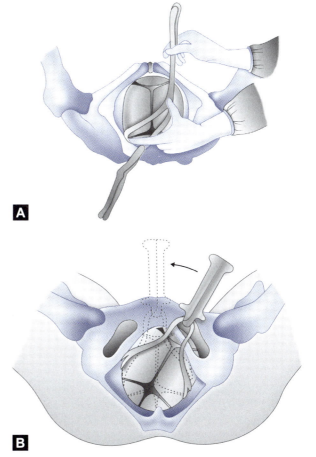

Figs 26.4A and B: Forceps application

rotated. When the head is sufficiently rotated, pelvic and cephalic applications should naturally coincide.

16. What is the technique of forceps application?

- *Identification of blades and their application:* The instrument should be placed in front of the pelvis with the tip pointing upwards and pelvic curve forwards. First, the left blade should be applied guided by the right hand and then the right blade with the left hand.
- *Locking of blades:* The blade handles should lock easily without applying any extra pressure. This indicates correct forceps application.
- *Clinical checks for correct forceps application (Fig. 26.5):*
  - Sagittal suture should lie in the midline of the shanks
  - The operator is unable to place more than a fingertip between the fenestration of the blade and the fetal head on either side
  - Posterior fontanelle is not more than one finger breadth above the plane of the shanks of the forceps.
- *Traction:*
  - Steady and intermittent traction should be given synchronizing with the uterine contractions, first downwards (horizontal), backwards, forwards and lastly upwards
  - In outlet forceps, only two fingers are to be introduced. Traction is applied in straight horizontal, upward, and then forwards direction
  - Removal of blades—right blade should be removed first followed by the left blade after delivery of the fetal head.
- *In occipitoposterior position:*
  - Blades are to be applied as usual but they should be equidistant from both the sinciput and the occiput
  - Traction should be in the horizontal direction till the root of the nose is under the pubic symphysis, then upward till the occiput emerges over the perineum and finally downwards.
- *In face presentation:*
  - Blades are to be introduced along the occipitomental diameter
  - Traction is applied downwards till the chin appears under the symphysis pubis and then upwards delivering the nose, eyes, brow, and occiput
- *Forceps for aftercoming head:*
  - Piper's forceps are especially designed for this purpose (Fig. 26.6)
  - Forceps to be applied when the occiput lies against the back of the symphysis
  - Blades should be applied from below after raising the legs
  - Traction should be maintained in an arc, which follows the axis of the birth canal.

17. What is the anesthetic requirement for forceps delivery?

- General anesthesia is not preferred because of its complexity. Moreover, it may lead to fetal distress. Its only rare indication is midforceps (But only outlet forceps are used in modern obstetrics)
- In most of the cases, local infiltration with vocal support is all that is needed, especially in cases of outlet forceps
- In few low forceps, pudendal block may become necessary.

Perineal infiltration

- Local infiltration of perineum is all that may be necessary for performance of episiotomy and outlet forceps delivery
- In fact when fetal head is low, down approach to the ischial spine is difficult
- Using a long fine needle, on a 20 mL syringe, 10–20 mL of 1% is injected fanwise from a point on fourchette.

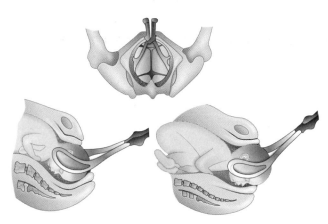

Fig. 26.5: Technique of forceps application

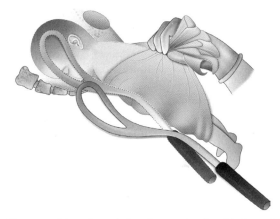

Fig. 26.6: Piper forceps for aftercoming head in breech

Pudendal block
Pudendal nerve may be approached by the transvaginal or the transperineal route. For either technique, 10–20 mL of 1% xylocaine can be used.

Transvaginal route: With patient in lithotomy position, the index and middle fingers of one hand are inserted into vagina in order to palpate ischial spine. The guarded needle is advanced between two fingers. The needle tip is advanced through vaginal wall until it lies below and beyond sacrospinous ligament. After aspiration to exclude blood, the pudendal nerve is blocked with 8–10 mL solutions.

Transperineal approach: Half way between fourchette and ischial tuberosity, while ischial spine is palpated per vaginally, needle is inserted through the wall attached to 10 mL syringe and advanced guided by finger in vagina to sacrospinous ligament and then the block is affected in the usual manner.

18. What are the advantages of forceps over vacuum?
- In suspected cases of pelvic contraction, where moderate traction is required, forceps is preferred
- Forceps can quickly expedite delivery in case of fetal distress where ventouse takes longer time
- Safer in premature baby
- It can be applied on face and aftercoming head in breech deliveries and when caput is present.

19. What are the advantages of vacuum over forceps?
- Same amount of traction can be applied with only ½ the rise in intracranial pressure resulting from the use of forceps
- It can be used before full dilatation of cervix
- The fetal head can be rotated easily
- It requires less skill than forceps delivery
- It can be applied when the station of the fetal head is high
- Maternal complications like cervical tears and vaginal lacerations are comparatively less.

20. What are the complications of forceps application?
Maternal:
- Soft tissue trauma
- Episiotomy extension, IIIrd degree perineal tear
- Vaginal and cervical lacerations
- Cervical tear with traumatic PPH
- Urethral/bladder/rectal injury/bladder injury
- Rarely rupture of the uterus may also occur
- Anesthesia hazards
- Postpartum hemorrhage and shock
- Sepsis
- Postpartum foot drop
- Long-term sequelae like chronic low backache and prolapse.

Fetal:
- Bruising, lacerations
- Cephalohematomas
- Facial nerve injury—due to pressure on the nerve, as it comes out of the stylomastoid foramen
- Less common are depressed skull fractures, intracranial, hemorrhage and tentorial lacerations
- Cerebral palsy.

21. What are contraindications of forceps applications?
- Pelvic inadequacy
- Cervix not dilated and effaced
- Inexperienced operator
- Any contraindication to vaginal delivery.

22. What is the role of forceps in modern obstetrics?
Forceps delivery has still got place in modern obstetric practice and should be considered in certain cases, which reduces unnecessary cesarean sections and prevents fetal and maternal complications due to prolonged labor. Proper selection of cases and careful and timely application is important (only outlet forceps are recommended).

OPERATIVE VAGINAL DELIVERY—VACUUM EXTRACTOR/VENTOUSE

1. What are the indications of vacuum extractor?
- *Maternal:*
  - Prolonged second stage—Nulliparous >2 hours without regional anesthesia, >3 hours with regional anesthesia
  - Multiparous >1 hour without regional anesthesia, >2 hours with regional anesthesia
  - Maternal exhaustion
  - Maternal disorders (cardiac, cerebrovascular, neuromuscular conditions) where voluntary efforts are contraindicated or impossible.
- *Fetal:*
  - Fetal distress
  - Failure of descent or rotation.

2. What are the contraindications for vacuum extraction?
- Operative inexperience
- Inability to achieve proper application
- Uncertainty of fetal position and station
- Fetopelvic disproportion
- High fetal head
- Malpresentation—breech, face, brow
- Prior failed forceps

- Fetal suspected or known coagulation defect, osteogenesis imperfecta (prone for fracture)
- Relative—prematurity of <36 weeks and prior scalp sampling.

3. **What are the types of vacuum cups and their sizes?**
- Rigid cup—stainless steel (Figs 26.7A and B)
- Soft cup—polyethylene, silicone
- Size—40 mm, 50 mm, 60 mm.

4. **What are the prerequisites of vacuum extraction?**
- Informed consent—the need for the operation, risks and benefits, alternative modes of treatment
- Physician should have knowledge of the instrument, indication and a willingness to abandon on operative difficulty
- Prepare patient—ruptured membrane, empty bladder, full cervical dilatation, engaged fetal head, no suspicion of fetopelvic disproportion
- In uncertainty of fetal position or station, transperineal or transvaginal scan is indicated
- Acceptable analgesia/anesthesia—local anesthesia, regional pudendal block, major conduction anesthesia like epidural, spinal, etc.

5. **What is trial ventouse?**
Vaginal route of delivery is a possibility, but outcome is uncertain, thus with initial traction, there is no descent and vacuum is abandoned for cesarean section.

6. **What is the procedure of vacuum extraction?**
- Ghosting—a ghost or phantom application done, which is an exact parallel in front of the perineum in the same angle and position once the extractor has been applied (Fig. 26.8)
- Insertion—lubricated rigid cut inserted sideways, soft cup collapsed
- Application on the cranial flexion or pivot point—which is an imaginary spot 6 cm from the center of anterior fontanelle, or 1-2 cm anterior to posterior fontanelle, 60 mm cup edge will be approximately 3 cm or 2-finger breadth from posterior fontanelle (Fig. 26.9).

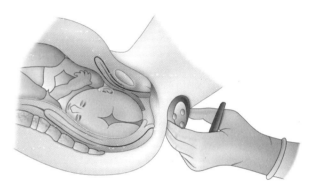

Fig. 26.8: Image showing ghosting

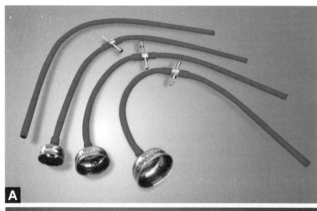

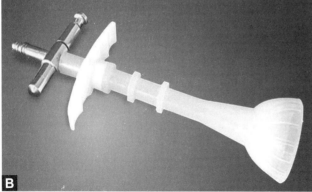

Figs 26.7A and B: Vacuum cups: (A) Rigid cup; (B) Soft cup

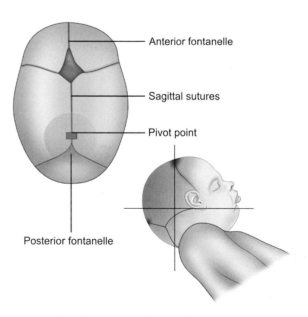

Fig. 26.9: Image showing the pivot point

Wrong application

- Vacuum of 500–600 mm Hg created by negative pressure of 0.2 kg/cm^2 every 2 minutes until 0.8 kg/cm^2 is reached in 8–10 minutes in rigid cup, in soft cup negative pressure increased to 0.8 kg/cm^2 over 1 minute. This creates an artificial caput succedaneum or 'chignon'
- Traction—pull coincides with uterine contraction, only 4–5 traction recommended, with 2 pulls descent of presenting part should be seen, overall duration of procedure is 20–30 minutes
- Documentation in detail (Fig. 26.10).

7. What is the rule of 3?

Vacuum should be abandoned in the following cases:
- 3 pulls, over 3 contractions without progress
- 3 pop offs, after one pop off, reassess carefully before reapplying
- After 30 minutes of application with no progress.

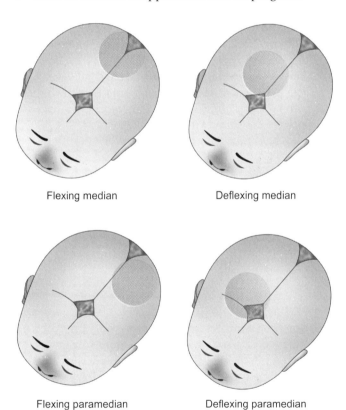

Fig. 26.10: Cup position on fetal head

8. What is the role of episiotomy for ventouse delivery?

Restrictive use of episiotomy using the operator's individual judgment is advised.

9. What is special application of ventouse?

Special application in assisting extraction of high head in cesarean section.

10. What are the complications of vacuum delivery?

- Maternal—soft tissue injuries to cervix, vagina, and traumatic PPH, dysfunction of perineum
- Fetal—sloughing of scalp, cephalohematoma, subaponeurotic hemorrhage, intracranial hemorrhage, retinal hemorrhage, and neonatal jaundice.

Injuries are less common with soft cup but detachments are more common.

11. Describe ventouse verses forceps.

- Maternal injury less common with ventouse
- Reduction in the requirement of anesthesia in ventouse
- Failure rate is high in ventouse as compared to forceps
- Neonatal subdural, intracranial hemorrhage is more common in ventouse whereas facial nerve injury is more common in forceps.

MUST REMEMBER

- Forceps assisted is an instrumental delivery and carried out only when contracted pelvis and CPD is ruled out.
- It can be applied under local anesthesia.
- It is a skilled procedure and should be carried out by trained personnel.
- Before application of forceps, all the prerequisite conditions must be fulfilled.
- Successful application of forceps results into more number of vaginal deliveries, thereby decreasing incidence of cesarean section.
- After delivery of baby cervix and vagina should be explored for any extension of episiotomy or tears.
- Prophylaxis for PPH is mandatory after application of forceps.
- Ventouse can be applied even in nonrotated head but the time required for creation of negative pressure is more so cannot be applied in emergency conditions like fetal distress.
- Ventouse cannot be applied without suction so electricity is must.
- Following ventouse application, there is swelling over scalp (Chignon), which disappears within 3–5 days.

Contraception

Haresh U Doshi, Sonali Deshpande

Contraception is a mean for promoting global health. When contraception is not used by presumably fertile partners, approximately 90% of women will conceive within 1 year. Current methods include oral steroidal contraceptives, injected or implanted steroidal contraceptives, intrauterine devices, barrier techniques, withdrawal, sexual abstinence around the time of ovulation, breastfeeding and permanent sterilization.

1. Which are the different methods for contraception?

Methods of contraception: (A) Temporary; (B) Permanent
- *Temporary contraception:*
  - *Natural and behavioral family planning methods:*
    a. Total abstinence
    b. Coitus interruptus
    c. Fertility awareness based methods
    d. Lactational amenorrhea method.
  - *Barrier contraceptives:*
    a. *Mechanical:*
       i. Male-condom
       ii. Female-condom, diaphragm, cervical cap, dumas cap, etc.
    b. *Chemical:* Spermicidal substances in the form of foam tablets, creams, jellies, etc.
    c. *Combined:* Mechanical plus chemical.
  - *Intrauterine contraceptive devices (IUCD)*
  - *Steroidal contraceptives:* Oral contraceptives (OCs), injectables and others
  - *Emergency contraception*—postcoital contraception
  - Uterotubal junction devices—sialistic or ceramic plugs
  - *Miscellaneous:*
    - Male pill—Gossypol
    - Immunological (under research)
- Permanent contraception
  - *Male:* Vasectomy operation
  - *Female:* Different sterilization operations.

2. Which are the natural and behavioral methods for contraception?

They are as follows:
- *Total abstinence*
- *Coitus interruptus*
- *Calendar or rhythm method:* Record the number of days for previous 6 menstrual cycles. Subtract 18 from the length of her shortest cycle.
  This is first day of her fertile period. Then subtract 11 days from the length of her longest cycle. This is the last day of her fertile period.
- *Cervical mucus (Billing's method):* Here the fertile period starts from the first day of any cervical secretions or feeling of vaginal wetness until the 4th day after the peak day of slippery secretions.
- *Symptothermal method:* At least 2 indicators are used to identify fertile period, i.e. BBT + cervical mucus or BBT + calendar rhythm.
- *Hightech hormonal monitoring:* Here small electronic devices detect urinary metabolites of LH and estrogen, estrone-3-glucuronide (E3-G). Threshold level of estrogen determines the beginning of the fertile period and 4 days past a threshold level of LH marks the end of fertile period. "Persona" and "Clearpan" are such personal hand held devices with test strips. In last 4 methods which detect fertile period, the couple avoids sex, uses a barrier method, or uses withdrawal during the fertile time.
- *Lactational amenorrhea method:* This is most useful when mother is doing exclusive breastfeeding and she is not menstruating (first 6 months).

3. What is the history of condom? What precautions are taken while using condom?

The origin of word "condom" is believed to have come from the Latin word "condom" meaning a receptacle. Its invention is also attributed to physician Dr Condom who recommended it to king Charles II to prevent illegal offspring.

Condom should be applied on erect penis and prelubricated one is preferred. If there is no teat, some space pressed empty of air, is left at the end. During sexual act, after ejaculation has occurred, one should be sure that condom does not get dislodged from the penis, i.e. penis should be withdrawn while still erect and condom should be held firmly at the root of the penis. Chemical contraceptive (spermicidal jelly) used along with it gives extra protection and lubrication. Do not use lubricants made with oil. Most of them damage condoms. Store condoms in a cool, dark place, if possible. Heat, light and humidity damage condoms. Handle condoms carefully. Fingernails and rings can tear them. Do not unroll condoms before use. This may weaken them. Also, an unrolled condom is difficult to put on.

Check the condom for tear before throwing it away and if it has torn, use one of the emergency contraceptive method. Do not reuse the condom.

4. What are the advantages and disadvantages of condom?

Advantages:
- Easy to use
- Relatively cheap
- Freely available without medical supervision and prescription
- Failure rate is low as compared to physiological and chemical methods
- Protects against common vaginal infections including human immunodeficiency virus (AIDS) infection
- Protects against carcinoma cervix. Because carcinoma cervix is promoted by sexually transmitted agent. Suggested agents are: (i) Human papillomavirus, (ii) Herpes virus, and (iii) Sperm
- Safe. No hormonal side effects
- It can be used at any age
- Often helps prevent premature ejaculation.
- It can be used where pills and IUCD are contraindicated, i.e. follow-up of vesicular mole, diabetes, valvular heart disease.

Disadvantages:
- Failure rate is high as compared to IUCD and pills
- Because it prevents full genital contact, it may decrease sensation making sex less enjoyable for either partner
- Couple must take sometime to put the condom on the erect penis before sex. Hence motivation in each act is required. In male partner, rarely it causes psychological disturbances and even impotence
- Disposal is a social problem, it may embarrass some one to buy condoms
- Hypersensitivity reaction to either of the partners.

5. What is the failure rate of condom? Why it is high?

Failure rate of condom is 3–18/100 women years observation (3–8/HWY if used with chemical contraceptive). This is also known as pearl index.

Causes of failure are:
- Incorrect use
- Inconsistent use. Not used with each sexual act, e.g. patient under effect of alcohol
- Used without chemical contraceptive
- Defect in condom
- Tearing or bursting of condom during sexual act (4%).

6. Which are the other uses of condom?

Other uses of condom:
- In transvaginal sonography, it is applied over the vaginal probe
- For preparation of mold in vaginoplasty
- Immunological cervical factor in infertility. Husband should use it for 3 to 6 months so that antibody level against the sperms in cervical mucus decreases. Then chances of pregnancy increase
- *Threatened abortion:* After few weeks of abstinence, if couple resumes sexual relations. Male partner should use condom, because semen contains prostaglandins which may cause abortion.

7. Describe female condom.

Female condom is a newly developed female barrier contraceptive. It has combined features of diaphragm and condom. It consists of two flexible polyurethane rings located at the either end of a 15 cm soft loose fitting polyurethane sheath. The inner end is closed. The inner ring is placed high in vagina, while outer ring covers the labia and base of penis. It is prelubricated with silicone-based lubricant. It is available with different names, e.g. reality, femidom, femshield.

Advantages:
- Controlled by woman
- It prevents STDs more effectively than condom as it covers some perineal area also
- No allergic reactions
- More convenient than male condom as it can be inserted precoitus
- Less chances of breakage.

Disadvantages:
- Expensive at present
- Some women have difficulties in insertion.

It is meant for single time use, however WHO recommends reuse for maximum 5 times with proper care for disinfection, washing and drying. Its failure rate reported in various studies range from 6.8 to 15.1/HWY in first year of use.

8. Why female condom is better than male condom?

Female condom is better than male condom because:
- Controlled by woman
- It covers some perineal area also
- More convenient to use as it can be inserted precoitus
- Less chances of breakage
- Reusable for few times.

9. What are the contraindications, advantages and disadvantages of vaginal diaphragm?

Contraindications
- Cystocele or rectocele
- Uterine prolapse
- Local infection, ulceration
- Allergy to rubber
- Severe retroversion
- VVF or RVF.

Advantages:
- Relatively cheap
- Effective as compared to physiological and chemical methods
- Used by female so cooperation of male partner is not required
- It does not interfere with natural coitus or orgasm of either of the partners and it is relatively harmless
- It also gives some protection against PID.

Disadvantages:
- In sensitive patients, it may cause embarrassment and some women may consider diaphragm unaesthetic. Use of spermicide is messy
- Failure rate is high as compared to IUCD and pills
- High degree of motivation of the patient is required for its use
- Allergic reactions to rubber may occur
- Vaginitis, UTI and rarely toxic shock syndrome are reported.

10. Tell everything about "Today".

Today available as a vaginal sponge made of polyurethane containing one gram of the spermicidal nonoxynol-9. The sponge is shaped like mushroom cap with the concave side covering the cervix. It is 2" in diameter, 1.25" thick and loop is attached to the bottom. It has 3 actions:
1. It releases spermicide during coitus.
2. It absorbs the ejaculate.
3. It blocks the entrance to the cervical canal.

It is effective for 24 hours regardless the frequency of coitus, but then it is discarded. It releases 125–150 mg nonoxynol in 24 hours. Its failure rate ranges from 9 to 27 per 100 users.

Today is now available in small pessary form 'Today premium' containing 5% nonoxynol-9. It dissolves within 10 minutes and is effective for one hour only. Its efficiency rate is more than 99%.

Nonoxynol has bactericidal and virucidal activity so it protects against AIDS. Usually, there are no major side effects. It may produce allergic type reactions and vaginal or penile irritation. Patient may have vaginal discomfort like soreness, itching, stinging. Rarely toxic shock syndrome can occur.

11. Which are the different IUCDs you know?

Grafenberg ring, a silver coiled wire ring was the first popular IUCD widely used in the past. It was introduced by Grafenberg of Germany in 1929. Since then many different types of devices are invented. They are divided into two groups.
1. First generation or inert or unmedicated devices, e.g. Lippes loop, Saf-T-coil
2. Second generation or bioactive or medicated devices containing metals like copper (Cu-T, Cu-7) zinc, silver or containing hormones, e.g. progestasert, Mirena or containing drugs like tranexamic acid or epsilon aminocaproic acid.

Various IUCDs were used in past, e.g. Grafenberg ring, Chinese ring, Ota ring, Birnberg bow, Margulies coil, Soonawala loop, Saf-T-coil, Dalkon shield, Hall-stone ring, Antigon-F, Dana super.

12. What is the difference between Cu-T 200B and Cu-T 380A?

Copper T (Cu-T 200B) is T-shaped device made up of polyethylene which is a biologically inert plastic. It is impregnated with barium sulfate to make it radiopaque. It has 2 monofilament polypropylene threads attached to its lower end. Copper wire is wound around the vertical limb. Surface area of copper is 200 sq mm, weight is 120 mg and diameter of wire is 0.25 mm. It daily releases 50 µg of copper in first year. Its applicator, made up of synthetic plastic consists of cannula with guard and a plunger rod. Guard is blue and mobile. Cu-T along with its applicator is supplied in a plastic pack presterilized by gamma radiation. Cu-T 200B has a small ball at its lower end to prevent cervical perforation. Lifespan is 3 years. Needs to be change after 3 years.

Specifications:
Length—36 mm, width—32 mm, weight—120 mg.
Surface area of copper—200 sq mm, diameter—0.25 mm.
Cu-T 380 A is a T-shaped device with 2 solid copper sleeves on transverse arms and copper wire on vertical stem. Total surface area of copper is 380 sq mm (314 sq mm of copper wire and 33 sq mm of each copper sleeve). It has 2 monofilament white threads. Its effective life is estimated to be 6–10 years, in Cu-T 380 Ag copper wire on the vertical stem has a silver core. The silver core prevents fragmentation of copper and lengthens the effective life of the device.

13. Describe the time and technique of IUCD insertion.

Time of insertion:
- During menstrual period from second day onwards or within 10 days of menstruation (during menses, it is easy to insert and bleeding related to insertion is masked).

- Immediately after first trimester MTP or spontaneous abortion.
- Postpartum—after normal or preterm delivery, it can be introduced immediately or at the end of 6 weeks. In fact if insertion is done within first 48 hours, there are less chances of perforation. But more chances of spontaneous expulsion.
- At the time of cesarean section.
- Postcoital—within 5 days of unprotected intercourse in a fertile period.

    Technique of IUCD insertion— 'Withdrawal technique':
    - Patient is explained about the type, principles, side effects and failure rate, etc. of the device and informed consent is taken.
    - Detailed history is elicited and complete pelvic examination is done to rule out contraindications.
    - Full aseptic and antiseptic precautions are observed.

Guard is adjusted at the total uterocervical length of that patient after measuring the uterocervical length by sound. Loaded applicator is introduced so that when guard is at external os, tip of the applicator with Cu-T is at fundus. Now plunger is fixed by one hand and cannula is withdrawn over it, so Cu-T is released high up at fundus without being pushed. Then plunger is withdrawn, cannula is withdrawn and threads are cut for 2 to 3 cm from external os so that patient can easily feel it by self-examination. The Cu-T should not be loaded for >2–5 minute as they tend to lose their memory.

14. What are the contraindications to IUCD insertion?

Contraindications are:

Absolute:
- Abnormal menstruation—irregular heavy or prolonged
- Suspected pregnancy
- Recent or past pelvic infection
- Suspected malignancy of genital tract
- Uterine anomalies, e.g. bicornuate uterus
- Uterine pathologies, e.g. fibroid
- Bleeding disorders
- History of ectopic pregnancy.

Relative:
- *Nulliparous patient:* Difficult to insert, expulsion rate is high and if infection occurs it can lead to infertility
- Previous cesarean section or other scar on uterus
- Primary dysmenorrhea
- Local infection, i.e. cervicitis, vaginitis
- Moderate or severe anemia
- Patients on corticosteroid or anticoagulant therapy
- Recently terminated vesicular mole
- Valvular heart disease, diabetes
- Wilson's disease.

15. What is the mechanism of action of Cu-T 380A?

Mechanism of action: It works primarily by preventing fertilization contrary to the popular belief that it prevents implantation.
- Presence of device with its nylon thread occupies some space in the uterus and causes mechanical obstruction to ascent of sperms.
- Transcervical threads cause changes in the cervical mucus and make it hostile to sperms.
- IgM level in serum is increased so antifertility action is in part to their ability to produce antibodies.
- *Actions of copper:*
    - Directly damages sperms and fertilized ovum
    - Causes biochemical changes in cervical mucus and renders it hostile.
        Sperm motility and capacitation are affected.
    - Changes in the endometrium: (a) Enzymatic inhibition, i.e. carbonic anhydrase (copper replaces zinc), alkaline phosphatase, glycogen synthetase, etc. (b) Intense leukocytic infiltration. (c) Changes in DNA constituent of endometrial cells. (d) Decrease in glycogen content of cells. (e) Increase in fibrinolytic activity of endometrium and (f) Endometrial vasoconstriction and ischemic damage.
- Increase in tubal motility so fertilized ovum, before it is mature enough for implantation, reaches the uterus which is also unprepared.
- Increase in uterine contractions which result in expulsion of newly implanted ovum
- Device causes low-grade tissue reaction (i.e. inflammatory changes) in the endometrium making it unreceptable for implantation. It also attracts macrophages to its site which engulf the sperms as well as fertilized ovum by phagocytosis.

16. What are the side effects and complications of IUCD?

Side-effects and complications:
- *Menstrual problems:* Spotting, heavy periods and prolonged periods frequently occur in first 2–3 months.
- Cramps like pain in lower abdomen. Removal due to excessive bleeding and pain occurs in 5–15/100 users.
- *Dysmenorrhea:* Spasmodic type, with infection there can be congestive type also.
- *Leukorrhea.*
- *Pelvic infection:* Risk is more in first month of insertion. Ascending infection can occur at any time as nylon threads constantly project in vagina. Flaring up of already existing infection can also occur.
- *Displacement:* Device may penetrate the uterine wall or perforation of uterus and migration into pelvis or upper abdomen. Perforation commonly occurs at the

time of insertion. Common sites of perforation are fundal and isthmic region. Incidence of perforations is 1 to 3 per 1000 insertions.
- *Spontaneous expulsion:* During first menstrual period or within the first year of insertion. The rate is 5–15/1000 insertions.
- Failure, i.e. pregnancy.
- *Ectopic pregnancy:* 5% of pregnancies with IUCDs are ectopic, but as the failure rate is very low, overall there is protection as compared to no contraception used. Risk is more with progestasert.
- Fracture or breaking of IUCD and embedding in the endometrium resulting in decreased efficacy and difficulty in removal. Removal due to excessive bleeding and pain occurs in 5–15/100 users.
- Rarely fainting and collapse at the time of insertion, if patient is not properly motivated.

17. What advises are given to the patient after IUCD insertion?

Advice to the patient:
- Patient is taught to feel the thread by self-examination and should regularly check the thread and particularly after the first menstrual period
- She is informed about possible initial reactions: Increased bleeding, pain for first 2–3 months, etc. They are treated symptomatically. They gradually disappear with time
- She should come for follow-up after first menstrual period and then yearly
- She should consult the doctor immediately if she misses a period, if she develops any complications, or if she does not feel the thread
- The device should be replaced, when time limit is over
- She should not use intravaginal sanitary measures (menstrual tampons) for few menstrual periods.

18. How will you compare other methods with IUCDs?

Advantages of IUCDs over other measures:
- Simplicity in insertion
- No loss of time
- Return of fertility is immediate on removal of device
- Cheap (supplied free by Government)
- Does not interfere with sexual act
- No systemic side effects
- Less failure rate (except pills)
- Long-term—lasts for 10 years
- No effect on breastmilk, can be inserted immediately after child birth.

Disadvantages:
- *Side effects:* As mentioned in Question 16.
- Does not prevent HIV/STDs

- Patient cannot use on her own or stop on her own. Some medical help required for insertion and removal
- May come out without women's knowledge
- Male partner can feel the strings rarely.

19. What are the other uses of Cu-T?

Other uses of Cu-T are:
- After breaking of adhesions in a case of uterine synechia (Asherman syndrome) to prevent refusion of walls. Cu-T after removal of copper wire is used
- After Strassman operation—to prevent fusion of anterior and posterior walls.

20. How will you manage the patient who does not feel the thread?

Management of a patient who does not feel the thread:

Possibilities:
- Mistake of the patient
- Indrawing of threads inside the uterine cavity or cervix, or it is torn and expelled out
- Perforation of uterus and migration in the peritoneal cavity
- Spontaneous expulsion
    - Do per speculum examination, if the thread is seen, everything is all right and make the patient to palpate it
    - If thread is not seen, USG (TVS) is done, if the device is inside the uterus it is easily seen on USG. But if it has migrated in the peritoneal cavity it is not seen on USG. Take simple X-ray abdomen, if device is not seen anywhere in the X-ray, it is expelled out
    - But if it is seen in the X-ray, it is displaced device
    - IUCD whether it is intrauterine or extrauterine can also be checked by one of the following: (i) AP and lateral X-ray abdomen and pelvis with uterine sound in cavity. (ii) HSG.

Treatment: Any displaced IUCD requires removal either by laparoscopy or laparotomy. Medical devices cause adhesions and ring-shaped cause intestinal obstruction, loop is relatively inert but it also should be removed as patient may be disturbed psychologically.

If it is intrauterine, it can be removed by different instruments like simple curette, long artery forceps, uterine dressing forceps, Shirodkar hook or with the help of hysteroscope. It may be badly embedded.

21. How will you manage patient having pregnancy with Cu-T *in situ*?

Management of patient having pregnancy with Cu-T *in situ*: Advice should be given for termination of pregnancy with removal of Cu-T because of following risks: Increased risk of abortion, septic abortion, premature rupture of membranes, premature labor, IUGR, accidental hemorrhage, puerperal sepsis and ectopic pregnancy. But it does not produce any congenital malformation.

With all risks explained, if patient is keen to continue her pregnancy, at least Cu-T should be removed—if uterus is less than 12 weeks, if threads are seen and if device can be removed easily without disturbing the pregnancy. Otherwise leave it. Cu-T may be retrieved at the time of delivery.

22. Tell something about other IUCDs you know.

Other IUCDs:
- *Multiload-Cu 250 (or Multiload-Cu 375):* It is made of mixture of high density polypropylene and ethylene vinyl acetate copolymer impregnated with barium sulfate. Its shape is different from Cu-T, i.e. side arms of T are bent with small outer projections (serrated fins) which help to hold the device in place without stretching the uterine cavity. Copper wire with 250 sq mm (or 375 sq mm) surface area is wrapped around vertical arm. Both are 36 mm long and 21 mm wide, but multiload-Cu 375 has copper-wire of 0.4 mm diameter. Effective life recommended for Cu-250 is 3 years while that of Cu-375 is 5 years. Its inserter has no plunger and it is introduced by withdrawal technique. It has 2 nylon threads at its lower end, perforation and expulsion is less with multiload as compared to Cu-T.
- *Cu-7 (Gravigard):* It is "7" shaped device made of polypropylene impregnated with barium sulfate. Copper wire is wrapped around vertical arm. Surface area of copper wire is 200 sq mm. It is 36 mm long and 26 mm wide. It has only one (instead of usual two) polypropylene thread, blue in color. Its proven lifespan is 3 years. It is inserted by withdrawal technique.
- *Cu-T 220:* It is T-shaped device with 7 solid copper sleeves, 2 on transverse arm and 5 on vertical stem. Total exposed surface area of copper is 220 sq mm. It is developed by Population Council and its effective life is estimated to be 15–20 years. It has 2 threads and it is introduced by withdrawal technique.
- *Nova-Cu-T 200 and 200 Ag:* It is T-shaped device made of polyethylene with barium sulfate impregnated. The fine copper wire is wrapped around the vertical stem. The surface area of copper is 200 sq mm. In 200 Ag variety, a silver core has been added to the copper wire to reduce its fragmentation. It has 2 white threads and it is inserted by withdrawal technique. As compared to other copper devices, it is slightly short (32 mm long instead of 36 mm).
- *Zicoid:* It is T-shaped deviced with flexible and resilient side arms with small projection on the inside of the side arms. This prevents irritation of the cervical canal during insertion. Its surface area is 350 sq mm and copper wire is placed in the upper part of the stem. Diameter of wire is 0.5 mm. Plunger with special stop at proximal end ensures high fundal placement of the device. Failure rate is 0.2/HWY. It is effective for 5 years.
- *Flexigard:* It is a frameless device which has a nylon 2 suture with which it is anchored to the uterine musculature. There are 6 copper sleeves on the nylon thread. Total surface area of copper is 390 mm^2. Device is flexible because the sleeves are not connected to each other. It is effective for 5 years.

23. What do you know about progesterone containing IUCDs?

Progesterone containing devices:
- "Progestasert" is a T-shaped device, made up of ethylene vinyl acetate copolymer. Barium sulfate impregnated. It has two monofilament threads, black in color. It has its special inserter without a plunger and introduced by modified withdrawal technique. It contains 38 mg progesterone in vertical arm, dispensed in silicon oil and daily releases 65 μg progesterone. Progesterone has added contraceptive effect. It causes decidual changes in the endometrium and glandular atrophy which interfere with normal reproductive process. It is useful where use of another device has caused excessive bleeding or cramping which may be relieved by progestasert, but spotting is increased. Incidence of ectopic pregnancy is increased with it. Unlike Cu-T, it is to be replaced every year.
- *LNG 20:* (Mirena, LNG—intrauterine system) T-shaped device with flexible arms. The shape is that of Nova-T but it has capsule on the stem. The core of the capsule contains a mixture of silicone rubber and 60 mg levonorgestrel, which is released at 20 μg/day. It is 32 mm long and 32 mm wide. Its inserter is withdrawal type and it is effective for 5 (possibly 8) years. Apart from contraception, it helps in treatment of DUB and fibroids.

24. Which are the different types of steroidal contraceptives?

The different types of steroidal contraceptive types:
- Oral—commonly known as pills
- Injectable—intramuscular
- Newer sustained release systems.

Oral pills are of different types:
- Combined
- Phasic
- Minipill
- Newer pills.

(Sequential pill has been withdrawn from the market because of high incidence of endometrial carcinoma and thromboembolic complications).

25. What do you know about combined oral pills?

Combined oral pill:
- They are combination of estrogen and progesterone-21 such tablets. Ethinyl estradiol is the estrogen commonly used
- Supplied in a pack of 28 tablets, where last 7 tablets are placebo containing iron and vitamins, to complete the menstrual cycle
- Newer pack is started immediately after first pack is over, irrespective of onset or stoppage of menstruation
- In a Family Planning Program, it is supplied free of charge by Government: Mala-N
- Commonly used market preparations are ovral, ovral-L, duoluton L, novelon, etc.
- Preparation estrogen progestogens
- Mala D EE 30 μg, norgestrel 0.3 mg
- Mala-N EE 30 μg, norethisterone 1.0 mg
- Ovral EE 50 μg, levonorgestrel 0.25 mg
- Ovral L EE 30 μg, levonorgestrel 0.15 mg
- Duoluton-L EE 50 μg, levonorgestrel 0.25 mg
- Novelon EE 30 μg, desogestrel 0.15 mg
- Femilon EE 20 μg, desogestrel 0.15 mg.

26. What do you know about phasic pills and minipill?

Phasic Pills

Biphasic or triphasic:
- Biphasic-All 21 tablets contain E + P but dose of progesterone is doubled after first 10 days, dose of estrogen remaining constant (ethinyl estradiol 35 μg. Norethindrone 50 μg and 100 μg). It has slightly high failure rate and not popular in India.
- Triphasic—All 21 tablets contain E + P but dose varies in 3 phases, e.g.
  - *Triquilar:*

Ethinylestradiol	Levonorgestrel	Days
30 μg to	50 μg	1-6
40 μg to	75 μg	7-11
30 μg to	125 μg	12-21

    Triquilar is started from the 5th day of cycle while second pack is started after 7 days of pack free interval.
  - "Cyclessa" contains ethinyl estradiol 25 μg and triphasic desogestrel and "tricyclen" contains EE 25 μg and triphasic norgestimate. They are not yet available in India.

Minipill
- Contains only progesterone, i.e. Norgestrel 75 μg or Norethisterone 350 μg or Levonorgestrel 30 μg

- Estrogen-free pill now available in India is Cerazette containing 75 μg desogestrel
- To be taken daily one throughout the cycle for 28 days.
- It inhibits ovulation and also acts locally by making endometrium unreceptable for implantation and renders cervical mucus hostile to sperms
- Failure rate is comparable to combined OC pills
- It avoids undesirable side effects of estrogen found with combined pills and sickle cell patients or lactating mothers can take it.

Contraception:
- Menstrual irregularities and amenorrhea are common with its use
- Side effects contributed to progesterone content can occur, i.e. alopecia, loss of libido, weight gain, nervous irritability. Androgenic side effects are less with cerazette.

27. Which are newer pills now available?

Newer pills
- *Femilon:* It contains only 20 μg ethinyl estradiol (as compared 30 μg in Novelon) and 150 μg Desogestrel. Due to lowest dose of estrogen, estrogen-related side effects like nausea, breast tenderness and headache are very low. Desogestrel, a newer progestogen which has minimal androgenic side effects: Reduces the risk of cardiovascular disease and cures acne and hirsutism.
- *Postcoital pill:* Discussed in details under emergency contraception.
- *Pill with antiandrogenic effects:* "Diane 35" contains ethinyl estradiol 35 microgm + cyproterone acetate 2 mg and "Yasmin" contains EE + Drospirenone (aldosterone derivative). Due to antiandrogenic effects, they are useful in patients with acne and hirsutism. Yasmin due to its antimineralocorticoid activity, also decreases BP and weight in the users.
- *Once a month pill:* Each pill contains 3 mg of Quinestrol (long-acting estrogen) and 12 mg megesterol acetate (progesterone). It is not available in India.
- *Pills with extended cycle length:* Seasonale is monophasic pills (EE + LN) for 84 days with one week off.
- *Nonestrogen combined pill:* Containing RU-486 (mifepristone) in first half of the cycle and progesterone (MPA) in second half of the cycle is under study.

28. What is the mechanism of action of pills?

Mechanism of action: Pills containing estrogen and progesterone work in following ways:
- Their main action is inhibition of ovulation. They act at hypothalamic level inhibiting release of gonadotropin releasing hormone (GnRh). Secretion of FSH and LH from pituitary are thus suppressed, so there is no follicular growth. As there is no LH surge, ovulation is suppressed. It is also suggested that they directly

inhibit pituitary as there is no response to exogenous GnRh administration in pill users.
- They alter the maturation of endometrium making it unsuitable for implantation. Under the effect of progesterone, there is stromal edema with glandular exhaustion and atrophy.
- Progesterone makes cervical mucus thick, viscid, scanty and impermeable to sperms.
- Effect on tubal motility by progesterone is also suggested.

29. What are the contraindications to pills?

Contraindications:

Absolute:
- Thromboembolic disease
- Acute or chronic disease of liver
- Cancer of breast or genitals
- Pregnancy known or suspected
- Focal migraine.

Relative:
- Hypertension
- Valvular heart disease
- Epilepsy
- Smokers over 35 years
- Nursing mothers
- Sickle-cell anemia, thalassemia
- Asthma
- Allergic disorders
- Herpes gestation alies
- Porphyria
- Pruritus of pregnancy
- Varicose veins
- Obesity
- Elective surgery
- Diabetes
- Crohn's disease.

30. Which are other uses of pills?

Other uses of pills:
- Regularization of cycles
- DUB
- Endometriosis
- Postponement of menstrual period
- Amenorrhea to test for withdrawal bleeding
- Primary dysmenorrhea
- Suppression of functional ovarian cysts.

31. What are the side effects and complications of pills?

Side effects and complications:
- *Nausea and vomiting:* It is very common side effect. It appears to be related to the estrogen content of the pill. It is managed by: (i) reassurance that it subsides as therapy continues (ii) taking the pill after food or with cup of milk (iii) taking the pill at bedtime so that the individual is sleeping during peak concentrations of drug in the blood (iv) changing over to another compound and (v) reducing the estrogen content of the pill.
- *Breakthrough bleeding:* It occurs in almost half of all patients at some time. It may be due to failure to take the pill at the same time each day. It is more common with low dose pill. However, with newer pills, cycle control is good. It diminishes after first 3–4 pill cycles.
  Management: Double up of pills in an attempt to stop the bleeding and discontinuing the pills to restart them on the fifth day of bleeding are now considered ill-advisable. Following measures should be taken:
  - Switching to another low dose compound
  - Increase in the estrogen dose of the pill temporarily or taking short course of additional estrogen temporarily
  - A search for pathological cause of bleeding must be made.
- *Absence of withdrawal bleeding (Pill amenorrhea):* As high as up to 22% of women experience it at some time.
  Management: After ruling out the pregnancy, either of the following options is given to the patient:
  - Reassuring the patient of the benign nature of the amenorrhea and the likelihood of regular menstruation when the pills are discontinued and second pack is started from the seventh day of last pill
  - If withdrawal bleeding is desired, switching to a pill with higher estrogen activity or adding tablet of estrogen, i.e. EE 0.02 mg last 7 days for few cycles is advised. Amenorrhea and oligomenorrhea are less common with triphasic pills.
- *Hypertension:* It is 3 times more common in pill users. Both systolic and diastolic BP rises. It is minimal with triphasic pills.
- *Cardiovascular diseases:*
  - *Venous thromboembolism:* Deep vein thrombosis is 5–6 times more common in users, while superficial vein thrombosis is 2–3 times more common in users. It is due to estrogen and it is dose-dependent.
  - *Myocardial infarction:* It is 2–3 times more common in pill users. It is due to both estrogen as well as progesterone. The incidence is now decreasing with greater care in selecting the patients and due to low dose pills.
  - *Cerebrovascular stroke:* Cerebral thrombosis is more common than cerebral hemorrhage. It is not dose-dependent so it is not decreased with low dose pills.

- *Weight gain, fluid retention:* 5–50% of women gain weight. Both estrogen and progesterone are responsible and tendency is more in first 6 months of use. Weight gain is negligible with low dose pills.
- *Breasts:* Pain, tenderness, engorgement are common side effects.
- *Carbohydrate metabolism:* Glucose tolerance is impaired in pill user, latent diabetes may become symptomatic. This is less with low dose pill.
- *Liver and gallbladder:* Altered liver functions noted in pill users. Cholecystic jaundice can also occur. Gallstones and infection of gallbladder are found in young women on pills.
- *Post-pill amenorrhea:* It is found in 3–5/1000 users. It is not related to duration of use and it is common in women having oligomenorrhea before starting the pill.
- *Neoplasia:*
  - *Cervix:* There is higher incidence of dysplasia and carcinoma in situ cervix reported in pill users. Little increase in the risk of cervical cancer is reported in women who use OCs for >5 years.
  - *Breast:* Risk of breast cancer is not convincingly proved. It is very slightly increased only in young women, nulliparous patient, after prolonged use and with positive family history.
  - *Liver:* For hepatic adenoma (benign), there is unequivocal evidence. The risk is rare (3–4/lacs) but condition may be fatal due to severe, intraperitoneal hemorrhage. With long-term use (8 years or more), there is a risk of hepatocellular carcinoma.
  - *Malignant melanoma:* Controversial.
- *Teratogenicity:* If pregnancy occurs during the course of pill or immediately after stopping the pill, there is a very small but definite risk to the fetus.
- *Miscellaneous:* These include melasma, headache, giddiness, leukorrhea, acne, change in libido, mental depression, alopecia, leg cramps and some ophthalmic complications like retinal vascular disease, corneal edema or diseases of eyelids and conjunctiva.

32. Which drugs cause drug interaction with OC pills?

They are Rifampicin, Penicillin, Tetracycline, Ampicillin, Barbiturates, Phenytoin, Sulfonamides.

33. How will you manage forgotten pill?

It patient forgets to take one tablet white (hormonal), she should take it as soon as she remembers and 2nd pill is taken as usual. If she misses for consecutive two days then for 7 days, she should avoid sex or use condoms. If 7 or more white tablets are left in the pack, she should take all the rest of the pills as usual. But, if <7 tablets are left in that pack, take rest of the white pills as usual. Do not take brown tablets and start a new pack after the last white tablet of previous pack. She may miss a period. This is okay. Missing of 1 or more brown pills is of no importance, take the rest of the pills as usual, one each day.

34. What are the beneficial side effects of pills?

Beneficial side effects:
- *Menstrual comforts:* Regularization of cycle, blood loss is controlled (cure of anemia), relief from primary dysmenorrhea and premenstrual tension.
- *Prevents pelvic inflammatory diseases:* Cervical mucus is thickened, menstrual blood loss is reduced, uterine contractions are inhibited (so spread of infection to tubes prevented). Prevents pregnancy and abortion which provide opportunity for infection.
- *Prevents ectopic:* As it is highly effective contraception method and also as it prevents PID (except mini pill).
- *Lowers risk of endometrial cancer:* Because of progesterone component. Upto 50% reduction in risk of endometrial cancer and protection persists up to 20 years after discontinuation.
- *Lowers risk of ovarian cancer:* Because of suppression of pituitary secretion of gonadotropins and ovulation. There is 40–80% overall decrease in risk of ovarian cancer among users. Protection lasts for 15 to 20 years after discontinuation.
- *Protection against benign breast diseases:* Thirty to fifty percent decrease in the incidence in current and recent long-term users.
- Protection against functional ovarian cysts, i.e. follicular cysts, granulose lutein and thecalutein cysts due to suppression of ovulation (except multiphasic preparation), 50 to 80% reduction.
- Some studies have shown reduced risk of uterine fibroids, colorectal cancer, rheumatoid arthritis and benign thyroid conditions. However, this is not unequivocally proved.
- Improvement in bone mineral density also occurs.

35. What do you know about nonsteroidal oral contraceptive pill?

Centchroman (centron, Saheli) is nonsteroidal oral contraceptive pill. It exhibits weak estrogenic and potent antiestrogenic (5 times) activity. It is started in a dose of 30 mg (1 tablet) on the first day of menstruation, given twice a week for the first 3 months and then once weekly. It is safe and reliable and with correct use its failure rate (1.6 HWY) is comparable to OC pills. It has no effect on HPO axis, so it does not inhibit ovulation. The contraceptive mechanism is local either by defective implantation of blastocyst due to abnormal decidualization or blastocyst abnormality itself. Added effects are antiestrogenic effects on altered tubal motility and poor cervical mucus sperm penetration. Return of fertility is reported within 6 months of discontinuation. As it is nonsteroidal, all the major side effects of steroidal contraceptives are avoided. Menstrual disturbances like coligomenorrhea and amenorrhea are found in >1/3rd users. Because of these side effects it could not gain much acceptance. It has been successfully used in treatment of DUB. Clinical trials are on for its use in treatment of breast cancer and for HRT.

36. Which are the injectable steroidal contraceptives available?

Injectable contraception are as follows:

- *Long-acting progestins:*
  - Depot-medroxy progesterone acetate (DMPA)—150 mg every 3 months (Depo-provera).
  - Norethisterone enanthate (NET-EN)—200 mg every 2 months (Noristerate).
- *Combined injectables (estrogen + progesterone):*
  - DMPA 25 mg—estradiol cypionate 5 mg (Lunelle, Cyclofen)—monthly.
  - NET-EN 50 mg + estradiol valerate 5 mg (Mesigyna)—monthly.
  - Dihydroxy progesterone acetophenide 150 mg + estradiol enanthate 10 mg (Deladroxate)—monthly.

37. What is DMPA? What are the advantages and disadvantages of DMPA?

DMPA

- It is highly effective, long acting, safe, reversible injectable contraceptive.
- It is given as 150 mg IM every 3 months with a grace period of 2 weeks late or early.
- It should be given deep IM in gluteus or deltoid muscle with all aseptic precautions. Injection into the fat (decreases absorption) or rubbing the injection site (increases absorption), changes the efficacy.
- *Time:* It is given within 7 days of menstrual cycle. It can also be given immediately after abortion and MTP. In postpartum patient also it can be given immediately within 7 days, however in breastfeeding patient one can wait for 6 weeks postpartum.
- Failure rate is very low and it is <1/100 women years.
- Mechanism of action is same as that of OC pills and it also hinders the rate of ovum transport.
- Return of fertility after DMPA is about 9 months after the last injection (i.e. 5.5 months after the effect of last injection is over). There is no long-term impairment of fertility.

Advantages:

- Very effective
- Long-term—3 monthly injections
- Does not interfere with sex
- Reduces the incidence of PID and conidial vulvovaginitis
- Flexibility in return visit due to 2 weeks grace period
- It can be used at any age
- No estrogen-related side effects
- Makes sickle cells crisis less frequent and less painful
- Decreases seizure frequency in epileptics
- It can be used in nursing mothers. It increases milk production
- It helps in preventing endometrial cancer and uterine fibroids.

Disadvantages:

- Delayed return of fertility—7-9 months after last injection
- Menstrual irregularity and ammenorrhea occurs in 10 to 15% of women
- Weight gain of 1-2 kg each year may occur
- Decrease in HDL and increase in LDH cholesterol is reported so women with severe vascular disease should not use it.
- May cause headache, breast tenderness, mood swings, nausea, hair loss, less sex drive.

38. What is norplant?

Norplant:

- The norplant contraceptive is a long-acting, low-dose, progestin only contraceptive system for women. The drug is delivered by means of 6 silastic capsules implanted subdermally in the woman's arm employing a minor surgical technique. It is highly effective and highly reversible.
- Previously available in 6 capsules (36 mg each), norplant-2 rod system comprises 2 silastic rods containing a total of 140 mg of levonorgestrel (70 mg/rod). The rods are implanted subdermally in the women's arm employing a minor surgical technique.
- *Time:* Within 7 days after the onset of menstruation or immediately after abortion or first trimester MTP. The implants become effective within 24 hours of placement.
- Mechanism of action is mainly local on cervical mucus and endometrium but it also inhibits ovulation in about 50% of the cycles.
- *Failure rate:* Less than 0.5 per hundred women years.
- *Contraindications:* Anticoagulant therapy, undiagnosed abnormal uterine bleeding, known or suspected pregnancy, hemorrhagic diathesis, liver diseases.
- *Side effects:* Bleeding disorders, amenorrhea, nausea, loss of appetite, dizziness, headache, changes in libido, depression, acne, infection at implant site.
- *Removal:* Implants work up to 5 years, after that they should be removed employing a minor surgical technique.

39. What is implanon?

Implanon is a newer implant which consists of an ethinyl vinyl acetate copolymer device (single rod—4 cm long, 2 mm in diameter) containing 68 mg of progestogen 3-ketogestral also known as etonogestrel. It releases 30–40 μg of drug/day. It is effective for 3 years. Other single rod devices are Nestorone for 2 years and Uriplant (nomegestrol acetate) for 1 year and ST-1435.

40. What do you mean by biodegradable devices?

Biodegradable devices: They deliver progesterone from a carrier that gradually dissolves and disappears. Compared with norplant, they are easier to insert and need not be removed. Two are under trial—Capronor (40 mm rod) containing levonorgestrel (effective for 1.5 years) and norethindrone pellets (1 year).

41. What do you mean by emergency contraception?

Emergency contraception means a particular type of contraception that is used as an emergency procedure to prevent pregnancy following an unprotected but possibly fertile intercourse.

Indications for emergency contraception include unprotected intercourse, failure of barrier method, unsuccessful withdrawal (coitus interruptus), missed oral contraceptive pills and sexual assault.

42. Which are the different methods of emergency contraception?

Methods

- *Yuzpe method:* It was introduced by a Canadian physician Albert Yuzpe in early 1970s. Combined oral contraceptive pills containing ethinyl estradiol 50 μg and norgestrel 500 μg (or levonorgestrel 250 μg) are taken
- Pills as early as possible and 2 after 12 hours of first dose. The treatment is most effective if first dose is taken within 12–24 hours of intercourse but it can be taken up to 72 hours. OC pills containing lower dose of estrogen (30 μg) should be taken as 2 doses of 4 pills 12 hours apart. Failure rate ranges from 0.2 to 2%.
- *Progesterone only pill:* Levonorgestrel 0.75 mg 2 doses 12 hours apart. First dose should be started as early as possible but within 72 hours. It is available as Ecee 2, Pill 72, preventol Norlevo, etc.
  It is useful when estrogen is contraindicated.
- *IUCD:* Insertion of copper IUCD within 5 days intercourse (later than hormonal method). It can be kept inserted if couple wants to continue with it as method of temporary contraception.
- *Antiprogesterone:* Mifepristone (RU-486) 600 mg oral single dose within 72 hours after unprotected intercourse. Doses as low as 50 and even 10 mg are found effective. Failure rate reported for different hormonal methods are <2% while for IUCD.

43. Tell something about silastic vaginal ring and contraceptive patch.

Silastic vaginal rings: These have advantage over previous methods that women can insert and remove themselves and they are immediately reversible. Progesterone is slowly released from the ring and can be absorbed through the vaginal epithelium. Most rings are between 50 and 60 mm in outer diameter and 7.5–9.5 mm thick. They are pliable and similar to the inert pessaries used for prolapse. The ring containing levonorgestrel 5 mg releases 20 μg per day and can be left in place for 3 months. The ring containing estro + prog (Nuva ring) have also been found useful. Like OCs, they are worn for 21 days and then again inserted after 7 days ring-free period. Failure rate is less (1.8/HWY) but breakthrough bleeding is a problem.

Contraceptive patch: Combined estrogen + progesterone patch is under trial. It delivers in the blood stream 20 μg of ethinyl estradiol and 150 μg norelgestromin. New patch is worn every week. After wearing for consecutive 3 weeks, 4th week is patch free. It may be applied-abdomen, buttocks, thigh or upper outer arm. Failure rate is less than 1/HWY.

44. What are the prerequisites for locational amenorrhea methods?

No return of menses, child less than 6 months of duration and exclusive breastfeeding.

45. What are newer pills?

Newer pills are combined oral contraceptive pills to suit the needs and lifestyle of different women. This has been possible by reduction of estrogen dose, use of newer progestins or by change in cycle duration, e.g.
EE + drosperinone
EE + cyproterone acetate
Extended cycle combined regimen.

46. What are the benefits of extended use regimen?

Women have vaginal bleeding only 4 times a year or not at all. Reduces PMS, mood swings, heavy painful menses.

47. What is essure?

Essure is a device which is delivered into the Fallopian tube under direct visualization with hysteroscopy. After insertion, it stimulates inflammatory response characterized by macrophages, fibroblasts, foreign body giant cells and plasma cells. This reaction requires 3 months' time for occlusion of tube. For these months, use of alternative method for contraception is must. At the end of 3 months, HSG is performed to confirm the occlusion of tubes.

48. Which contraceptive is used in seropositive women?

IUDs are efficacious and do not increase risks to women with HIV and their partners. Hormonal contraceptives probably do not increase disease progression or risk of transmission. Caution should be used in prescribing COCs to women on antiretroviral medications, which increase or decrease contraceptive steroid or antiretroviral area under the curve. Barrier contraceptives are the choice.

49. Contraception in obese woman?

Although obesity decreases the efficacy of COCs, they are still likely to be more effective than barrier methods alone. Counsel women regarding moderate decrease in efficacy and the increased absolute risk of venous thromboembolism in small group of patients. The LNG-IUS may provide protection against pregnancy and obesity associated endometrial hyperplasia.

MUST REMEMBER

- Who can use COC pills—from adolescent age to women over 40 if no contraindication.
- Contraindication to COC pills—Migraine, diabetes with vasculopathy, severe hypertension, IHD, cholestasis, abnormal liver function, major surgery requiring immobilization, smokers >35 years of age.
- Indications of minipills—Lactating mothers, history of hypetension, thrombosis, indications of injectable progesterone, lactating mothers, endometrosis.
- Mechnism of action of LNG-IUS—Endometrial atrophy, changes in cervical mucus and may inhibit ovulation.
- Clinical uses of LNG-IUS—Contraception, DUB, endometriosis, endometrial hyperplasia, anovulation.

Ultrasonography in Obstetrics

Kanan Yelikar, Jayprakash Shah

1. What are the indications of USG in obstetrics?

There are 'n' number of indications. USG has become an integral part of examination and plays vital, diagnostic role in obstetrics.

Recommended scan during pregnancy:
- 11-14 weeks scan—genetic scan (NT+NB scan)
- 18-20 weeks scan—anomaly scan (Ideal is 22-24 weeks, but in India due to termination limit up to 20 weeks this is recommended)
- 32-34 weeks scan—growth scan.

First trimester (AIUM Guidelines—effective since 2003):
- Confirm the presence of an intrauterine pregnancy
- Evaluate a suspected ectopic pregnancy
- Define the cause of vaginal bleeding
- Evaluate pelvic pain
- Estimate gestational (menstrual) age
- Diagnose or evaluate multiple gestations
- Confirm cardiac activity
- As an adjunct to chorionic villus sampling, embryo transfer, and localization and removal of an intrauterine device (IUD)
- To evaluate maternal pelvic masses and/or uterine abnormalities
- To evaluate suspected hydatidiform mole.

2. What do you mean by viable pregnancy on USG?

Viability in ultrasonic language means:
- Presence of cardiac activity
- Normal embryo with normal anatomy
- Presence of normal yolk sac/fetal pole
- Normal amniotic cavity with CRL > Mean amniotic diameter
- Homogeneous trophoblast.

3. What are the normal findings in first trimester USG?

Following structures to be identified:
- Number of gestational (G) sac
  - Single—monochorionic pregnancy
  - Two—dichorionic pregnancy
- Position of G sac—fundal, mid, low in uterus, corneal. Ectopic position is different than normal intrauterine position
- Number of embryos
- Number of yolk sac
  - Two yolk sac in one G sac—MCDA twin
  - Two yolk sac in two G sac—DCDA twin.
- Trophoblast—homogeneous, heterogeneous (suggest poor trophoblast)
- Amniotic cavity—normally CRL > mean amniotic diameter
  - When flushed amnion—CRL < mean amniotic diameter—marker for chromosomal abnormality
- Uterus—mass lesion and malformation
- Ovaries—mass lesion and malformations.

4. What are the abnormal ultrasonic findings in first trimester?

- *Blighted ovum:* It is empty gestational sac, i.e. gestational sac without embryo. It is also called embryonic pregnancy.
- *Missed abortion:* EP with embryo without cardiac activity.
- *Threatened abortion:* EP with embryo with cardiac activity and bleeding P/V.
- *Inevitable abortion:* Embryo with cardiac activity <90 beats/minute—absolute bradycardia.
- *Ectopic gestation:* Pregnancy at other site than normal habitate (uterus).
- *Molar pregnancy:* Molar changes in placenta. May be complete or partial (with embryo with/without cardiac activity).
- *Heterotopic pregnancy* = intrauterine pregnancy + ectopic pregnancy.

5. Which fetal anomaly can be diagnosed in first trimester? (Not all can be diagnosed with 100% accuracy. They can be diagnosed and stamped at 12-14 weeks in confirmed cases).

- Chorionicity and amnionicity with 100% accuracy at 8-9 weeks (Not abnormal finding but has poor outcome based on chorionicity)
- Anencephaly
- Holoprosencephaly
- PUV

- Diaphragmatic hernia
- Pentalogy of Cantrell
- Ectopia cordis
- Conjoined twin
- Encephalocele
- Dandy-Walker
- Complex cardiac malformations (Suspected)
- Skeletal abnormality with limb involvement.

6. Which route of sonography is preferred in first trimester?

Transvaginal sonography is the preferred route. It is high frequency probe so gives better resolution and practically gives 1 week early detection of the findings.

7. How do you decide gestational age?

- CRL is best parameter during early pregnancy
- Criteria for ideal CRL
- Neutral mid-sagittal position with spine away from transducer or towards it
- Maximum length to be measured
- G sac—mean sac diameter is useful before 8–9 weeks
- BPD, AC and FL can be used as added parameter at 11–14 weeks scan.

8. How do you diagnose ectopic pregnancy?

Positive pregnancy test with:
- *Uterine findings:*
  - Empty uterus
  - Decidual reaction (echogenic endometrium)
  - Uterus with pseudosac (in midline in endometrium)
  - Intrauterine pregnancy (heterotopic ectopic pregnancy)
- *Adnexal findings:*
  - Normal adnexa
  - Adnexal mass
  - G sac in adnexal mass with yolk sac
  - G sac in adnexal mass with yolk sac with live embryo
- *Cul de sac findings:*
  - Normal POD
  - Free fluid in POD.

9. What are indications for ultrasonography in second trimester (AIUM Guidelines)?

- Estimation of gestational age
- Evaluation of fetal growth
- Vaginal bleeding
- Abdominal/pelvic pain
- Incompetent cervix
- Determination of fetal presentation
- Suspected multiple gestation
- Adjunct to amniocentesis
- Significant discrepancy between uterine size and clinical dates
- Pelvic mass
- Suspected hydatidiform mole
- Adjunct to cervical cerclage placement
- Suspected ectopic pregnancy
- Suspected fetal death. Suspected uterine abnormality
- Evaluation of fetal well-being
- Suspected amniotic fluid abnormalities
- Suspected placental abruption
- Adjunct to external cephalic version
- Premature rupture of membranes and/or premature labor
- Abnormal biochemical markers
- Follow-up evaluation of a fetal anomaly
- Follow-up evaluation of placental location for suspected placenta previa
- History of previous congenital anomaly
- Evaluation of fetal condition in late registrants for prenatal care.

Recommended Suggestion for Mid Trimester Anatomical Survey (ISUOG)

Head:
- Intact cranium
- Cavum septi pellucidi (CSP)
- Midline falx
- Thalami
- Cerebral ventricles
- Cerebellum
- Cisterna magna.

Face:
- Both orbits present
- Median facial profile
- Mouth present
- Upper lip intact.

Neck:
Absence of masses (e.g. cystic hygroma, thyroid and other neck tumors).

Chest/heart:
- Normal appearing shape/size of chest and lungs
- Heart activity present
- Four-chamber view of heart in normal position
- Aortic and pulmonary outflow tracts
- No evidence of diaphragmatic hernia.

Abdomen:
- Stomach in normal position
- Bowel not dilated
- Both kidneys present
- Cord insertion site.

Skeletal:
No spinal defects or masses (transverse and sagittal views).

Extremities (all 12 long bones to be visualized)
- Arms and hands present, normal relationships
- Legs and feet present, normal relationships.

Environment:
- Placenta
  - Position
  - No masses present
  - Accessory lobe
- Umbilical cord—three-vessel cord
- Amniotic fluid.

10. What are common anomalies?

- Most commonly detected anomaly are of neural tube.
- But most common anomaly are of heart—1% of live birth
  - Head—anencephaly, hydrocephus (aqueduct stenosis, ACC, Dandy Walker, schizencephaly, porencephaly, lissencephaly), encephalocele
  - Congenital heart disease VSD, truncal anomaly (TOF, DORV, truncus arteriosus, transposition of great vessel), hypoplastic heart, cardiac tumor
  - Renal anomalies—obstructive (hydronephrosis, hydroureter, PUV) parenchymal (multicystic kidneys, polycystic kidney) anomaly (absent kidney, horse shoe kidney) renal tumors
  - GIT esophageal atresia, duodenal atresia, intestinal obstruction, echogenic bowel (marker for chromosome abnormality)
  - Facial anomalies cleft lip/palate
  - Musculoskeletal anomalies—osteogenesis imperfecta, dwarfism.

11. What are the indication of USG in third trimester (growth scan)?

- *Growth:* BPD, FL, AC, HC. Growth charts are recommended for comment on type of growth.
- *Amniotic fluid:*
  - AFI <5 cm oligo, >25 cm polyhydramnios.
  - *Goldstein criteria:*
    - Visual impression less with largest pocket <2
    - Visual impression more with largest pocket >7.
    - Largest pocket <2 cm oligohydramnios
    - Largest pocket > 8 cm polyhydramnios.
- Placenta
  - *Location:* In relation to cervix
  - *Echogenicity:* Homogeneous
  - *Seperation:* Retroplacental—Accidental hemmorhage.

12. What are indications of Doppler in obstetrics?

- In IUGR to understand fetal hypoxia and acidemia and decide the time of delivery and fetal outcome
- At 22–24 weeks—uterine artery for screening for PIH and IUGR
- In fetal malformation like fetal echocardiography, vein of Galen's aneurysm, DV agenesis as a confirmative, and diagnostic tool
- In Rh isoimmunization—to decide the degree of anemia.

13. Which blood vessels are significantly studied?

- *Uterine artery:* Information of maternal side of placenta screening for PIH and IUGR.
- *Umbilical A:* Information of fetal side of placenta. Helps to understand development of fetal hypoxia.
- *Middle cerebral artery:* For understanding the degree of fetal hypoxia.
- *Ductus venosus:* For understanding degree of fetal acidemia and heart decompensation.

14. What are the parameters of biophysical profile (BPP)?

Biophysical profile (BPP) is now with availability of color Doppler and has limited application: It is also known as Manning score. It can analyse:

- Fetal breathing movement
- Fetal movements
- Fetal tone
- Fetal reactivity
- Amount of AF.

Score between 6 and 10 indicates a good fetal outcome.

Modified BPP:
- AFI largest pocket > 2 cm
- and NST.

MUST REMEMBER
- Ultrasonography in obstetrics has almost become mandatory investigation in each and every patient
- First trimester ultrasonography is done to diagnose early pregnancy, to know the location whether intrauterine or extrauterine. If intrauterine to know number of gestational sacs, i.e. single or multiple, to know the viability of fetus by looking at cardiac activity, to know the gestational age.
- Second trimester ultrasonography is mainly dedicated for anomaly scan, cervical length especially before encircalage operation.
- Third trimester ultrasonography is required to confirm the gestational age, for placental localization, to diagnose fetal growth restriction, to measure amniotic fluid index, and to perform biophysical profile (BPP) for fetal well-being.

Intrauterine Growth Retardation

Pankaj Desai, Kanan Yelikar

CASE STUDY

Mrs A, 28 years, middle socioeconomic status, history of pregnancy 34 weeks, G2P1A0, first full-term vaginal delivery, was admitted with complaints of swelling over limbs, transient headache and complication of breathlessness. On examination, pulse—84/min, 140/90 BP, pallor present, pedal edema ++, facial puffiness +, CVS and respiratory system examinations, normal, maternal weight gain 10 kg in last month.

On obstetric examination, per abdomen 28 weeks, liquor adequate for the gestational age, cephalic presentation, fetal heart sounds 142/min regular, abdominal wall edema + EBW 1.2–1.4 kg.

Investigations

- Hb—8 g%
- T and D—10,500/mm^3, VDRL—nonreactive
- HIV—nonreactive, RBS—70 mg%
- Urine—R/M—protein traces, no pus cells/no RBC
- Fundus—WNL
- Serum creatinine—0.7 mg%
- BUN—18 mg%
- Serum proteins (total)—5.8 g%.

1. What is your provisional diagnosis in this case?

34 weeks pregnancy with IUGR with mild degree of anemia with pregnancy-induced hypertension.

2. What are the different types of growth restriction?

Asymmetrical, symmetrical, unclassified, and idiopathic.

3. How do you differentiate small-for-date an IUGR?

By history, clinical examination, and biometry.

4. How far your gestational dating is correct on history taking?

Patient is educated, aware of her cycles, her previous cycles have been regular 3/30 days and so, her dates can be said to be "excellent."

5. What are the substrates for normal fetal growth?

Most important being oxygen, glucose, and amino acids.

6. Which of the two types of IUGR, you think are prognostically bad?

Symmetrical variety, as it reflects some congenital defect or intrauterine infection or chromosomal problem.

7. What maternal condition in your case, can be correlated as cause for IUGR?

Anemia and mild PIH as the cause of IUGR.

8. What are other common causes of IUGR?

Pre-eclampsia chronic hypertension, diabetes, cardiac disease, placental causes like abnormal placentation, chronic villitis, placenta previa, and placenta infarcts. Fetal causes like chromosomal abnormalities, infections, and multifetal pregnancies.

9. What other investigations you will like to do, for confirming the diagnosis?

Sonography to do gestational dating (fetal/biometry).

10. What parameters on sonography are taken under consideration for gestational dating?

Biparietal diameter, femur length, abdominal circumference, head circumference, HC/AC and estimated fetal weight.

11. How will you manage this case?

As patient is diagnosed as a case of IUGR (history and examination), we will admit her for rest and further investigations. Improve her nutrition and control her blood pressure. After optimum maturity of fetus, deliver her.

12. How will you assess her while admitted in hospital?

By clinical examination, gravidogram, maternal weight gain, AFI, fetal heart sound record by serial USG, Doppler, CTG, etc.

13. What is the importance of weight gain?

Decreased maternal weight gain during pregnancy is a relatively insensitive sign of inadequate fetal growth. A gain of 12 kg is ideal during pregnancy and if weight gain is suboptimal, fetal growth can be hampered.

14. What other treatment to you suggest for management of IUGR?

Rest in left lateral position, oral and IV hydration, amino acid supplementation and aspirin. However, none of these have been proved to be conclusively helpful.

15. What is the incidence of IUGR in developing country like India?

40–45%.

16. What is Ponderal index?

- PI = Fetal weight/L3. It is an index for measurement of fetal malnutrition
- Normal value is 8.325 + 2.5 (2 SD). If PI <7, it is indicating IUGR.

17. Is any other radiological investigation helpful in diagnosis of IUGR?

Color Doppler study, to know the resistance and pulsatility index.

18. What is trisomy 21?

It is also known as Down syndrome, and a cause of IUGR, it is a chromosomal abnormality (8–12% of growth retarded infants are due to chromosomal abnormality).

19. What does the pneumonic "TORCH" stands for?

Toxoplasma, rubella cytomegalovirus and herpes simplex. Intrauterine infection caused by these organisms can cause IUGR.

20. In which conditions, you will like to deliver the patient before term?

Anhydramnios (no pockets of fluid that are clear of cord loops at 30 weeks), gestation or beyond. Repetitive fetal heart rate decelerations. Lack of growth over 3 weeks period and mature lung studies. Abnormal umbilical Doppler velocity (UAD).

21. On what parameters, your decision to delivery such a patient depends?

- Gestational age
- Underlying etiology
- Probability of intact extrauterine survival
- Level of expertize
- Available technology
- NICU—neonatologist availability.

22. When would you deliver her?

As she is admitted, we will like to wait for pulmonary maturity to be achieved, which can be indirectly judged by fetal biometry, lecithin sphingomyelin ratio. If liquor volume is adequate, management can be continued till optimum fetal growth is achieved.

23. As she has a previous normal delivery, no adverse factor can we try for a vaginal delivery?

It depends on whether the fetus is acidotic or otherwise. If on basis of color Doppler the fetus is acidotic then vaginal trial should not be given. If not, with continuous intrapartum fetal monitoring and preparation of immediate intervention, a vaginal trial can be given.

24. What are the neonatal complications of IUGR baby?

The IUGR infant shows signs of soft tissue wasting. The skin is loose, thin and there is little subcutaneous fat. They are susceptible to hypoglycemia, hyperbilirubinemia, necrotizing enterocolitis, hyperactive viscosity syndrome.

25. What other neonatal problems are specific to an IUGR?

Perinatal asphyxia, acidosis, persistent fetal circulation, MAS, hypoxic ischemic encephalopathy and hypothermia.

26. What are the clinical indices that the fetus is developing fetal distress?

Decreased fetal movements, bradycardia or tachycardia, and if in labor then meconium stained liqor.

27. Can liquor be increased in cases of oligohydramnios?

Yes, by amnioinfusion procedure (In idiopathic IUGR).

28. How does one differentiate IUGR/preterm baby?

IUGR—neonate has an old man's look, loss of subcutaneous fat, thinned skin, gestational maturity is ahead of the preterm neonate. Neurological reflexes are well-developed.

29. What do you mean by placental insufficiency?

Placenta is the main supportive organ for growth of fetus. Fetoplacental circulation can be hampered due to decreased blood flow, placental aging, reduction in villi and stem capillaries and decrease in stroma and parenchyma, poor trophoblastic invasion.

30. What is the role of dexamethasone and when it should be administered (Liggins regimen)?

Dexamethasone therapy is given to accelerate pulmonary maturation when gestational age is less than 34 weeks.

Dose
- Betamethasone 12 mg—24 hours apart
- Dexamethasone 4 mg—6 hourly to 24 hours.

31. What advise you would give regarding feeding of an IUGR neonate?

Early feeding within 1–2 hours is to be started, with 5–10 mL of 10% glucose. The feeding is to be repeated at 2 hourly intervals. If baby can tolerate it, expressed breastmilk or humanized milk may be given 2 hourly in small amount for 48 hours.

32. What is biophysical profile? Who devised it?

It is scoring system to assess fetal well-being. It takes fetal movements, NST, fetal tone, amount of amniotic fluid, and fetal breathing movements. A total score of movements (10) is given. In account, lower score suggests fetal distress. Amniotic fluid index is the most sensitive parameter of all.

Manning, et al. devised the score, which was later on modified by Vintzeleous et al. (AFI + NST).

33. Which antihypertensive drugs are used in pregnancy? How will you manage this case?

Tablet Methyldopa (250 mg qid) and then taper to (250 mg tds) over a period, to buy time for gaining pulmonary maturity. Nifedepine can be used for acute hypertension. It has quick action, but can interfere in induction of labor and can cause postpartum hemorrhage due to its relaxant effect on uterus.

MUST REMEMBER
- Fetal growth restriction is defined as sonographic estimated weight less than 10th percentile.
- SGA is the term applied to newborns with weight less than 10th percentile.
- PFGR pathological growth restrictions are where pathological condition prevails.
- Antepartum complications are increased incidence of stillbirth, oligohydramnios and antepartum fetal distress.
- The common causes of IUGR are placental vascular insufficiency, fetal genetic conditions, and maternal conditions.
- Intense fetal monitoring is required in these cases, BPP, Doppler.
- Intrapartum amnioinfusion with saline may be required in severe oligohydramnios.
- The worst prognosis is for IUGR secondary to congenital anomalies, congenital infections, and chromosomal defects.

Maternal Mortality

Milind Shah, Ashwini Talpe

1. How would you define maternal mortality?

Maternal mortality is the death of a woman while pregnant or within 42 days of termination of pregnancy, irrespective of the duration or site of the pregnancy, from any cause related to or aggravated by the pregnancy or its management, but not from accidental causes.

2. What are the indicators of maternal mortality?

Indicators of maternal mortality

The most common indicators of maternal mortality are:
- *Maternal mortality ratios:* The number of maternal deaths per 100,000 live births.
- *Maternal mortality rates:* The number of maternal deaths per 100,000 women aged 15-49 per year.
- *Lifetime risks:* The probability of maternal death faced by an average woman over her entire reproductive life-span.

3. Why is measuring maternal mortality difficult?

- *Maternal deaths are frequently underreported and misidentified:* This is especially true in many developing countries, where people often die outside the formal healthcare system and subsequently where the family must assume the responsibility of registering the death with the responsible local authorities. In this type of environment, such a death is often left unrecorded or information related to the cause of death and the temporal relationship to pregnancy is not recorded. Studies conducted in developed and developing countries indicate that underreporting of maternal deaths is significant. Some studies have shown that the actual number of maternal deaths for the period under study was double or triple what was initially reported.
- *Maternal deaths are often misclassified:* In many situations, the medical "cause of death" of the woman might not be known and/or noted properly by health professionals or other officials at the time of registry. As mentioned above, omission of the information related to whether the woman was pregnant or had recently delivered, might also be omitted, thus further obscuring the possible causes of death. In some countries, the cause of death can also be intentionally misclassified, especially when it is related to complications of clandestine abortions. The most recent estimates developed by WHO, UNICEF, and UNFPA on the maternal mortality rates worldwide relate that:

- 515,000 women die each year—one every minute-from complications of pregnancy and childbirth
- Of these deaths, over half (273,000) occurred in Africa, about 42% (217,000) occurred in Asia, about 4% (22,000) in Latin America and the Caribbean, and less than 1% (2,800) in the more developed regions of the world
- Twelve countries account for 65% of all maternal deaths worldwide. These include India (110,000), Ethiopia (46,000), Nigeria (45,000), Indonesia (22,000), Bangladesh (20,000), Democratic Republic of Congo (20,000), China (13,000), Kenya (13,000), Sudan (13,000), United Republic of Tanzania (13,000), Pakistan (10,000) and Uganda (10,000)
- The lifetime risk of maternal death varies widely from one region of the world to another. For example, in Africa it varies from 1 in 11 in Eastern Africa, to 1 in 65 in Southern Africa, from 1 in 55 in South-Central Asia to 1 in 840 in Eastern Africa, and in Latin America from 1 in 85 in the Caribbean to 1 in 240 in Central America. Within specific regions of the world, it varies from country to country, and further from region to region within each country.

4. Which method would be better to measure maternal mortality according to you?

Methods of measuring maternal mortality

The most accurate method of monitoring maternal mortality is through vital registration. Vital registration registers all births and deaths and for death statistics, it provides medical certification of the causes. To be efficient, the method must ensure the complete or near-complete reporting of all births and deaths within a specific region or country.

Although considered the most efficient method to track maternal mortality trends, the vital registration approach relies on the proper registration and classification of all deaths, including maternal deaths.

Unfortunately, the vital registration approach is not possible in many developing countries where vital registration systems are lacking or incomplete and causes of death are more often than not incorrectly attributed or are unreported. In response to this reality, alternative methods of determining the level of maternal mortality have been used to estimate maternal mortality.

The most well-known include:

- *Reproductive age mortality surveys (RAMOS):* This approach consists of in-depth reviews of deaths among all women of reproductive age. Although RAMOS can provide useful data for program planning, monitoring and evaluation (e.g. not only maternal mortality ratio, but also causes of deaths, high-risk groups and avoidable factors), they are considered complex, time-consuming and costly to conduct.
- *Household survey using direct estimations:* The household survey method consists of visiting a large number of households for the purpose of seeking data related to maternal deaths. Overall, this method is also considered expensive for most countries, due to the large sample of households that need to be surveyed to ensure reliable and representative results.
- *Sisterhood method:* This third method of estimating maternal mortality is based on the collection of information provided by siblings (usually sisters). Although it requires much smaller sample sizes, it is considered a more cost-effective method, especially when conducted in conjunction with existing household surveys. Its major disadvantage lies in the fact that the data collected is usually ten years old and thus, provides little insight of the changes that may have occurred over the recent past.
- *WHO/UNICEF/UNFPA estimates:* In 1996, WHO and UNICEF, with the participation of UNFPA developed estimates of maternal mortality for the year 1990. The approach developed consisted of a "dual strategy" method where; (i) for countries where maternal mortality estimates already existed, the figures were adjusted to account for under-reporting and misclassification and (ii) for countries where no reliable estimates were available, a model which permitted the calculation of estimates based on fertility rates and the proportion of births assisted by skilled personnel was used. The exercise (with some adjustments) was repeated in 2001 for the purpose of establishing maternal mortality estimates for 1995. Although this approach provides some sense of the magnitude of the problem, the figures generated are not intended to serve as precise estimates.

5. Though woman survives what are other complications often not accounted properly in obstetrics and what is their impact on maternal health?

In addition to these maternal deaths, as many as 50 million women—more than one quarter of all adult women now living in the developing world—experience maternal health problems annually. These include uterine rupture, prolapse, hemorrhage, vaginal tearing, urinary incontinence, pelvic inflammatory disease, and obstetric fistula, a muscle tear that allows urine and feces to seep into the vagina.

- It is estimated that as many as 300 million women—more than one quarter of all adult women now living in the developing world—currently suffer from short- or long-term illnesses and injuries related to pregnancy and childbirth
- Adolescent girls (15-19 years of age) are at a greater risk during pregnancy and childbirth. In fact, they are twice as likely to die from childbirth as women in their twenties, and if under 15 years of age, five times more likely to die
- Unwanted pregnancies, which often lead to unsafe abortions, continue to be a major preoccupation for women worldwide. It is estimated that 50 million unwanted pregnancies are terminated each year, and some 20 million of these are deemed unsafe and thus, a threat to women's health and lives. Furthermore, as with maternal deaths, approximately 95% of unsafe abortions occur in developing countries, causing the deaths of more than 200 women daily.

6. What are the causes of maternal death and how far they can be predicted or prevented?

Main causes of maternal death and injury:

During the last 10 years, much has been learned about the main causes of maternal death and injury and a women's chances of experiencing some complications during labor and delivery.

Research in the field of maternal death and injury has confirmed that:

- The direct causes of maternal deaths are similar throughout the world. They include hemorrhage (25%), sepsis (14%), hypertensive disorders (13%), complications due to unsafe abortions (13%) and obstructed labor (7%)
- An additional 20% of maternal deaths in developing countries are attributed to preexisting medical conditions such as anemia, malaria and HIV/AIDS that are aggravated during pregnancy

- Obstetrical complications can neither be predicted nor prevented, except those related to unsafe induced abortion. It is estimated that for every 100 women who become pregnant, 15 will develop life-threatening complications mostly around the time of birth.

7. Which are other social and medical factors that influence complications during pregnancy?

Birthing mothers' capacity to survive complications is also influenced by a number of others factors, such as:

- Women's poor health and nutrition from childhood as well as during pregnancy
- Inadequate, inaccessible, or unaffordable healthcare services
- Poor hygiene and care during childbirth
- Socioeconomic and cultural factors, such as poverty, women's unequal access to resources—including healthcare, food and preventive services, their heavy physical workload and their lack of decision-making power in families, communities, and societies
- In summary, it is now recognized that maternal death and injury "are rooted in women's powerlessness and unequal access to employment, finances, education, basic healthcare and other resources. These factors set the stage for poor maternal health even before pregnancy occurs, and make it worse once pregnancy and childbearing have begun." It is for this reason that maternal death and injury are considered a matter of social injustice.

8. What is 3 delay model? Which delay do you feel is more commonly seen in our country or other countries where maternal mortality is very high?

The 3 Delay Model

- When looking at the issue of access to essential obstetrical care (or medical care at the time of complications), the 3 delay model is often used. This concept may be useful in helping to identify which delays, or barriers, prevented the birthing mother from accessing appropriate healthcare when complications arose. They include:
  - The delay to seek care
  - The delay to reach proper medical services
  - The delay in accessing quality care when she reaches the medical facility.

Delay 1: Deciding to seek care

- When complications arise, the decision to seek care is the first step which must be taken by the birthing mother, her family and/or her attendant(s) to ensure access to the appropriate medical care needed. This decision may be influenced by many factors, such as:
  - The ability of the birthing mother and her family or attendants to recognize obstetrical complications
  - Who decides when to seek care: The birthing mother herself, her family (husband, mother-in-law) or the assistants
  - Knowledge as to where to go to seek appropriate medical assistance, and
  - Cultural factors, such as the way society views delivery and childbirth (e.g. women are expected to labor in silence).

Delay 2: Reaching the proper medical services

Once the decision has been made to seek medical care, the issue of transportation and/or communication often comes into play. A woman who lives in a rural area, far from health facilities, can face difficulties accessing transportation to get to a health center, especially if she or her family have no means of transportation and/or little financial resources. Furthermore, once at the community clinic, the birthing mother may need to be transferred to a higher level medical facility for services, such as blood transfusion or cesarean section. The delays in accessing transportation to ensure timely access to health services is thus extremely important to consider when trying to this barrier is: "Is there a village or subcounty plan for emergency transportation in case of obstetrical emergencies?"

Delay 3: Accessing quality care

Once the birthing mother arrives at the healthcare, it is thus just as important that she accesses the required emergency care services. Access to care delays are usually dependent on a number of factors, such as the number and skill level of staff, availability of drugs, supplies and blood and the general condition of the facility. They may also include:

- Delay in the arrival (time wise) of the nurse, midwife or physician attending the patient
- Delay in accessing, in a timely fashion, the needed medical procedure (e.g. cesarean section, blood transfusion).

A good way to gain insight on the quality of this care is to survey the patients on their perception of the care they received. It is usually recognized that the quicker each delay is dealt with, the greater the chances that a birthing mother and her newborn will survive and be able to live free of any long-term injuries.

9. What is impact on families of maternal death or injury?

- Women are not the only victims of maternal death and injury. A women's death affects her infant and often her other surviving children, her family and her community at large. Maternal injury can also impact on her families' "economic status."

- It is internationally recognized that the impact of maternal death on families and communities are the following:
  - In developing countries, a mother's death during childbirth means almost certain death for a newly born infant and severe consensus for her surviving children. Studies have shown that there is an increased probability of older children, especially daughters, dying and of their absenteeism from school. Without education, the cycle of poverty continues
  - Women are more likely than men to spend their income on family welfare. Consequently, when a mother dies during childbirth, the family may lose an important, or its only, financial contributor
  - Within the family, the mother usually assumes the main responsibility for maintaining the home and caring for society's dependents—children and the elderly. The loss of a mother thus affects the well-being of the family as a whole
  - When a mother dies, the community loses a vital member whose unpaid labor is often central to community life.

10. Which essential services for safe motherhood are must to reduce maternal mortality and morbidity?

Essential services for safe motherhood
In light of the above, much has also been learned as to safe motherhood programming. It is internationally recognized that the essential services for safe motherhood include:
- Community education on safe motherhood
- Antenatal care and counseling, including the promotion of maternal nutrition
- Skilled attendance during childbirth
- Care for obstetric complications, including life-threatening emergencies
- Postpartum care
- Services to prevent and manage complications due to unsafe abortion
- Family planning counseling, information, and services
- Reproductive health education and services for adolescents.

11. That's how this concept of reproductive health has come, what is it?

Reproductive health
A reproductive health approach means that:
- People have the ability to reproduce and regulate their fertility
- Women are able to go through pregnancy and childbirth safely
- The outcome of pregnancy is successful in terms of maternal and infant survival and well-being
- Couples are able to have sexual relations free of the fear of pregnancy and of contracting disease (Fathallah, 1988).

The reproductive health approach extends beyond the narrow confines of family planning to encompass all aspects of human sexuality and reproductive health needs during the various stages of the life cycle.

12. We are failing in implementation due to several reasons. So what should be rational for recommending a package of services?

The rationale for suggesting a package approach is to enable program planners to (i) assess the feasibility and management implications for implementing various combinations of health services at different levels of the health service system in diverse settings and (ii) examine the cost, financing and sustainability implications of implementing these health services.

As there is enormous diversity in India among the regions and states as well as between rural and urban areas, no single package of services can be recommended for nationwide implementation. While in underserved areas such as in the Northern states of India, there is a continuing need to strengthen the health infrastructure and improve service access, in states with better developed programs, such as Tamil Nadu and Kerala, efforts should be now made to expand the range and quality of services provided.

The following services are included in a comprehensive reproductive health services package:
- Prevention and management of unwanted pregnancy
- Services to promote safe motherhood
- Services to promote child survival
- Nutritional services for vulnerable groups
- Prevention and treatment of reproductive tract infections and sexually transmitted infections
- Prevention and treatment of gynecological problems
- Screening and treatment of breast cancer
- Reproductive health services for adolescents
- Health, sexuality and gender information, education and counseling
- Family planning services
- Establishment of effective referral systems.

The last two services, health, sexuality and gender information, education and counseling, and the establishment of effective referral systems, are not separate services but are critical for the effective implementation of all the other reproductive health services within the service system.

The following package of essential reproductive health services is recommended for nationwide implementation:
- Prevention and management of unwanted pregnancy
- Services to promote safe motherhood
- Services to promote child survival
- Nutritional services for vulnerable groups
- Prevention and treatment of reproductive tract infections and sexually transmitted infections
- Reproductive health services for adolescents
- Health, sexuality and gender information, education and counseling
- Establishment of effective referral systems.

All the services included in this package are presently recommended as a part of the government's health and family welfare program.

13. Various levels of health service systems have their own problems while executing these services. Which are these problems?

While all the services are theoretically included in the national program and are specified in the various policy and program documents, there have been serious problems with their implementation at various levels of the health delivery system.

The discussion focuses on interventions within each service component that can be implemented at various levels of the health service system. Health interventions that can be implemented at the community, subcenter, primary health center (PHC), and community health center (CHC)/district/subdistrict hospital levels are as follows:

The PHC is the weakest link in the chain. While one PHC catered to a population of about 100,000 in the past, according to the present norms, there is one PHC for a population of 20,000–30,000 population. In fact, the new PHC is often an upgraded subcenter.

According to the government's prescribed norms, in addition to a voluntary worker who is paid on honorarium, there is a provision for one male and one female multipurpose worker at each subcenter. The female health worker is an auxiliary nurse midwife (ANM). A subcenter caters to 5000 population in the plains and to 3000 population in hilly and tribal areas. The staffing norms for the new PHC that cater to 30,000 population in the plains and 20,000 population in tribal and hilly areas include one medical officer, a pharmacist, a nurse midwife, a health educator, one male and one female health assistants, and one male and one female health workers. The old PHCs have 1–3 physicians and more paramedical staff. The prescribed norms for staff at the CHC include: Five qualified or especially trained doctors—a surgeon, an obstetrician gynecologist, a physician, a pediatrician, and a public health physician. In addition, there should be seven nurse midwives, a dresser, a pharmacist/compounder, a laboratory technician, and a radiographer at this facility. A CHC covers approximately 100,000 population (Government of India, 1995). The CHC is expected to have facilities for managing obstetric emergencies. Currently, there are very few CHCs with prescribed staff and facilities.

In many areas, staff are not in place at PHCs and CHCs according to prescribed norms. There are particular gaps in the case of women physicians and male multipurpose workers. It is difficult to recruit women physicians for rural facilities. The government proposes to contract private physicians for PHCs and CHCs.

However, community health workers, such as traditional birth attendants (TBAs), who are not a part of the formal health system, play an important role in providing reproductive health services at the community level. Urban health in India has been neglected even though the urban poors are growing in number and are increasingly exposed to serious health risks.

14. Prevention and management of unwanted pregnancies itself would lead to marked reduction in maternal mortality. What are hurdles we face while advocating contraception and what could be solution for it?

For ensuring contraceptive safety, the program must focus on all clinical procedures especially aseptic techniques and on screening clients for contraindications and preexisting health problems.

Developing effective outreach programs should be a high priority if counseling and follow-up services are to be provided, especially in rural areas.

15. One of the definitely preventable cause of MM is providing services for safe abortions. How to go about it? And are safe abortions really safe in India?

- The Medical Termination of Pregnancy (MTP) Act was passed by the Indian Parliament in 1971 but what was thought to be a landmark in social legislation, has failed to translate into reality for the majority of Indian women, particularly in rural areas. Today, there are more illegal abortions in India than there were prior to the MTP Act with about 15,000–20,000 abortion-related deaths occurring annually, mainly among married, multiparous women
- Services for first trimester abortion should be made available at PHCs and facilities for second trimester abortions at CHCs. Unsafe abortion is an important cause for maternal mortality and results in high levels of maternal morbidity in India.

- About 11-12% of maternal deaths in rural India are due to septic abortion (Government of India, 1990). Septic abortions account for up to 25% of all maternal deaths in hospital studies in India.
- Although unsafe induced abortion is the greatest single cause of mortality for women, it is also the most preventable. Women need not die or suffer medical consensus from abortions because abortions do not kill women; it is, rather, unsafely performed abortions which kill.
- Expanding family planning services is an important strategy for decreasing pregnancy-related mortality and morbidity.
- Unsafe abortion is an important cause of maternal mortality and results in high levels of maternal morbidity in India. While public sector programs should be strengthened to provide safe abortion services, there is an urgent need to improve the quality of services provided by the private sector as private practitioners are by far the most important providers of abortion services in the country.
- While public sector programs should be strengthened to provide safe abortion services, there is an urgent need to examine the quality of services provided by the private sector and to organize training programs for private practitioners, as they are by far the most important providers of abortion services in the country.

16. Coming to maternity health services, it is debate nowadays as far as usefulness of antenatal services is concerned. What is your comment? How do you get about ideal ANC services?

Services for maternal care should be designed to ensure timely detection, management and referral of complications during pregnancy, delivery and the postpartum period.

Antenatal services should be organized to detect and manage complications related to pregnancy, such as anemia, infection, preeclampsia, malpresentation, and obstructed labor. Women should be educated about the danger signs of pregnancy and provided information on where to seek help. Antenatal visits should provide an opportunity to offer advice and counseling on hygiene, breastfeeding, nutrition, family planning and immunization as well as to treat preexisting conditions such as diabetes and infections, such as malaria and tuberculosis that are commonly prevalent, may be aggravated by pregnancy, and may complicate pregnancy (World Bank, 1994).

There should be at least 3-4 antenatal examinations by a healthcare provider. The first visit should take place as soon as pregnancy is detected, preferably before 10 weeks to confirm the pregnancy; provide nutritional advice and supplements; and provide the first dose to tetanus toxoid immunization. A second visit is recommended at 20-24 weeks to detect and treat abnormalities; to identify and refer cases with complications; and to provide the second tetanus toxoid injection. A visit at 28-32 weeks would enable the service provider to detect malpresentation and to diagnose and treat maternal illnesses. An antenatal visit should be made at 36-38 weeks to confirm the position of the fetus; to make an assessment of cephalopelvic disproportion; and to manage maternal illnesses.

The subcenter must be equipped for examining hemoglobin, blood pressure, urine albumin, and sugar, and for checking body weight and height.

17. Safe delivery services would be definite solution in avoiding many deaths. But again so many difficulties we face for it. How to overcome it?

All deliveries must be managed by trained birth attendants. Because complications can develop without warning, it is critical to put in place effective systems to ensure timely referral and management of emergency complications. However, the vast majority of births in India take place at home. The National Family Health Survey shows that in 1992-93 only 25.6% of all births and 16.1% of all rural births were conducted in institutions and as many as 65% were delivered by traditional birth attendants (International Institute of Population Studies, 1994). The need for conducting clean home deliveries using safe delivery kits and the importance of recognizing danger signals for emergency obstetric care should be highlighted.

18. Postpartum period is the period during which maximum maternal deaths take place. Why is it so and what is solution for it?

To date, postpartum programs in India have focused primarily on providing family planning services. Postpartum programs should include services for the early detection and management of infection and hemorrhage; support for breastfeeding for at least six months; nutrition counseling; and family planning services. Antibiotic treatment is sufficient to cure infection in more than 80% of cases if taken within four days of the onset of fever.

19. Now, in spite of this, if maternal death takes place, How it should be faced or rather what lessons we should take?

Maternal death case reviews
A maternal death case review is defined as a qualitative, in-depth investigation of the causes of and circumstances surrounding maternal deaths occurring at health facilities. Maternal death case review focuses on with identifying the factors at the facility and in the community that contributed to the death, and which ones were avoidable".

Usually carried out by facility staff, maternal case reviews provide valuable information on the circumstances—in the facility and in the community—surrounding a death. They are considered affordable and because of their participative approach (e.g. they involve health professionals and at levels and community people) further, they can offer good opportunities for sensitizing and educating people to the issue of maternal mortality.

Verbal autopsy of maternal deaths
Verbal autopsies consists of "a method of finding out the medical causes of death and ascertaining the personal, family or community factors that may have contributed to the deaths in women who died outside of a medical facility." They consist of inquiries collected from lay reporters and relatives to establish the cause of death. The data is usually collected outside the health facilities.

Verbal autopsies are a useful tool for identifying maternal deaths and collecting valuable information about deaths that have occurred outside the health facilities. Further, they provide a great opportunity to obtain family and community members' opinions on issues related to access to and the quality of health services.

Confidential enquiry into maternal deaths
A confidential enquiry into a maternal death consists of "an investigation undertaken by multiprofessional team that identifies weaknesses and deficiencies in the maternal healthcare system. It investigates individual maternal deaths, with the cooperation of all those involved in the care of the patient, yet removes all identifying details from individual case reports to ensure that information is used only for making recommendations for positive practice changes, and not for punitive action." Confidential enquiries are not interested in determining who is at fault, but more specifically in determining the deficiencies in the healthcare systems that may have contributed to the death for the purpose of instituting change as to ensure that future similar deaths are prevented.

Usually, more resource intensive (e.g. time, structure, and support system needed) than the other investigative tools, confidential enquiry methods can be instituted by public health authorities or by government and are usually undertaken and supported at national level by the Ministry of Health.

20. What is AMDD?

Averting maternal deaths and disability program (AMDD): This program has been funded by Bill and Melinda Gates foundation. This program aims at reducing maternal mortality by improving emergency obstetric care (EMOC) in India.

21. What is WHO near-miss criteria?

A women presenting any of the life-threatening conditions and surviving a complication during pregnancy, childbirth, or within 42 days of termination of pregnancy should be considered a near-miss case (Table 30.1).

Table 30.1 Management of various dysfunction of systems

Dysfunctional system	Clinical criteria	Laboratory markers	Management based proxies
Cardio-vascular	Shock, cardiac arrest	PH <7.1, lactate >5 mEq/mL	Use of continuous vasoactive drugs, CPR
Respiratory	Acute cyanosis gasping, RR <6, >40	O_2 saturation <90% for >60 min PaO_2/FiO_2 <200 mm Hg	Intubation and ventilation not related to anesthesia
Renal	Oliguria nonresponsive to fluids or diuretics	Creatinine 300 μmol/L or >3.5 mg/dL	Dialysis for acute renal failure
Hematologic/coagulation	Failure to form clots	Acute severe thrombo-cytopenia (< 50,000 plates/mL)	Transfusion of >5 units of blood/red cells
Hepatic	Jaundice in the presence of preeclampsia	Bilirubin >100 μmol/L or >6.0 mg/dL	
Neurologic	Any loss of consciousness lasting >12 hours Stroke uncontrollable fit/status epilepticus Total paralysis		
Alternative severity proxy			Hysterectomy following infection or hemorrhage

22. What are strategies to reduce maternal mortality?

- Strengthening outreach services and community-based approaches
- Improving education for girls and women
- Targeting public sectors subsidies to poor families and disadvantaged areas
- Developing effective "poor-friendly" referral systems
- Improving quality and availability of essential and emergency obstetric care services (EOC) for the poor
- Promoting affordable maternal health services. Scale up adolescent sexual and reproductive health information and services
- Strengthening monitoring and evaluation of practices for improved maternal survival.

MUST REMEMBER
- Postpartum hemorrhage.
- Active management of the third stage of labor, including administration of uterotonic agents.
- Hypertensive disorders.
- Magnesium sulfate for women with eclampsia.
- Calcium supplementation for women with low dietary calcium intake.
- Labor induction using extra-amniotic saline infusion or very low dose misoprostol for severe cases.

Obstetric sepsis
- Clean birth practices.

HIV
- Primary prevention (lifestyle changes, condom use).
- Antiretroviral treatment for immunocompromised women.

	Scores			
	0	1	2	4
Age (years)	<40	>40	-	-
Antecedent pregnancy	Mole	Abortion	Term	-
Interval (end of antecedent pregnancy to chemotherapy) in months	<4	4-6	7-13	>13
Human chorionic gonadotropin (hCG) (IU/L)	<10^3	10^3-10^4	10^4-10^5	>10^5
Number of metastasis	0	1-4	5-8	>8
Site of metastasis	Lung	Spleen, kidney	Gastro-intestinal tract, liver	Brain, liver
Largest tumor mass	-	3-5 cm	>5 cm	-
Previous chemotherapy	-	-	1 drug	>2 drugs

14B. What is FIGO staining of GTN?

Stage I	Disease confined to the uterus
Stage II	GTN extends outside of the uterus but is limited to the genital structures (adnexa, vagina, broad ligament)
Stage III	GTN extends to the lungs, with or without known genital tract involvement
Stage IV	All other metastatic sites (brain, liver)

The combination of FIGO staging and risk factors scoring is currently used for management of GTN.

15. What are the chemotherapy regimens for low-risk patient?

Chemotherapy regimens for low and medium risk patients includes:
- Methotrexate (MTX)—50 mg by IM injection repeated every 48 hours × 4
- Tab folinic acid—15 mg orally 30 hours after each injection of MTX (Folinic acid)
- Courses repeated every 2 weeks, i.e. days 1, 15, 29, etc.

16. What is the chemotherapy regimen for high-risk patients?

EMACO regimen
EMA
Day 1	Etoposide
	Actinomycin D
	Methotrexate
Day 2	Etoposide
	Actinomycin D
	Folinic acid rescue starting 24 hours after methotrexate infusion

CO
Day 8	Vincristine
	Cyclophosphamide

17. What is the management of drug resistant disease?

- *Low-risk disease:* Decision to alter treatment are made on progressive hCG trend over 2-3 values. Low-risk and medium risk patients failing methotrexate whose serum hCG is >100 IU/L, disease can be cured by substituting actinomycin D hCG >100 IU/L EMA/CO.
- *High-risk disease:* Most patients who have failed EMA/CO can still be salvaged by further chemotherapy and/or surgery.

18. Outline follow-up after chemotherapy, hCG.

	Urine	Blood
Weekly for the first 6 weeks	✓	✓
Then every 2 weeks until 6 months	✓	✓
Then monthly × 12 months	✓	×
Then 2 monthly × 6 months	✓	×
Then 3 monthly × 4 months	✓	×
Then 4 monthly × 3 months	✓	×
Then 6 monthly for life	✓	×

19. What is placental site trophoblastic tumor (PSTT)?

PSTT is a rare form of GTD that develops where the placenta attaches to the uterus. Most PSTTs do not spread to other sites in the body. They are not chemosensitive and must be completely removed by surgery.
- Relative to their mass, these tumors produce small amount of hCG and human placental lactogen (HPL). They tend to remain confirmed to the uterus and metastasizing late in their course

- USG, hCG estimation, color Doppler, CT mainstay for investigation
- hCG regression curve helps to monitor the patients and to decide the chemotherapy regime
- Chemotherapy (single drug therapy/multiple drug therapy) forms the mainstay of treatment
- Future pregnancies are unaffected
- Molar pregnancies should be monitored and managed in specialized clinics.

Choriocarcinoma
- Metastatic GTT occurs in about 4% of patients after molar evacuation, but it is seen more commonly when GTT develops after nonmolar pregnancy
- Choriocarcinoma has high tendency to early vascular invasion within widespread dissemination
- Symptoms of metastasis may result from spontaneous bleeding at metastatic foci.

The common sites for metastasis are:
Pulmonary—80%, vaginal—30%, hepatic—10%, cerebral—10%.

Invasive mole
Locally invasive GTT, occurs in almost 15% patients after molar evacuation and infrequently after other gestations. Metastatic tumor occurs in 4% of cases.

Clinical Features
- Vaginal bleeding—most common symptom (84%)
- Excessive uterine size relative to gestational age of patients (50%)
- Pre-eclampsia (27%)
- Hyperemesis (25%)
- Trophoblastic embolization (2%)
- Theca lutein cysts 6 cm in diameter.

20. What are the risk factors for development of GTD?
Maternal age < 20 or > 35 years, previous history of V mole, vitamin A deficiency, Asian race, low socioeconomic status are the risk factors for development of GTD.

21. What are the complications of invasive mole/choriocarcinoma?
Uterine perforation profuses vaginal bleeding and sepsis. Patient may die due to hemorrhagic shock.

22. What is the role of methotrexate in management of GTD?
- Most common drug used in the treatment of GTN: It is folic acid antagonist. It inhibits DNA and RNA synthesis and thereby inhibits rapidly dividing cells.
- Nausea, diarrhea, stomatitis alopecia, bone marrow suppression and hepatotoxicity are adverse effects.

23. What are the indications for hysterectomy?
Placental site trophoblastic tumor, perforating mole with intraperitonial hemorrhage, uncontrolled vaginal bleeding, chemoresistant disease confined to uterus.

24. What is phantom β-hCG?
Phantom β-hCG results from the presence in serum of heterophilic antibodies that interfere with the β-hCG immunoassay and cause a false positive result. Phantom β-hCG can be demonstrated by a negative urine pregnancy, but only patient's serum β-hCG level is significantly higher.

25. What is quiescent GTD?
If patient's true serum β-hCG level shows persistent mild elevation in absence of tumor on clinical or imaging studies, patient may have dormant premalignant condition. This is called quiescent hCG.

MUST REMEMBER
- The term GTD includes hydatidiform mole, invasive mole, choriocarcinoma and placental site trophoblastic tumor.
- GTN includes invasive mole, choriocarcinoma and placental site trophoblastic tumor. All GTDs secrete hCG.
- All GTDs secrete hCG.
- Diagnosis is by symptoms, signs and USG snowstorm appearance.
- Management of hydatidiform mole is suction evacuation.
- Postmolar follow-up consists of history, serial estimation of β-hCG and chest X-ray.
- Contraception with combined oral contraceptive pills or DMPA/progesterone only pills is recommended.
- Choriocarcinoma develops after term pregnancies, abortions or ectopic pregnancies and spreads by hematogeneous route.
- Chemotherapy is the mainstay of the disease.
- Monitoring for 12–24 months is must in the management of GTD.

Ectopic Pregnancy

Kamini Rao, Sonali Deshpande

DIAGNOSIS AND TREATMENT (FLOW CHART 32.1)

- Abdominal pain—95%
- GIT symptoms—80%
- Amenorrhea with uterine bleeding—60–80%
- Dizziness—58%
- Per vaginal examination
  - Enlarged uterus
  - Pelvic pain with movement of cervix
  - Palpable adnexal mass
  - Hypotension/tachycardia
  - Abdominal tenderness with guarding and rebound tenderness.

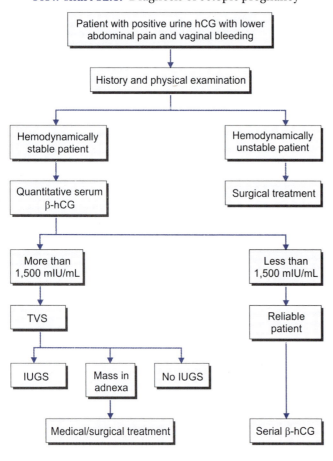

Flow chart 32.1: Diagnosis of ectopic pregnancy

DEFINITION (FLOW CHARTS 32.2A AND B)

- Fertilized ovum is implanted and develops outside the normal uterine cavity
- Incidence of ectopic pregnancy in natural conception and IVF conception
- Natural conception—incidence-1%
- IVF conception—2–8%
- ICSI-1—2%
- Reasons for increased incidence of ectopic in ART
- Increased incidence of tubal damage in infertile patients
- Larger volume of media used during transfer
- Fundal placement of embryos during transfer.

ETIOLOGY OF ECTOPIC PREGNANCY

Factors which are responsible for the fertilized ovum to remain in the tube are:
- Chronic inflammatory disease of the tube
- Excessive elongation of the tube. Diverticulae, accessory ostium
- Distortion of tube by fibroid
- Intrapelvic adhesions, tubal surgeries IUCD, minipills.

REASONS FOR INCREASED RATES OF ECTOPIC PREGNANCY

- Increasing STD/chronic PID
- Increased contraceptive use/tubal surgery
- Increasing abortion with postabortal infection
- Increasing ART
- Better diagnostic techniques
- Is there any relation between incidence of ectopic pregnancy and age
- Highest rate of ectopic pregnancy occurs between 35 and 44 years of age 4-fold increased risk in this age group compared to 15–24 years
- Proposed explanation is aging which may result in progressive loss of myometrial activity along the Fallopian tube
- Probable mechanism by which smoking can cause 1.6–3.5 fold increased in risk of ectopic pregnancy in smokers compared to nonsmokers

Flow charts 32.2A and B: Treatment of ectopic pregnancy

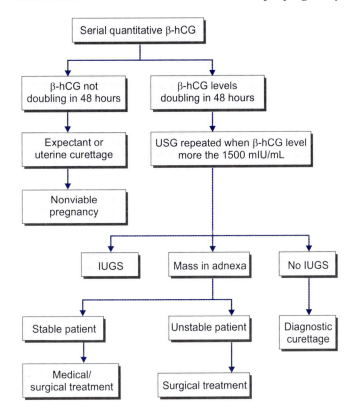

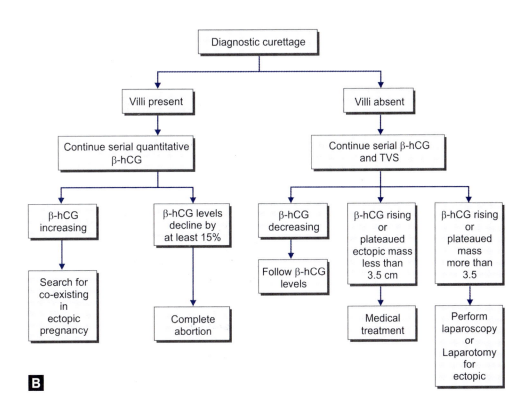

- Probable mechanisms are delayed ovulation, altered tubal, uterine motility, and altered immunity
- Role of estrogen and progesterone in ectopic incidence
- Estrogen and progesterone can slow the normal movement of the fertilized egg through the tubal epithelium and result in implantation in the tube
- Women who became pregnant despite using progesterone only OCP have 5-fold increased risk of ectopic pregnancy.

Relation between IUCD and Ectopic
- Incidence of ectopic with non-medicated IUCD—5%
- Incidence of ectopic with progesterone bearing IUCD—15%
- Incidence of ectopic after tubal sterilization—60%
- After tubal coagulation, 51% of pregnancies are ectopic
- After non-laparoscopic tubal ligation, 12% of pregnancies are ectopic
- General rules often used for hCG to diagnose ectopic
- hCG level should rise at least 66 percent in 48 hours and at least double in 72 hours, Kadar principle.

1. **What are the fates of tubal pregnancy?**
- Tubal mole
- Tubal abortion
- Tubal rupture.

2. **What are the clinical varieties of ectopic pregnancy?**
- Acute
- Subacute/chronic.

3. **What are the clinical features of acute ectopic pregnancy?**
- Short period of amenorrhea
- Pain in abdomen
- Vaginal bleeding
- Fainting attack.

This is usually associated with signs of hemorrhagic shock (tachycardia, pallor and hypotension).

4. **What are the clinical features of chronic ectopic pregnancy?**
- Apart from the short period of amenorrhea, pain in abdomen, vaginal bleeding dysuria, tenesmus
- Ill-looking patient, varying degree of pallor with persistent tachycardia
- Features of shock are absent.

5. **What is the diagnosis of ectopic pregnancy?**
- Clinical features
- Serum β-hCG—1500 MIU with midline echo on TVS confirms—diagnosis
- USG—midline echo, with adnexal mass and hemoperitoneum
- Paracentesis positive.

6. **How will you treat ruptured ectopic?**

Laparotomy—quick in and quick out, salpingectomy is the procedure of choice.

7. **Will you give anti-D prophylaxis in Rh-negative mother?**

Yes, 50 μg IM should be given.

8. **What is culdocentesis?**

Aspiration of collected fluid, from posterior fornix, i.e. fluid from POD.

9. **What is the interpretation of culdocentesis?**
- Negative—clear fluid (peritoneal fluid)
- Dry tap—indeterminate (wrong plane)
- Positive—bloody tap—(confirms ectopic or hemoperitoneum).

Indications for MTX use
- Unruptured tubal pregnancy
- GA <6 weeks
- Tubal mass not more than 3.5 cm
- Fetus not alive.

Methotrexate regimen
- Multiple dose regimen
- MTX 1 mg/kg IM on day 0, 2, 4, 6, followed by leucovorin 0.1 mg/kg on day 1, 3, 5, 7
- Increased adverse effects with multiple dose regimen— Hence not followed
- Single dose regimen—MTX 50 mg/m² IM
- Both methods are similar in efficacy.

Follow-up after MTX injection
- β-hCG on day 4 and day 7 after MTX injection
- A decline in β-hCG at least 15 percent from day 4–7 postinjection indicates a successful medical response
- β-hCG/weekly until they become undetectable.

Success rate of MTX regimen
88–94%.

Contraindication of medical management of ectopic pregnancy—hemodynamically unstable, immunodeficiency, preexisting blood dyscrasia.

10. **What is the future pregnancy outcome?**
- Eighty-five percent will have normal intrauterine pregnancy
- Recurrent ectopic rate—10–20%

- Recurrence after 1st ectopic—15%, and after 2nd ectopic is 30%.

Future fertility rate with laparoscopy/laparotomy
- Laparotomy salpingectomy intrauterine pregnancy rate—25–70%
- Laparoscopic salpingectomy—50–60% (similar rates)
- Rate of persistent ectopic in both groups—5–20%
- Higher rate of recurrent ectopic in laparotomy group (7–28%) compared to laparoscopic group (6–16%), this is due to adhesions after laparotomy group.

Recurrence rate of ectopic with milking of the tube 33%.

Criteria to diagnose primary abdominal pregnancy (Studdiford's criteria)
- Normal tubes, ovaries
- No evidence of uteroplacental fistula
- Pregnancy exclusively in the peritoneal surface.

Sonographic criteria to diagnose abdominal pregnancy
- Visualization of sac separate from the uterus
- Failure to visualize uterine wall between the fetus and urinary bladder
- Close approximation of fetal parts to the abdominal wall
- Eccentric position/abnormal attitude.

Spiegelberg criteria (ovarian pregnancy)
- Intact tube
- Fetal sac must occupy the position of the ovary
- Ovary must be connected to the uterus by the ovarian ligament
- Definitive ovarian tissue in the sac wall.

USG criteria for cervical pregnancy
- Gestational sac or placental tissue visualized within the cervix
- Cardiac motion noted below the level of the internal os.
- No intrauterine pregnancy
- Hourglass uterine shape with ballooned cervical canal
- No movement of the sac with pressure from TVS
- Closed internal os.

MUST REMEMBER
- Incidence of ectopic pregnancy is increased in past century due to increase in pelvic inflammatory disease.
- The classic triad—pain, amenorrhea, vaginal bleeding.
- Serial hCG levels will help to differentiate it from intrauterine pregnancy.
- Transvaginal sonography plays a pivotal role in the diagnosis.
- Positive UPT, adnexal mass on USG and midline endometrial echo on USG is diagnostic of ectopic pregnancy.
- Medical management is helpful in hemodynamically stable patients with sac size <3.5 cm.
- Laparoscopy/laparotomy are the options for management of ectopic pregnancy.
- Small unruptured tubal pregnancies can be managed with laparoscopy.

Vaginitis

Varsha Deshmukh

Any excessive vaginal discharge that is physiological, i.e. premenstrual or midcycle is known as leukorrhea. The discharge is from the cervix as the vagina contains no glands. Inflammation of vagina is called vaginitis.

DIFFERENT TYPES OF VAGINITIS

1. *Candidal vaginitis:* Most common type of vaginitis. Predisposing factors are diabetes mellitus, pregnancy, OC pills, steroids, HIV and STD. It is characterized by scanty thick, curdy white, discharge, which on removing with swab leaves bleeding points, (strawberry appearance). Pruritus is present. Specific culture media is Nickerson's medium. Clotrimazole is the drug of choice. It can be used in the form of cream (1%) 5 g vaginally for 7–10 days OR vaginal pessary 100 mg for 6 days OR tab fluconazole 150 mg single dose orally.
2. *Trichomonal vaginitis:* It is characterized by copious thin and greenish, frothy, foul-smelling discharge. Specific culture medium is Stuart's medium. In trichomonal infection, pear-shaped motile organisms can be seen in a wet mount preparation. Both partners should receive treatment. Condom should be essentially used during intercourse. Regimes recommended are: (a) Tab metronidazole 200 mg TDS for 7 days OR (b) Tab metronidazole 400 mg BD for 5 days OR (c) Single dose 2 g tab metronidazole. Repeat same dose after one week.
3. *Bacterial vaginosis:* It represents the disturbed vaginal microbial ecosystem rather than true infection. There is no vaginal inflammation. It has a polymicrobial etiology. It is diagnosed after ruling out *Candida* and *Trichomonas* infection. *Gardnerella vaginalis*, *Mycoplasma hominis*, *Bacteroides*, etc. are the organisms responsible for bacterial vaginosis. Copious, malodorous thin white homogeneous discharge paravaginally at the labia and fourchette is diagnostic of bacterial vaginosis. When KOH solution is added to the slide, there is fishy amine odor. This is a diagnostic test for *Bacterial vaginosis*. In *Gardnerella* infection, clue cells can be seen on wet mount preparation. Tab metronidazole 400 mg BD for 7 days is used for treatment of *Gardnerella vaginalis*.

CRITERIA FOR CLINICAL DIAGNOSIS OF VAGINAL DISCHARGE

Variables	Normal	Bacterial vaginosis	Candidal vaginitis	Trichomonal vaginitis
Symptoms	None	Malodorous discharge	Vulval itching, irritation	Itching
Amount of discharge	Scanty	Excessive	Scanty	Profuse
Color	Clear	Gray or milk	White	Yellow
Consistency	Non homogeneous	Homogeneous, non-adherent	Curdy, adherent	Frothy

1. What is the most common type of vaginitis?

Candidal vaginitis is the most common type of vaginitis.

2. What is pruritus vulvae?

Itching of the local genital parts is pruritus vulvae.

3. What systemic disorders are associated with pruritus?

Hepatitis, diabetes and chronic renal failure are associated with pruritus.

4. How is pregnancy responsible for increased incidence of vaginitis?

The increased estrogen level during pregnancy makes the vaginal pH favorable for the vaginitis.

5. What lesions will you rule out on the cervix in case of excessive vaginal discharge?

Chronic cervicitis, cervical polyp, CIS, cervical erosion are some of the lesions on the cervix to be ruled out.

6. What investigations will you do on the PV discharge?

Microscopy and culture are done on the discharge.

7. Would you like to take a Pap smear of the patients with PV discharge? Why?

Yes; because excessive vaginal discharge can be associated with CIS.

8. What is added to the slide to observe *Candida albicans*?

Ten percent KOH solution is added to the slide. It dissolves the debris and makes the fungus seen.

9. What does Gram staining of the vaginal discharge show?

Gram-positive spores indicate candida infection and Gram-negative diplococci indicate gonorrhea infection.

10. What culture media is specific for Candida, Trichomonas, Gonococci?

- Candida—Nickerson's medium
- Trichomonas—Stuart's medium
- Gonococci—Thayer-Martin medium.

11. What is the role of blood sugar estimation in case of recurrent vaginitis?

Recurrent vaginitis is seen in patients of diabetes mellitus. The glycogen content of the vaginal cells increases thereby predisposing for vaginal infection. Hence, diabetes should be ruled out.

12. What is the treatment of Chlamydia infection?

Cap Doxycycline 100 mg BD for 10–14 days.

13. What is the treatment of Gonorrhea?

Tab norfloxicillin 800 mg orally for 5 days OR tab ciprofloxacillin 500 mg orally for 5 days.

14. What is the treatment of senile vaginitis?

Local estrogen cream is used in the treatment of senile vaginitis dose EE 0.01 mg/day 3 weeks.

15. What are the factors causing vaginal candidiasis in India?

Improper hygiene, untidy undergarments, unclean nailbeds, use of tepid water for washing the urogenital parts as well as defecation.

16. What are the other factors causing *Candida vaginitis*?

Hot and humid atmosphere, ignorance about the local hygiene and noncompliance of the male partner in the treatment of vaginitis lead to repeated attacks of vaginitis.

17. What are the IDSA guidelines for the classification of vaginitis?

Complicated and uncomplicated are the two types of vaginitis according to the IDSA guidelines.

18. What are the clinical features of vaginitis?

Vulval pruritus, soreness, burning, dyspareunia, dysuria, erythema, noneffective and irritating discharge paravaginally are the symptoms of vaginitis.

19. What is recurrent vaginitis?

When there are 4 episodes of vaginitis in one year or 3 episodes with prolonged antibiotic therapy within one year, it is known as recurrent vaginitis.

20. What is the difference between recurrent vaginitis and persistent vaginitis?

There is no symptom-free interval in persistent vaginitis.

21. How OC pills are responsible for increased incidence of vaginitis?

The more the concentration of estrogen in the pill, more are the chances of vaginitis. Estrogen encourages the increased level of glycogen in the vaginal cells which favor the growth of organisms in the vagina.

22. What is the disadvantage of topical therapy over oral therapy?

Topical therapy is messy, lasts for 7 days and is applied only at night whereas oral therapy is single dose, convenient and with equally good results.

23. What is the treatment of recurrent vaginitis?

The principle of treatment of recurrent vaginitis is induction therapy with oral or topical azole followed by maintenance therapy for 6 months.

24. After how many days of intercourse with an infected partner, the lady gets *Trichomonas vaginitis*?

Four to twenty-eight days is the time required to contract the infection.

25. How does *Trichomonas* infection present in males?

In males, this infection is mostly asymptomatic. However, it can present as urethritis, prostitis or epidymitis.

26. What are the complications associated with bacterial vaginosis?

Preterm labor, chorioamnionitis, postpartum endometritis, PROM, sexual dysfunction and psychological upset are some of the complications associated with bacterial vaginosis.

27. What is clue cell?
Clue cells are the vaginal squamous cells showing stippling of cytoplasm due to adherent coccobacilli.

28. Why *Trichomonas* is sexually transmitted?
As *Trichomonas* harbors in the male urethra, it is sexually transmitted.

29. What is "strawberry sign"?
It is seen in the Trichomonal vaginalis infection. "Strawberry vagina" is a naked eye finding where petechial lesions in the vagina appear as strawberry like in candidial vaginitis.

30. What is "Nugent criteria" in bacterial vaginosis?
It is the assessment of relative concentration of bacterial morphophytes (anaerobes than *Lactobacillus*), characteristic of altered flora called "Nugent criteria" in a Gram-stained smear.

31. What is Whiff's amine test?
The addition of KOH 10% to vaginal discharge produces fishy odor. Used in Amsel's criteria for diagnosis of bacterial vaginosis.

Amsel's criteria:
- Homogeneous vaginal discharge
- Vaginal pH ≥ 4.5
- Amine-like odor on addition of KOH (Whiff test)
- Clue cells on wet smear

Any 3 out of 4 should be present.

MUST REMEMBER

Vaginitis is inflammation of vagina. Candidal, *Trichomonas*, *Gardnerella* and senile are the different types of vaginitis. Candidal vaginitis is the most common type of vaginitis. Diabetes mellitus, pregnancy, OC pills, steroids, HIV, STD are the predisposing factors for candidial vaginitis. Specific culture media for Candida is Nickerson's medium, Trichomonas—Stuart's medium, Gonococci—Thayer-Martin medium. Clotrimazole is the drug of choice for treatment of candidiasis. Tab metronidazole 200 mg TDS for 7 days *OR* Tab metronidazole 400 mg BD for 5 days is recommended for treatment of *Trichomonal vaginitis*. Both partners should receive treatment. Tab metronidazole 400 mg BD for 7 days is treatment for *Gardnerella vaginitis*. Local estrogen cream is used in the treatment of senile vaginitis. Bacterial vaginosis represents the disturbed vaginal microbial ecosystem rather than true infection. There is no vaginal inflammation. Copious, malodorous thin white discharge paravaginally at the labia and fourchette is diagnostic of bacterial vaginosis.

Sexually Transmitted Infections

Jayantdeep Nath, Pralhad Kushtagi

34

1. Which are the different organisms that cause STI?

Infection	Organism	Disease
Bacterial	Neisseria gonorrhoeae	Gonorrhea
	Chlamydia trachomatis (D-k serotype)	Non-gonococcal urethritis
	Treponema pallidum	Syphilis
	Chlamydia trachomatis (L type)	Lymphogranuloma venereum
	Haemophilus ducreyi	Chancroid
	Donovania granulomatis	Granuloma inguinale
	Haemophilus vaginalis	Non-specific vaginitis
	Mycoplasma hominis	Mycoplasma infection
Viral	Human immunodeficiency virus (HIV-1 and 2)	AIDS
	Herpes simplex virus (HSV-2)	Genital herpes
	Human papillomavirus (HPV)	Condyloma acuminata
	HPV-16, 18, 31	CIN (cervical intra-epithelial neoplasia), Cancer cervix
	Pox virus	Molluscum contagiosum
	Hepatitis B virus	Viral hepatitis
Protozoal	Trichomonas vaginalis	Trichomonas vaginitis
Fungal	Candida albicans	Monilial vaginitis
Parasitic	Crab louse (Phthirus pubis)	Pediculosis pubis
	Sarcoptes scabiei	Scabies

2. What are the non-sexual means of STI transmission?

STI can transmit through:
1. Placenta — HIV, syphilis
2. Infected nodule, blood transfusion — Hepatitis B, HIV, syphilis
3. Inoculation to infants mucosa — Gonococcal, chlamydia, herpes simplex, candidiasis

3. What are the effects of STI in women?

STI may produce adverse effect in several ways in a woman:
- PID, tubal block, infertility, ectopic pregnancy, abortion, chronic pelvic pain
- HPV virus may cause oncogenesis of cervical, vulval, vaginal and anal epithelium. Herpes simplex is involved in oncogenesis
- Hepatitis B and C may cause jaundice.

4. Can STI affect pregnancy outcome?

Various effects of STI in pregnancy are:
- Abortion, PROM, preterm labor, chorioamnionitis, IUGR, IUD
- Congenital anomalies particularly by syphilis, herpes simplex, etc
- Postabortal and puerperal infection
- Difficulties in deliveries. Elective CS is recommended in herpes simplex infection
- Obstruction or excessive bleeding during delivery in large genital warts
- Vertical transmission from mother to fetus like HIV, syphilis.

5. Is the incidence of STI rising? What are the reasons for this epidemiologic change?

The incidence of STI is rising due to several reasons:
- Increasing promiscuity and permissiveness
- Change of sex partner
- Better understanding of mode of transmission
- Antibiotic resistance
- Increasing DNA viral infection
- Lack of sex education
- Increased use of pill and IUCD.

6. What are classic venereal diseases?

Classic venereal diseases are those which are recognized as such long since like syphilis, gonorrhea, chancroid, lymphogranuloma venereum, granuloma inguinale.

7. What are the principles of management of a case of STI?

The detailed history taking, adequacy of clinician's knowledge and maintenance of confidentiality are vital in the management of STIs. The clinical features should be properly evaluated. Suspicion of the diagnosis should be confirmed and adequate treatment with appropriate antimicrobial should be immediately started. The sexual partner should be treated. The effect on pregnancy should be evaluated in detail and counseled.

8. Which are the three main strategies to reduce incidence of STI?

As a health problem, STI needs to be prevented. In the light of AIDS epidemic, the prevention and control of STI are highly essential. The sex education, advocating barrier contraceptive and screening of high-risk cases can reduce STI.

9. What is normal vaginal flora?

The normal vaginal flora is predominantly aerobic with an average of six species of bacteria, most common is hydrogen peroxide (H_2O_2) producing lactobacilli.

10. What is the normal pH of vagina?

The normal pH of vagina is below 4.

11. Which is the second generation STI?

Most of the recently recognized STIs are now known as second generation STIs. For example, AIDS is most recently recognized as second generation STI.

12. What do you understand by internal and external dysuria?

Pain during micturition is known as dysuria.
- *Internal dysuria:* Symptomatic urethritis caused by *C. trichomatis*, *N. gonorrhoeae* and occasionally HSV infection. Here, dysuria is without urinary urgency and frequency and pain occur during micturition due to some lesion internal to the labia or introitus.
- *External dysuria:* Pain occurs during micturition due to contact of urine with the inflamed or ulcerated labia or introitus. This external dysuria is associated with vulvar herpes or vulvovaginal candidiasis.

13. How color of vaginal discharge is best determined?

Color of discharge is best determined by examination against the white background of a swab.

14. Which sexually transmitted infections are associated with gynecological cancers?

The STDs associated with gynecological cancer are HPV, HIV, HSV, hepatitis B virus infection.

SYPHILIS

15. What is the indication for retreatment in case of syphilis?

Treated women whose titer rise by four-fold (two dilutions) or who do not show a four-fold (two dilutions) decrease in titer over 3 months period, should be subjected to retreatment.

16. What is the most important diagnostic test for asymptomatic *Trichomonas vaginalis* infection?

Polymerase chain reaction (PCR) test is confirmative test for asymptomatic *Trichomonas vaginalis* infection.

17. What concentration of treponemes in tissue results in appearance of clinical lesions?

Clinical lesions appear when the concentration of *Treponema pallidum* is 107/g of tissue.

18. What is the most sensitive test for syphilis?

Venereal disease Research Laboratory test (VDRL) is the most sensitive test.

19. VDRL test becomes positive after how many days of appearance of lesions?

VDRL test becomes positive after 7 days of appearance of lesions.

20. What are the causes of false positive VDRL test?

False positive VDRL test reactions can be grouped into acute and chronic false positive reactions based on the duration of positivity and disease.
- *Causes of acute false positive (<6 months) reaction:*
  - Recent viral illness or immunization
  - Genital herpes
  - HIV infection
  - Malaria
  - Parenteral drug use
- *Causes of chronic false positive (>6 months) reaction:*
  - Aging
  - Autoimmune disease
  - Systemic lupus erythematosus (SLE)
  - Rheumatoid arthritis
  - Parenteral drug use.

21. When should VDRL test be requested during antenatal care?

VDRL test should be done at first prenatal visit. Women at high-risk of exposure should have a repeat test in the third trimester and at delivery.

22. What are the causes of painful genital ulcer?

Causes of painful genital ulcer are:
- Herpes simplex infection
- *H. ducreyi* infection
- Traumatic ulcer.

23. What are soft and hard chancre?

Hard chancre: These are painless, relatively avascular, circumscribed, indurated and superficially ulcerated lesions. Lesions are covered by thick, glairy exudates very rich in spirochetes. The regional lymph nodes will be swollen, discrete and non-tender.

Soft chancre 'Chancroid': These are tender, non-indurated, irregular, ulcerated lesions. The regional lymph nodes will be enlarged and painful. It is caused by *H. ducreyi.*

24. What are the different laboratory tests used in the work-up of case with syphilis?

Various tests used in the diagnosis and screening for syphilis are:
- Dark ground illumination (DGI)
- VDRL—Flocculation test; positive after 6 weeks of initial infection; screening test
- Complement fixation Wassermann test (PTI test)
- Specific tests
    - *Treponema pallidum* hemagglutination (TPHA)
    - *Treponema pallidum* immobilization test (TPI)
    - Fluorescent treponemal antibody absorption test (FTS-abs)
    - ELISA test for IgG or IgM
    - Immunoblotting and PCR—confirmatory and sensitive.

25. What are the effects of syphilis on pregnancy and fetus?

The syphilis may cause late abortion, preterm labor, congenital abnormalities and IUFD. The fetal effects include fetal ascites, placentomegaly hepatic dysfunction, anemia, thrombocytopenia and hydrops.

26. At which period of gestation do the maternal syphilis affect fetus and what are the influencing factors?

The spirochetes can cross placenta and infect the fetus from about 14–16 weeks of pregnancy and the risk of fetal infection increases with gestational age. The manifestations of congenital syphilis are influenced by gestational age, stage of maternal syphilis, maternal treatment, and immunological response of the fetus. Because of its immunocompetence prior to approximately 18 weeks, the fetus generally does not manifest the immunological inflammatory response characteristic of clinical disease before this time. Although transplacental transmission is the most common route, neonatal infection may follow after contact with spirochetes through lesions at delivery or across the membranes. Implication of this knowledge is appropriate and adequate treatment of the mother before 14th week of pregnancy should prevent fetal damage.

27. What are the manifestations of syphilis in newborn?

The syphilitic baby may appear normal at birth. It may develop weeks, months or years later mucocutaneous lesions, anemia, edema, maculopapular rash, pemphigus on soles and palms, purulent nasal discharge (hemorrhagic sometimes, hoarse cry, failure to thrive, pyrexia, and widespread osteochondritis).

28. What is the radiological evidence of congenital syphilis?

The radiological examination may reveal subperiosteal thickening and patchy rarefaction near the ends of the shaft.

29. How is syphilis treated?

The treatment schedules are the same as for nonpregnant adults (Table 34.1). The objectives of treatment in pregnancy are to eradicate the maternal and to prevent congenital syphilis. Parenteral Penicillin G remains the preferred treatment for all stages of disease in pregnancy.

Table 34.1: Recommended treatment for pregnant women with syphilis

Category	Treatment
Early syphilis (< 1-year duration)	Benzathine penicillin G, 2.4 million units intramuscular, single dose; some recommend a second dose 1 week later
Late syphilis (>1-year duration)	Benzathine penicillin G, 2.4 million units intramuscular, weekly for 3 doses
Neurosyphilis	Aqueous crystalline penicillin G, 3–4 million units intramuscular, every 4 hours for 10–14 days OR Aqueous procaine penicillin, 2.4 million units, intramuscular, daily and probenecid 500 mg orally 4-times a day, both for 10–14 days

Source: Centers for Disease Control and Prevention: Sexually Transmitted Diseases Treatment guidelines, 2006. MMWR 55:1

For treatment of congenital syphilis:
- Procaine penicillin 0.5 million units/kg body weight daily for 10 days or
- Benzathine penicillin 0.05 million units/kg body weight.

30. What is Jarisch-Herxheimer reaction?

This is a focal and systemic reaction which sometimes follows first dose of antisyphilitic treatment. It is attributed to the release of destructed and disintegrated treponema products.

31. What is the plan for follow-up of the cases treated for syphilis?

The follow-up in the treatment of syphilis is essential.
a. *Early syphilis*
   - First 6 months   Monthly
   - Next 18 months   3 monthly
   - After two years   If CSF analysis is negative, consider cure (Wassermann test; quantitative serological tests)

b. *Late syphilis*
- Initial   CSF - Wassermann
- After 1 year CSF - FTA-abs

c. *Neurosyphilis*
- 6 months   CSF – cell count
- 2 years   CSF – cell count

32. What is the alternative to penicillin treatment for syphilis in pregnancy?

There is no satisfactory alternative to penicillin for treating syphilis in pregnancy. If sensitive, desensitization should be done. Alternative drugs may not prevent congenital syphilis.

33. What is the impact of HIV infection on clinical manifestations of syphilis?

Infection with HIV increases chances of early CNS involvement. Morbidities due to neurosyphilis—meningitis, optic neuritis, deafness, etc. become all the more common. Necrotizing encephalitis is also seen. Concomitant HIV infection suppresses manifestations of secondary syphilis.

GONORRHEA

34. Which is the oldest known venereal disease? What is the causative organism?

Gonorrhea is the oldest known venereal disease described by Hippocrates as stannary in 400 BC. It is caused by *Neisseria gonorrhoea* which is a Gram-negative diplococci found intracellularly in groups of 4 to 8.

35. What is transmission rate between male and female?

The transmission rate of gonorrhea is 75% from male to female and 25% from female to male.

36. What are the symptoms and signs of gonorrhea?

The symptoms and signs of gonorrhea include:

1. Local	Asymptomatic (50%); in others symptoms pertaining to lower genital tract infections like urethritis, bartholinitis, vulvitis, skenitis, cystitis, proctitis, vaginitis, cervicitis; in some features of pharyngitis may occur
2. Pelvic infection	Salpingitis with tubo-ovarian abscess, menstrual irregularity, menorrhagia, dyspareunia, infertility
3. Metastatic	Arthritis, endocarditis, septicemia, perihepatitis

37. What is Fitz–Hugh–Curtis syndrome?

In gonococcal and chlamydia salpingitis, perihepatitis is reported in 5% cases. It is called Fitz-Hugh-Curtis syndrome.

38. How will you diagnose chronic gonorrhea?

The chronic gonorrhea is difficult to diagnose in the absence of positive history; positive gonococcal complement fixation test are of presumptive value.

39. Any precautions to be taken while collecting sample from endocervix to diagnose gonorrhea?

Collect the endocervical swab with the help of large cotton tipped swab containing calcium alginate or synthetic fibers as raw cotton or wood may be toxic to *Gonococcus*.

40. What is the most sophisticated method of diagnosing gonococcal infection?

Presence of *Gonococcus* without polymorphonuclear cells does not necessarily indicate gonococcal infection. Detection of gonococcal ribosomal RNA in the test specimen with the help of standard DNA probe is the most sophisticated with sensitivity as that of culture positivity and specificity of 99%.

41. What is the primary site of infection of gonorrhea in women?

In women with uterus, the primary infection occurs in endocervix; in women after hysterectomy, urethra is the primary site for infection.

42. What is the most common presentation of disseminated gonococcal infection?

Acute asymmetric polyarthritis and dermatitis are the common presentations.

43. Which are the investigations to be carried out in a case suspected to have gonorrheal infection?

The following investigations are advised to confirm gonorrhea:
- Smear
  - Acute phase   Reliable
  - Chronic phase   10%
- Culture (combined urethral and cervical culture)—97%
- Complement fixation test—positive after ten weeks
- Fluorescent test—specific.

44. What are the treatment regimens followed to treat gonococcal infection?

A recommendation for treatment of gonococcal infection during pregnancy is as under:

a. Uncomplicated gonococcal infections

Ceftriaxone, 125 mg intramuscularly as a single dose
or
Cefixime, 400 mg orally in a single dose
or
Spectinomycin, 2 g intramuscularly as a single dose
plus
Treatment for chlamydial infection unless it is excluded

Source: Centers for Disease Control and Prevention: Sexually Transmitted Diseases Treatment Guidelines, 2006. MMWR 55:1

b. In complicated disseminated gonococcal infection

Ceftriaxone, 1 g intramuscularly or intravenously daily
or
Cefixime, 1 g intravenously, every 8 hours

c. In patients allergic to beta-lactam drugs

Ciprofloxacin (500 mg IV q 12h)
or
Ofloxacin (400 mg IV q 12h)
or
Spectinomycin (2 g IM q 12h)

d. Continuation therapy

Cefixime (400 mg orally, twice daily)
or
Ciprofloxacin (500 mg orally, twice daily)
or
Ofloxacin (400 mg orally, twice daily)

45. What is the test of cure for gonococcal infection?

Three negative smears at weekly interval is considered as indicative of permanent cure.

46. What are the effects of gonorrhea on pregnancy?

Gonorrhea may result in prelabor rupture of membranes, gonococcal ophthalmia neonatorum (causing blindness), postpartum endometritis.

CHLAMYDIAL INFECTION

Chlamydia trachomatis is an obligate intracellular bacterium. It is not stable outside the cells. If untreated chlamydia infection can persist for years without much discomfort. One out of 10 infected will be symptomatic of infection. Highest rate of infection is found in sexually active adolescents.

47. What are the available tools for diagnosing chlamydia infection?

Direct and indirect means of diagnosis of chlamydia infection are:
- *Direct:*
  - Isolation in a tissue culture medium
  - 80–90% sensitive in expert laboratories.
- *Indirect:*
  - Direct fluorescent antibody detection—sensitivity 80%, specificity 97–98%
  - Enzyme immunoassay
  - DNA probe (ii, iii less efficient than i)
  - PCR very sensitive test on urine specimen.

48. Which specimen is collected for mass screening program for chlamydia?

Testing first catch urine specimen of high-risk population is used in screening.

49. What is the incubation period for infection with *Chlamydia trachomatis*?

The incubation period of *Chlamydia trachomatis* is 7–14 days.

50. What are the clinical features of chlamydia infection?

In 75% cases, the infection is asymptomatic. The symptoms of chlamydia infection include dysuria, dyspareunia, post-coital bleeding, and intermenstrual bleeding. The findings include mucopurulent cervical discharge, cervical edema, ectopy and friability.

51. What are the effects of chlamydial infection?

Chlamydial infection is an ascending infection causing endometritis, salpingitis, and PID. It leads to infertility, and may result in ectopic pregnancies. It is also associated with Fitz-Hugh–Curtis syndrome.

52. Which antimicrobials are effective against chlamydial infection?

The following antimicrobials are used for the treatment of chlamydia:
- *Tetracycline:* 500 mg 4 times a day × 7–14 days *or*
- *Erythromycin:* 500 mg 4 times a day × 7–14 days *or*
- *Doxycycline:* 100 mg 2 times a day × 7–14 day *or*
- *Azithromycin:* 1 g orally single dose
- The treatment of sexual partner is necessary.

BACTERIAL VAGINOSIS

53. What is bacterial vaginosis?

It is not actual vaginal infection but a rather a clinical syndrome resulting from replacement of normal H_2O_2 producing lactobacilli with anaerobic bacteria.

54. What are the organisms involved in bacterial vaginosis?

The organisms involved in bacterial vaginosis are *Gardnerella vaginalis, Prevotella*, Molrilencucess, *Mycoplasma hominis*—to name a few.

HERPES VIRUS INFECTION

55. Which organism causes Herpes genitalis?

The Herpes genitalis is caused by Herpes simplex viruses (type 1 and 2). The incubation period is 3–6 days, about 80% lesions are caused by type 2 HSV.

56. How do Herpes genitalis present?

Vesicles appear on an erythematous base. The Herpes genitalis starts with red painful inflamed area over clitoris, labia, vestibule, vagina, cervix and perineum. The lesions progress to shallow ulcer and heal up by crusting. There may be fever, malaise, dysuria or retention of urine with enlarged tender inguinal lymph nodes.

57. What are different types of HSV infection?

The different HSV infections are:
a. Primary   – No prior infection
b. Non-primary   – First episode of HSV-2
                          – Previous HSV-1 then HSV-2
c. Recurrent   – Previous HSV-1 or 2 infection
                          – Repeated infection.

58. How is the diagnosis of HSV infection confirmed?

The diagnosis, is confirmed by:
- Tissue culture   – 95% sensitive
- Tzanck smear   – Alcohol fixation and Pap smear; 70% sensitive
- PCR   – Highly sensitive
- Viral detection   – ELISA or immunofluorescence

59. What are the problems associated with of HSV infection?

The problems associated with HSV infection are:
- Cervical dysplasia and cancer
- Adverse effect on pregnancy—abortion, preterm labor
- Antenatal fetal infection   –5%
- Perinatal transmission   –85%
  - Primary   50%
  - Recurrent   5%
- Effect on babies
  - Postnatal infection   10%
  - Localized   skin, eye, mouth (45%)
  - CNS   encephalitis (3%)
  - Disseminated disease   (25%)

60. What is the prognosis of babies affected by herpes virus?

The prognosis is determined by antiviral therapy.
a. *With antiviral therapy:* CNS involvement and disseminated—20–50%
  - Disseminated   30% mortality
  - Localized   Good

b. *Without antiviral therapy*
  - In disseminated infection   Mortality 90%
                                           Mental retardation 90%
  - Localized   Mortality 17%
                                           Morbidity 40%

61. What are the recommended principles of management for HSV disease?

The principles of management for Herpes simplex virus disease are:
- Antenatal   Start antiviral treatment from 36 weeks of pregnancy
- Mode of delivery   Cesarean delivery is recommended in active lesion, reduces perinatal risk by 85%
- Intrapartum   Vaginal delivery, if no active lesions; antiviral therapy after rupture of membranes suggested
- Postnatal   Good hygiene; no separation from mother or other neonates; no constraints on breastfeeding

62. What are the different ways the HSV infection can be treated?

The antiviral drugs used are inhibitors of DNA synthesis. Different ways the antiviral treatment is delivered to a woman with HSV infection are:
- Acyclovir
  - Oral   200 mg 5 times a day × 7 day
  - Local   5% tropical cream
  - Intravenous   5 mg/kg 8 hourly
- Valacyclovir   Orally, 500 mg BD × 7 days
- Famciclovir   Orally, 125 mg BD × 7 days.

63. Is there any vaccine against HSV infection?

The vaccine prepared from an HSV-2 glycoprotein is in use. D subunit is effective against seronegative. Claimed to be 75% effective against HSV I and II.

HUMAN PAPILLOMAVIRUS INFECTION

64A. What are genital warts?

The genital wart or condyloma acuminata are papillary genital lesions caused by human papillomavirus, types I and II in 90% cases, and HPV types 16, 18 and 31 are incriminated in 10% of cases. Women usually present with itching, vaginal discharge and vaginal pain. The warts are usually multiple with small stalk and cauliflower like growth and can cover whole vagina. They may spread up to cervix. Malignancy is rare in them.

64B. What are the vaccines used and their efficacy?
i. Bivalent vaccine cervarix with dosage schedule as given at 0,1, 6 months between the age of 9 and 25 years before the commencement of sexual activity. It is effective against HPV types 16,18 with an efficacy of 70–90% in seronegative individuals in preventing carcinoma cervix.
ii. Quadrivalent vaccine Gardasil-effective against HPV 16, 18, 6, 11. Hence, it provides protection against genital warts also.
   - It is given at 0, 2, 6 months
   - Dose 0.5 mL IM

These are contraindicated during pregnancy.

65. What are the clinical problems associated with HPV infection?

The problems associated with HPV infection are:
a. Oncogenesis HPV 16, 18, 31 can initiate carcinoma of cervix, vagina, vulva, anus
b. Outlet obstruction during delivery and severe hemorrhage
c. Laryngeal papilloma in infant and children
d. Poor episiotomy healing.

66. What are the different physical treatments offered for genital wart?

There are several treatment options available for management of genital warts. There is no single effective cure for their removal. Genital warts may go remit spontaneously in 10–20% of cases over a period of three to four months.

Cryotherapy: It is an excellent first-line treatment. The response rates are high with few side effects. The technique uses liquid nitrogen to freeze the wart.

Laser treatment: Destroys the HPV-induced lesions. It is used for extensive or recurrent genital warts. It may require local, regional, or general anesthesia. The disadvantages include increased healing time, scarring, and cost. The laser plume has the potential to let infectious viral particles in the air.

Electrodesiccation: Destroys the warts. It can be performed under local anesthesia. The resulting smoke fumes may be infectious.

67. What are the medications used for treating genital warts?

Several medications exist for treating genital warts and can be used as an alternative to other treatments.

Podophyllum resin	– It is topically applied
Podofilox	– Topically applied; has a higher cure rate than podophyllum resin is also useful for prevention contraindicated in first trimester as it is absorbed in circulation and is cytotoxic causing abortion and peripheral neuropathy
25% trichloroacetic acid or bichloracetic acid	– Topically applied; the response is often incomplete and recurrence is higher; may cause pain and burning
5% 5-fluorouracil	– Applied as a cream; has a long-treatment time; can cause burning and irritation
Interferon alpha-n3	– As cream or injectable; for refractory cases; has many side effects
Imiquimod	– Applied as a cream; local skin irritation is a common side effect.

The sexual partner should be treated. The biopsy and Pap smear should be taken.

68. What are the options for treatment of genital warts in pregnancy?

Spontaneous regression of warts after pregnancy is not uncommon. Hence, all warts in pregnancy may not need treatment. In pregnancy, the options for management of significant lesions are:
- BCA or TCA
- Cryotherapy
- Laser
- Diathermy.

TRICHOMONIASIS

69. Is trichomoniasis an STD?

Yes. Trichomoniasis accounts for 20–30% of vulvovaginitis and is an STD. Rate of transmission after single contact from woman to man is 70%, and that from man to woman is even higher.

70. What is the causative organism?

It is caused by *Trichomonas vaginalis*, a motile anerobic protozoan. Bacterial vaginosis is associated in 60% of cases.

71. What are the diagnostic features in a patient with trichomoniasis?

Trichomoniasis may be asymptomatic. Most common symptom is vaginal discharge.

- *Symptoms:*
  - Vaginal discharge—profuse, frothy, yellowish-greenish, malodorous
  - Vulval pruritus
- *Signs:*
  - Strawberry spots on cervix
  - Patch erythema of vagina
  - Postoperative cuff cellulitis may be seen in patients after hysterectomy.
- Investigations with discharge
  - Vaginal pH   > 5
  - Microscopy   Motile trichomonas; increase in leukocytes; Clue cell may be found when associated with bacterial vaginosis
  - Whiff test   May be positive

72. What is the treatment of *Trichomonas vaginalis*?

The following drugs are used for treatment of *Trichomonas vaginalis*.

- Metronidazole 200 mg orally 3 times a day × 7 days *or* 2 gm orally single dose
- Tinidazole 300 mg orally twice a day × 7 days *or* 2 gm orally single dose
- Secnidazole 100 mg orally once a day × 2 days
- Ornidazole 1.5 gm orally once a day × 5 days *or* 500 mg orally twice a day × 5 days

Partner treatment is necessary; use of condoms or abstinence is suggested.

73. How will you treat *Trichomonas vaginalis* in pregnancy?

The treatment of *Trichomonas vaginalis* infection in first trimester is best avoided.

Vinegar douche to lower pH and betadine gel for vaginal application may be used.

In second half of pregnancy, metronidazole treatment may be given. Teratogenic and mutagenic effects are not noted in fetuses.

74. What are the effects of *Trichomonas vaginalis* in pregnancy?

Trichomonas vaginalis infection may cause PROM, preterm labor, and LBW babies.

CANDIDIASIS

75. What is candidiasis?

The vulvovaginal candidiasis is caused by *Candida albicans*. Other candida species that affect are *C. glabrata* and *C. tropicalis*.

76. What is combination substance?

It is the resistance of growth of opportunistic fungi by lactobacillus.

77. What are the diagnostic features of candidiasis?

The features of vulvovaginal candidiasis are typical.
- *Symptoms:*
  - Vaginal discharge watery to homogeneously thick, curdy white
  - Vaginal sourness, dyspareunia, vulvar burning, irritation and external dysuria
- *Signs:*
  - Labia   Erythema and edema of labia; skin edema; pustule-papular peripheral lesions
  - Vagina   Edematous with adherent whitish discharge
- Cervix—normal
- *Investigations:*
  - pH of vagina   Normal
  - Microscopy   Fungus present
  - Whiff test   Negative
  - Fungal culture

78. What are the treatment regimens available for candidiasis?

The general treatment of candidiasis includes:
- Nystatin   1,00,000 units vaginally × 10–14 day
                  or
                  5,00,000 unit orally
- Imidazole derivatives
  - Miconazole   100 mg
  - Clotrimazole Vaginal pessaries/1% vaginal cream × 7 days
  - Terconazole   Vaginal cream or pessary
  - Ticonazole
  - Fluconazole   150 mg stat and repeat after 1 week; in recurrent cases, it can be repeated after 3 days; thereafter weekly for 6 months
  - Ketoconazole 400 mg/day until symptoms disappear.

CHANCROID

Chancroid, also known as 'soft sore' is caused by Gram-negative *Streptobacillus, Haemophilus ducreyi*.

79. How does a case with chancroid present?

The chancroids begin as a small tender papule with surrounding erythema that rapidly becomes pustular and then erodes to form an extremely painful and deep ulcer with soft-ragged margins. The ulcer base is composed of easily friable granulation tissue that is usually covered with malodorous yellow-gray exudates. Ulcers may be single or multiple varying in size from 1 to 20 mm, with 1-2 cm.

The lesions most commonly are found on the fourchette, labia, vestibule, clitoris, cervix, and anus.

Painful, usually unilateral, regional lymphadenopathy occurs in 50% of patients and 25% may progress to a suppurative bubo, which may rupture spontaneously and ulcerate. If untreated, chronic draining sinuses may follow.

80. What are the different types of chancroids?

The different types of chancroids are:
- *Transient chancroid:* Ulcer resolves in 4-6 days; suppurative lymphadenitis follows 10-20 days later.
- *Dwarf chancroid:* Manifests as one or several herpes like ulcerations, with or without inguinal lymphadenopathy.
- *Follicular chancroid:* Ulcerations of the pilar apparatus in hair-bearing areas.
- *Giant chancroid:* Multiple small ulcerations, which coalesce to form a single large lesion.

81. How will you confirm diagnosis of chancroid?

The chancroid is diagnosed by culturing *H ducreyi*.

82. What is the treatment for chancroid?

Patients suspected or diagnosed to have chancroid should undergo complete evaluation for other possible concomitant STDs and receive appropriate antimicrobial therapy for the eradication of *H. ducreyi* and the treatment of other more common STDs.

As per the recommendations by CDC, antibiotic therapy from any of the following agents is equally efficacious:
- Azithromycin—1 g orally (PO) as a single dose *or*
- Ceftriaxone—250 mg intramuscularly as a single dose *or*
- Erythromycin base—500 mg PO 3 times daily for 7 days *or*
- Ciprofloxacin —500 mg PO twice daily for 3 days
- Ceftriaxone is the treatment of choice in pregnant women.

Fluctuant lymph nodes may be drained by either needle aspiration or incision.
The partner should be treated.

LYMPHOGRANULOMA VENEREUM

83. What is lymphogranuloma venereum?

Lymphogranuloma venereum (LGV) is a sexually transmitted bacterial infection caused by *L. serotype* of *Chlamydia trachomatis*.

84. How will the lesion in LGV present?

The presentation of lesions in LGV varies according to their stage.
- Primary LGV (1st stage) begins as a small, painless papule or pustule that may erode to form a small, asymptomatic herpetiform ulcer that usually heals rapidly without scarring. The most common sites of infection include the posterior vaginal wall, posterior cervix, fourchette, and vulva. They often go unnoticed by the patient.
- Secondary LGV (2nd stage) consists of painful regional lymphadenopathy (usually in the inguinal and/or femoral lymph nodes); these coalesce to form buboes, which may rupture and those that do not rupture harden, then to resolve slowly; symptoms include fever, chills, myalgias, and malaise. Systemic spread may lead to arthritis, ocular inflammatory disease, cardiac involvement, pulmonary involvement, aseptic meningitis, hepatitis or perihepatitis.
- Tertiary LGV (3rd stage) is also termed as genitoanorectal syndrome which is characterized by proctocolitis.

85. What are the complications of LGV?

The complications of LGV include:
- Vulval elephantiasis
- Perineal scarring and dyspareunia
- Rectal stricture, sinus and fistula formation.

86. How will you diagnose LGV?

The diagnosis is mainly based on clinical findings. Confirmation is made by:
- Culture-needle aspiration of an involved bubo is the best method to obtain tissue for culture of *C. trachomatis*
- Compliment fixation test titers greater than 1:64, when coupled with the appropriate clinical scenario, is considered diagnostic of LGV
- Immunofluorescent testing with monoclonal antibodies and polymerase chain reaction (PCR) are also reported to be effective; however, these tests are not widely available for commercial use
- Nucleic acid amplification tests (NAAT) used to identify the presence of *Chlamydia* in urine demonstrated an increased sensitivity and specificity.

87. How will you treat LGV?

- The treatment of LGV involves drainage of infected buboes and appropriate antimicrobials
- Any of the following antimicrobials—Doxycycline 100 mg orally, twice daily, 21 days *or* Erythromycin 500 mg orally, 6 hourly, 21 days
- Partner treatment, if asymptomatic, should involve either Doxycycline 100 mg orally, twice daily, 7 days *or* Azithromycin 1 g, single dose

- Abscesses are aspirated and not excised
- If there are strictures dilatation may be required.

GRANULOMA INGUINALE

Granuloma inguinale (GI) is a chronic progressive disease usually involving vagina or cervix caused by Gram-negative bacillus of *Klebsiella* species, *Donovania granulomatis*.

88. How do patients with granuloma inguinale present?

The cutaneous lesions may appear as:
- *Nodular lesion:* A papule or nodule that arises at the site; nodule will be soft, often pruritic and erythematous; it eventually ulcerates; it may be mistaken for a lymph node (pseudobubo).
- *Ulcerovegetative lesion:* These develop from nodular lesions and consist of large, usually painless, expanding, suppurative ulcers; ulcers will have friable bases with distinct, raised, rolled margins with a tendency to bleed easily; ulcers are "beefy red" and slowly expand centrifugally, eventually becoming more granulomatous with serpiginous borders.
- *Cicatricial lesion:* Dry ulcers may become cicatricial plaques and may be associated with lymphedema.
- *Hypertrophic or verrucous lesion:* It is a proliferative reaction, with the formation of large vegetation resembling genital warts.

89. How is the diagnosis of GI confirmed?

Although isolation of *Klebsiella granulomatis* has been reported, the organism is difficult to culture in most laboratories.
- Biopsy-smear is made, stained with Geimsa and confirmed by demonstration of Donovan bodies—plasma cells with rod-shaped cytoplasmic inclusion bodies (Mikulicz cell)
- Polymerase chain reaction techniques—may be more sensitive; however, they are currently only used for scientific research.
- Indirect immunofluorescent technique is available to test serum; however, it is not accurate enough for confirmatory diagnosis.

90. What is the treatment for GI?

The recommended antibiotic for granuloma inguinale is either trimethoprim/sulfamethoxazole or doxycycline.
- Alternatives include ciprofloxacin, erythromycin, or azithromycin.
- The antibiotic should be given for at least a 3-week course and continued until reepithelialization of the ulcer occurs and any signs of the disease have resolved.
- Use of sulfonamides, doxycycline and ciplofloxacin is a relative contraindication during pregnancy.

Once the GI lesions are healed, the disfiguring genital swellings may require surgical correction. Excision and in some cases vulvectemy is performed.

VIRAL HEPATITIS

91. What are the effects of pregnancy on hepatitis B infection?

The course of hepatitis B infection is not affected by pregnancy in developed countries. Fulminant hepatitis may occasionally occur.

92. What are the effects of hepatitis B infection on pregnancy and neonate?

Risk of preterm delivery is increased. The hepatitis B transmission through placenta is rare. Ingestion of infected material during delivery and neonatal period may transmit the disease. The breastmilk may also transmit. The infant may be asymptomatic or may develop fulminant disease.

93. What is the recommendation for neonatal prophylaxis?

The immunoprophylaxis recommended for neonates mothers with hepatitis B infection varies according to maternal antigen status (Table 34.2).

Table 34.2: Neonatal immunization schedule against hepatitis B infection

Maternal HBsAg status	Vaccine and schedule	
	HBVV	HBIG
Positive	10 mcg, IM/Birth—12 hour, 1 month, 6 month	5 mL, IM/ Birth-12 hour
Unknown	10 mcg, IM/Birth—12 hour, 1 month, 6 month	5 mL, IM/ Birth-12 hour
Negative	10 mcg, IM/Before discharge, 1 month, 6 month	–

Abbreviations: HBVV, hepatitis B virus vaccine; HBIG, hepatitis B immunoglobin

Pregnant woman suspected of having been exposed to Hepatitis B Virus (HBV) should be treated with HBIG and inoculated with HBV vaccine. This therapy is safe and effective in pregnancy.

94. Is universal screening of pregnant woman for HBsAg necessary?

The universal screening of pregnant women for HbSAg is necessary. The vertical transmission is 10% with negative HBeAg. Rate of neonatal infection in the absence of prophylaxis and vaccination may be up to 40%.

95. What are the chances of fetal/neonatal affection in a maternal acute infection in pregnancy?

The degree of fetal affection increases as the duration of pregnancy increases:
- 1st trimester   rare
- 2nd trimester   6%
- 3rd trimester   67%
- Perinatal period   100%

96. Can the mother with hepatitis B infection handle the baby and breastfeed?

The mother with hepatitis B infection can handle the baby and she can also breastfeed once the immunoprophylaxis is begun.

97. What is the rate of vertical transmission from a mother with hepatitis C infection?

Maternal-to-fetal transmission rate of hepatitis C infection is reported to be up to 18%. Perinatal transmission is more when the titer is more than 1 million copies per mL.

MUST REMEMBER

- Sexually transmitted infections are transmitted predominantly through sexual intercourse with infected partner.
- Syphilis, gonorrhea, Chancroid, Lymphogranuloma venerum are the classical venereal diseases.
- Cervicitis is usually caused by *Chlamydia trachomatis* and *Neisseria gonorrhoea*. Both are sexually transmitted infections.
- Infections of vagina are Bacterial vaginosis, Trichomonas vaginitis and Candidal vaginitis.
- Bacterial vaginosis and Trichomonas vaginitis are treated with metronidazole. Candidial vaginitis is treated with intravaginal azole or oral fluconazole.
- Early diagnosis and management are crucial in preventing sequelae, the WHO has recommended syndromic approach.
- Counseling and treatment of partners regarding safe sex and use of condom is mandatory.

Abnormal Uterine Bleeding

Pralhad Kushtagi, Raina Chawla

Normal menstrual bleeding is considered to occur cyclically every 28 days (range 21–35 days), with the flow lasting for 4 days (range 2–7 days), resulting in a blood loss of 35 mL (range 10–80 mL) per cycle. Any deviation from the attributes of normalcy-cycle length, cyclicity, duration and/or amount of flow is considered as abnormal uterine bleeding (AUB).

HISTORY

Menstrual

a. Cyclicity—cycle length, regularity (preferably exact dates over 3–4 cycles)
   - if irregular, presence of pre- or postmenstrual spotting
   - if acyclic, postcoital bleeding
b. Flow—amount (change of diapers/pads in a day; if heavy, need for change at night, passage of clots). This information will help to know the pattern of bleeding (Table 35.1).

Presence of postcoital, acyclical or contact bleeding would indicate lesion on or in the cervix and/or vagina like cancer of cervix or vagina, erosion or ulcer on cervix, atrophic vaginitis.

c. Last menstrual period and exposure to pregnancy is important. With a sudden change from a regular menstrual history to abnormal bleeding pattern, pregnancy related causes are a possibility.

Anovulatory bleeding is typically non-cyclical with an unpredictable pattern ranging from prolonged bouts of spotting to outright hemorrhage. Conversely, predictable cyclic menses, especially with premenstrual molimina (suggestive of progesterone secretion) provides the possibility that a woman is ovulating.

Associated Problems

a. *Lower abdominal pain (dysmenorrhea):*
   - In relation to menstruation—before, during, after and midcycle
   - Intensity—vague, increasing with each cycle.
     Anovular DUB is usually painless. Congestive dysmenorrhea is associated with endometriosis and pelvic inflammatory disease. Spasmodic type is suffered by adolescents where no cause is found and also the women with submucous fibroid and those using intrauterine device. Patients with endometriosis may have progressive dysmenorrhea.
b. Dyspareunia is a common accompaniment with endometriosis and pelvic inflammatory disease.

Table 35.1: Patterns of abnormal uterine bleeding and their causes

Cycle length	Bleeding	Pattern	Cause(s)
Normal	Prolonged/excessive	Menorrhagia	Fibroids, adenomyosis, tuberculosis, endometrial dysfunction
Normal	Reduced	Hypomenorrhea	Tuberculosis, endometrial dysfunction
Shortened	Normal	Polymenorrhea	Pelvic inflammatory disease, endometriosis, endometrial dysfunction
Shortened	Excessive	Polymenorrhagia	
Prolonged	Normal/reduced	Oligomenorrhea	Polycystic ovarian syndrome, DUB, tuberculosis, long-acting progestins
Acyclical	Irregular, may be excessive	Metrorrhagia	Ulcer/growth on cervix, carcinoma–cervix/uterus/ovary, irregular ovarian hormone intake
Normal	Spotting	Premenstrual spotting; menorrhagia	(Irregular ripening) corpus luteum deficiency
Normal	Spotting	Postmenstrual spotting; menorrhagia	(Irregular shedding) Prolonged corpus luteum activity

c. Symptoms/features/indicators suggestive of:
   - Hypothyroidism
   - Bleeding diathesis
   - Tuberculosis.

Other Attributes

a. Age—some causes are more common in some age groups. In reproductive age group, pregnancy related and causes secondary to pelvic infection are more common. DUB will be the consideration in extremes of ages. However, one needs to exclude blood dyscrasias and endocrine-mediated etiologies in adolescents. In perimenopausal and women of later age, emphasis should be in excluding genital malignancies (Table 35.2).
b. Parity—adenomyosis and cancer cervix are more common in women with high parity, while fibroid, endometriosis and endometrial hyperplasia/cancer are associated with low parity.
c. Contraceptive use—IUCD, ovarian steroidal hormones.
d. Other drug use—exogeneous ovarian steroidal hormones, anticoagulants and salicylates.

1. What is dysfunctional uterine bleeding?

Dysfunctional uterine bleeding (DUB) is best defined as an abnormal uterine bleeding due to disorder in the endocrinal mechanisms of menstruation or physiological mechanisms responsible for arrest of menstruation. It is an abstract definition and the diagnosis of the entity is by process of exclusion of the causes of abnormal uterine bleeding. The working definition considered by many is 'abnormal uterine bleeding not due to organic disease or the iatrogenic cause'. The usage of the diagnosis as DUB is being discontinued since the hypothalamopituitary-ovarian (HPO) axis or endometrial dysfunction may coexist with the identifiable causes for AUB. Thus, it is thought to be more explicit to indicate the problem as AUB and specify whether it is due to ovulatory dysfunction (AUB-O) or endometrial cause (AUB-E). These causes may also be operating in a patient with fibroid uterus, adenomyosis, thyroid dysfunction and the like.

2. Can the terms 'menorrhagia' and 'heavy menstrual bleeding' be used interchangeably?

The patterns of the bleeding like menorrhagia, polymenorrhagia or a situation where the woman is having episode of continuous uterine bleeding—all lead to excessive blood loss. All such menstrual patterns could be grouped under 'heavy menstrual bleeding (HMB)'. Usage of this term will signify severity of the symptom and necessitate prompt attention.

3. Is there a basis for classification of AUB based on its onset?

It is necessary to triage to decide on which condition requires immediate attention to the symptom.
- *Acute AUB* is an episode of heavy bleeding that in the opinion of the clinician is of sufficient quantity to require immediate attention to prevent further blood loss.
- *Chronic AUB* is defined as bleeding from the uterine corpus that is abnormal in volume, regularity and/or timing and has been present for the majority of the past 6 months. Chronic AUB would not, in the opinion of the clinician require immediate attention and the etiology is meticulously looked into.
- *Intermenstrual AUB (IMB)* occurs between clearly defined cyclic and predictable menses. This terminology is preferred over the use of word 'metrorrhagia'.

4. Ovulation indicates functioning hypothalamo-pituitary-ovarian axis. Then despite ovulation why do some women have abnormal uterine bleeding?

The mechanism of AUB in ovulatory and anovulatory states is not fully understood. It is likely that local endometrial

Table 35.2: Causes of abnormal uterine bleeding in order of their occurrence in different age groups (years)

<20 years of age	20–40 years of age	>40 years of age
Coagulation defects	Pregnancy states	Ovulatory defects
Endocrinal defects	Infections	Malignancy and hyperplasia
Ovulatory defects	Polyp, leiomyoma, adenomyosis, endometriosis	Iatrogenic
Infections (Tuberculosis)	Coagulation defects	Polyp, leiomyoma, adenomyosis
Endometriosis	Endocrinal defects	Infections
Iatrogenic	Iatrogenic	Systemic (e.g. chronic liver/renal diseases)
Pregnancy states	Ovulatory defects	Endocrinal defects
Malignancy	Malignancy and hyperplasia	Coagulation defects

mechanisms are important in the pathophysiology of AUB. These local mechanisms probably involve uterine vasculature possibly influenced by prostaglandins and other vasoactive substances, altered mechanism of hemostasis, and changes in the process of tissue breakdown and remodeling. The influence of ovarian steroids upon these processes is likely to be indirect. Apart from the local menostatic mechanism, it is the function and longevity of corpus luteum that results in abnormal uterine bleeding (AUB) patterns.

5. What could be the mechanism for anovulatory AUB?

Menstrual cycles become irregular because of unopposed estrogen production and absence of progesterone withdrawal which leads to endometrial proliferation and eventual erratic breakdown. Estrogen may also stimulate excessive endothelial production of nitric oxide in endometrium.

6. Specify local endometrial mechanisms implicated in AUB?

The mechanisms considered could be grouped as vasculature related, due to vasoactive substances, and abnormalities of tissue breakdown and remodeling.

- Vasculature—morphometric analysis of uterine spiral arteriole density has shown no correlation with mean blood loss, but myometrial venous density can be increased in AUB-E. However, it can be functional rather than anatomical changes in the endometrial vasculature that are mainly responsible for excessive menstrual bleeding.
- Vasoactive substances—prostaglandins, endothelins and nitric oxide are the substances that could have a role in hemostasis.
    - *Prostaglandins:* AUB-E is associated with a shift in the ratio of endometrial vasocostricting PGF2α to vasodilatory PGE2 and an increase in endometrial concentration of prostaglandins. In persistently proliferative endometrium seen in AUB-O, the availability of arachidonic acid is reduced and prostaglandin synthesis is impaired. Endometrial tissues could be more responsive to the action of vasodilatory prostaglandins in AUB.
    - *Endothelins:* Receptors for endothelins are predominantly located at the endomyometrial junction and are present in increased concentration just before the menstruation. Sentinel estradiol and progesterone reduce receptor concentrations.
    - *Nitric oxide (endothelium derived relaxing factor):* Factors which modulate the synthesis and action of nitric oxide could lead to an increase in menstrual bleeding and might be an important mechanism in anovulatory bleeding.
- Abnormalities of tissue breakdown and remodeling may contribute to changes in the quantity and quality of menstrual loss. Endometrial breakdown and repair are largely controlled by local factors like lysosomes, matrix metalloproteinases, intercellular adhesion molecules, macrophages and other migratory leukocytes.
    - *Lysosomes:* Tissue hypoxia following spiral artery coiling and endometrial regression and vascular stasis stimulates lysosomal activation. Lysosomal enzyme activity in the endometrium is increased in women with ovulatory cycles but yet having AUB and that secondary to use of intrauterine devices.
    - *Matrix metalloproteinases* are a highly regulated enzymes that can degrade most components of extracellular matrix and are expressed cyclically consistent with ovarian steroid hormones. Menstruation is associated with change in balance between expression of these substances and their tissue inhibitors leading to tissue degradation.
    - *Macrophages and other migratory leukocytes* are increased premenstrually. Macrophages contain lysosomes and can release platelet activating factor and PGE2 that augment menstrual bleeding. Mast cells degranulate premenstrually to secrete heparin, histamine and other vasoactive substances. In cases with AUB, endometrial secretion of heparin-like substances is increased.
    - *Intercellular adhesion molecules and platelet:* Endothelial adhesion molecules are thought to control binding of leukocytes to endothelial cells and breakdown, these bonds may contribute to AUB.
- Endometrial repair and regeneration seem to be governed by local factors like cytokines through neutrophil chemotaxis, epithelial regeneration through vascular endothelial growth factor and endometrial hemostasis through balanced fibrinolysis. Over activation of the fibrinolytic system may unbalance the hemostatic system, causing early breakdown of thrombi in the endometrial vessels and excessive blood loss.

7. If there is a detectable fibroid, can the patient have AUB other than due to fibroid?

Fibroid, like AUB due to ovulatory dysfunction, like anovulation, is a result of hyperestrenic condition. Cervical, broad ligament and subserous fibroids do not produce menstrual abnormality through structural changes in uterus. AUB in such conditions could be due to dysfunction in endometrial hemostasis. Studies on myomata related bleeding suggest that it is not the increased surface area of the endometrium or local compression of vessels that causes bleeding. Nor does it seem that myomas have any effect on the hypothalamic pituitary ovarian axis. Instead the likely cause of the problem appears to be growth factor dysregulation causing uterine vascular dysfunction.

8. If a patient of uterine prolapse without decubitus ulceration has AUB, how to explain the cause for bleeding?

Apart from the obvious decubitus ulceration and vascular erosion, pelvic congestion in the early stages of prolapse following altered uterine and ovarian circulation (venous congestion) due to anatomic change may influence ovarian steroidogenesis and cause AUB. In the menopausal older age group, estatrophy could result in AUB.

9. What are the structural causes of AUB?

The structural causes of AUB are enlisted under the acronym 'PALM' by the new FIGO classification (Fig. 35.1) and these can most often be measured visually with imaging techniques and/or histopathology. The included causes are:

- *Polyp (AUB-P)*: These are proliferations of the endometrium or the endocervix and consist of varying amounts of vascular, glandular, fibromuscular and connective tissue. These are generally benign conditions with a few having atypical or malignant components. In the classification system, polyps are categorized as being either present or absent and are diagnosed by imaging (ultrasonography/hysteroscopy) or histopathology.
- *Adenomyosis (AUB-A)*: The presence of heterotopic endometrial tissue in the myometrium and the resulting myometrial hypertrophy is the main feature in adenomyosis and is also the basis behind its diagnosis by imaging (USG/MRI).
- *Leiomyoma (AUB-L)*: These are benign fibromuscular tumors. They vary in size and location (submucosal, intramural, subserous or a combination of these) and though many are asymptomatic, they are known to cause AUB. Leiomyomas, due to their spectrum of size and location have a separate classification system.
- *Malignancy and hyperplasia (AUB-M)*: Endometrial hyperplasia and malignancy are important causes of AUB and more common beyond 40 years. Both come under the category AUB-M.

10. Using FIGO classification system for AUB, how is presence of leiomyoma (fibroid) documented?

Leiomyomas are documented with three notations—primary, secondary and tertiary (Fig. 35.2).

- Primary notation reflects only the presence or absence of 1 or more leiomyomas, regardless of their

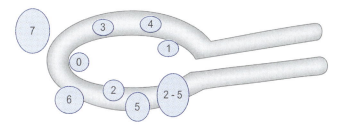

SM-submucous	0	Pedunculated intracavitary
	1	<50% intramural
	2	≥50% intramural
O-Others	3	Contacts endometrium, 100% intramural
	4	Intramural
	5	Subserosal ≥50% intramural
	6	Subserosal <50% intramural
	7	Subserosal pedunculated
	8	Others (specify, e.g. cervical, parasitic)
Hybrid leiomyomas (impact both myometrium and serosa)		Two numbers are listed separated by a hyphen. By convention, the first refers to the relationship with the endometrium while the second refers to the relationship with the serosa. One example is as shown below (and in the figure)
	2-5	Submucosal and subserosal, each with less than half the diameter in the endometrial and peritoneal cavity, respectively

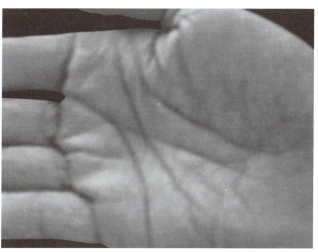

P Polyp
A Adenomyosis
L Leiomyoma
M Malignancy, endometrial hyperplasia

Fig. 35.1 Structural causes of AUB
(For color version, see Plate 1)

Fig. 35.2 Documentation of leiomyomas

location, number or size. The criteria for determining the presence of leiomyoma would require only sonographic examination determining the presence of such a lesion.
- Secondary notation requires the clinician to distinguish leiomyomas involving the endometrial cavity (submucosal – SM) from others (O). This emphasis is because submucosal leiomyomas are considered to contribute significantly to AUB.
- Tertiary notation describes the position of leiomyomas. This system is based on the classification of Wamstekar et al., for submucosal leiomyomas, and adds categorization for intramural, subserous and transmural lesions.

11. Which are nonstructural causes for AUB?

Nonstructural causes of AUB that cannot be defined by imaging and histopathology are grouped as such by the FIGO system of classification with acronym COEIN (Fig. 35.3).

Coagulopathy (AUB-C): This includes the various coagulation related disorders that can cause AUB. Caogulopathies like von Willibrand disease are known to be a cause of heavy menstrual bleeding. Similarly, women requiring chronic anticoagulation can also have HMB.

Ovulatory dysfunction (AUB-O): This generally manifests as variable menstrual flow and unpredictable timing of menstrual cycles. Under the olden terminology, 'DUB' ovulatory disorders constituted the majority of causes (being classified as ovulatory and anovulatory DUB). Most causes of ovulatory dysfunction cannot be defined though certain endocrinopathies like PCOS, hypothyroidism, hyperprolactinemia, obesity and anorexia can present with ovulatory dysfunction. Similarly, ovulatory disorders also occur at extremes of age (adolescence and the menopausal transition).

Endometrial (AUB-E): These include disorders which may be a manifestation of deficiency in the molecular mechanisms of endometrial repair. These could be secondary to endometrial inflammation or infection, abnormalities in the local inflammatory response or problems in vasculogenesis.

Iatrogenic (AUB-I): Use of gonadal steroidal therapy (breakthrough bleeding, included), oral or any other route of administration, intrauterine systems, tricyclic antidepressants, phenothiazines, etc. may result in AUB. Heavy menstrual bleeding resulting as a consequence of anticoagulant use are the women with systemic disorder of hemostasis, and they are included as AUB-I rather than AUB-C.

Not yet classified (AUB-N): Several uterine entities such as chronic endometritis, arteriovenous malformations and myometrial hypertrophy that might contribute to or cause, AUB have been poorly defined, inadequately examined, or both. In addition, there may be other disorders, not yet identified, that would be defined only by biochemical or molecular biology assays. They may be allocated a separate category or be placed into an existing category in the system. But until such time, they will be placed in this category.

12. What are the necessary investigations for the work-up of a case with AUB?

It is important to meticulously evaluate a patient presenting with AUB. There may be a single factor responsible or multiple causes identified in each case. Investigations are requested with the intention to know the effect, the type and to exclude the causes of abnormal uterine bleeding (AUB).
- Hemogram—at least hemoglobin estimate with hematocrit, in all cases. Anemia could be an effect as well as the cause. Local tissue anoxia may interfere with tissue regeneration and vascular hemostatic activity.
- Pelvic ultrasonography—will be of value for all cases in any age group to exclude pelvic causes of AUB and to note the endometrial pattern. Sonohysterogram will be an additional aid for ruling out intrauterine pathology.
- Coagulogram—restricted to bleeding/clotting time studies with platelet counts, especially in adolescents will reveal the cause for abnormal uterine bleeding patterns.

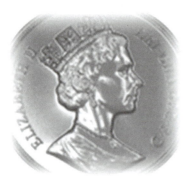

Coagulopathy
Ovulatory dysfunction
Endometrial
Iatrogenic
Not yet classified

Fig. 35.3 Nonstructural causes of AUB

- Thyroid function tests—the estimation of thyroid stimulating hormone for adolescents and perimenopausal groups will help to exclude subtle hypothyroid state which is not an uncommon cause for AUB.
- Uterine curettage—should be carried out in all cases of perimenopausal and menopausal age groups to over rule underlying neoplastic lesions. It will provide insight into type of endometrium and ovulatory status for specific hormonal manipulation when empirical treatment has failed in the mid reproductive age groups. It will not be required for adolescents since anovulation is more of a norm in them. Microbiologic analysis of menstrual blood of first day may help exclude genital tuberculosis in the latter.
- Other endocrine studies—like assay of follicular stimulating and luteinizing hormones are to be carried out, if the patient is obese or features of hirsutism, infrequent cycles are present in adolescents and early reproductive age. Prolactin estimation is ordered when the patient fails to respond to medical management or has galactorrhea.

13. If uterine curettage is advised, what is the basis?

Uterine curettage is advised in perimenopausal and menopausal women with recurrent episodes of AUB to rule out uterine adenocarcinoma. In younger women not responding as anticipated to the medical management, the curettage is timed to precede next menstrual period to obtain information about ovulatory status and the pattern of endometrium. In patients with continuous excessive bleeding, thorough curettage may have a therapeutic benefit. When carried out, curettage may curette out endometrial mucosal polyps, help diagnose submucous fibroid during the procedure and genital tuberculosis on histopathology.

14. What is 'threshold bleeding'?

It is the irregular bleeding because of thin endometrium due to poorly developed proliferative phase. In such cases, amount of estrogen is less-enough to reach threshold for bleeding, but not enough to produce a full proliferative phase. It is seen in young girls and in perimenopausal phase.

15. What is the mechanism of action of progestins for use in anovulatory AUB?

Apart from it being logical (the patient has AUB because she has not ovulated; and mimicking or inducing ovulation should set it right), the use of progestins help convert potent estradiol to less estrogenic estriol through stimulation of 17 beta-hydroxyl steroid dehydrogenase and sulfotransferases; hinder estrogen receptor replenishment by inhibiting estrogen's induction of its own receptor; suppress estrogen-mediated transcription of oncogenes, which property is harvested for reversing premalignant/malignant changes.

16. How do estrogens act to reduce bleeding?

Estrogens are used in the management of AUB because of their effect on capillary/small vessel bleeding by increase in fibrinogen, factors V and IX, and platelet aggregation on tissue reactions to bradykinin, mucopolysaccharides and capillary permeability of endometrial proliferation.

17. Can hysterectomy be avoided in patients not responding to medical management?

Levonorgestrel intrauterine systems (LNG-IUS), endometrial ablation methods and in some situations, uterine artery embolization may help avoid resorting to hysterectomy.

18. Does the knowledge of type of endometrium in AUB influence the management?

The histological type of the endometrium will reflect the hormonal influence and mostly helps in tailoring the management for the case. Anovulatory endometrial patterns can be undone by mimicking the ovulatory effect through supplementation of progestins in the latter half of menstrual cycle or in cases where fertility is also a concern by inducing ovulation. The ovulatory patterns may be set right by inhibiting ovulation or through altering the local menostatic mechanism (e.g. PGSIs, antifibrinolytics, vessel wall stabilizers, hematinics, etc.). It should be remembered that atrophic endometrium though is of anovulatory type would require estrogen supplementation; whereas, ovulatory endometrial patterns due to deficient corpus luteum activity would require progestins (Table 35.3).

19. What is the risk of progression of anovulatory endometrial patterns to endometrial carcinoma?

As the extent of unopposed estrogenic action increases, the risk of endometrial carcinoma increases (Table 35.4).

20. When will you consider that a patient has failed to respond to medical management?

A patient of AUB-O or -E is started and continued for 3 to 6 cycles on the initially planned medical management, hormonal or otherwise. They are then observed for about 3 cycles without any drugs. If the irregularity persists while on drugs or recurs after several attempts at the medical management, it can then be considered as treatment failure.

Amenorrhea

Bharati Shrihari Dhore Patil, Chandan Gupta

1. What is amenorrhea?
Complete absence of menstruation for a period of at least 6 months in a woman in reproductive age.

2. What are the most common physiological causes of amenorrhea?
Pregnancy, lactation and menopause.

3. What is the difference between primary and secondary amenorrhea?
Primary amenorrhea (incidence is less than 0.1%)
- The absence of menses in a female who has never menstruated by the age of 16 years regardless of the normal growth and development of secondary sexual characteristics, or
- The absence of menses in a female who has never menstruated by the age of 14 years in the absence of the normal growth or development of secondary sexual characteristics.

Secondary amenorrhea (incidence is about 0.7%)
- The absence of menses for longer than 6–12 months or
- The absence of menses for a total of three previous cycle intervals in previously menstruating women.

4. What are the most common causes of primary amenorrhea?
- Gonadal failure, such as Turner's syndrome
- Gonadal agenesis accounts for one-third of all patients with primary amenorrhea
- Müllerian anomalies, such as uterovaginal agenesis (Meyer-Rokitansky-Küster-Hauser syndrome-MRKH) are the second most common causes, accounting for 20% of primary amenorrhea
- Such anomalies occur in 1 per 4,000 female births
- One-third of patients with gonadal failure have associated cardiovascular or renal abnormalities.

5. A 14-year-old female patient comes with complaints of monthly abdominal pain but no menses. What is possible diagnosis?
Imperforate hymen or transverse vaginal septum also known as cryptomenorrhagia.

6. What is Kallmann's syndrome?
Primary amenorrhea that is secondary to inadequate GnRH release and insomnia. These patients have infantile sexual development.

7. Primary amenorrhea and normal breast development but absence of uterus occurs in which two syndromes?
a. Patients with androgen insensitivity or testicular feminization are XY genotype but phenotypically are females because an androgen intracellular receptor is not functioning (a maternal X-linked recessive gene). Androgen induction of the Wolffian duct system does not occur despite normal male levels of testosterone. Müllerian inhibiting factor (MIF) is still present, so the Müllerian system does not develop. These patients typically have large breasts with immature nipples but no axillary or pubic hair.
   Some incomplete testicular feminization does occur with some pubic hair, axillary hair, and phallic development in patients with Lubs, Reifenstein's, Rosewater's, and Gilbert Dreyfus syndromes. These patients should be allowed to reach normal sexual maturity. After age 20, the gonads should be removed because 20% of these patients will develop a gonadoblastoma or dysgerminoma.
b. Patients with Müllerian agenesis have sexual hair and mature nipples; 40% have associated renal anomalies, so an intravenous pyelogram or ultrasound should be performed.

8. Which rare enzyme defects can cause amenorrhea?
17-alpha-hydroxylase deficiency and 17–20-desmolase deficiency. 17-alpha-hydroxylase deficiency prevents the formation of sex hormones. In a 46 XX patient, this leads to the absence of breast development even though the uterus is present in a 46 XY patient, there is no breast development; the uterus is absent because of the presence of MIF. These patients also have hypernatremia, hypovolemia, and hypertension, because of increased mineralocorticoid production. There is excessive sodium

retention and potassium excretion. Cortisol production is decreased. Therefore, these patients require cortisol as well as sex hormone replacement to attain breast development and prevent osteoporosis. 17–20-desmolase deficiency also prevents the formation of estrogen and testosterone, but not aldosterone, cortisol, or progesterone. These patients do not have breast development.

9. A 15-year-old female patient gives history of amenorrhea. She is in the 25th percentile for height and weight. She is not an athlete and has an appropriate diet. On physical examination, she has no evidence of breast growth or pubic hair; vagina and uterus are present. What work-up will help determine the cause of amenorrhea?

The patient has no evidence of estrogenization. Serum gonadotropin levels will help to determine if the patient has gonadal failure or unstimulated gonads.

An elevated serum gonadotropin level indicates gonadal failure. A karyotype will usually show an X-chromosome abnormality, causing gonadal dysgenesis. If the patient has an XY chromosome, the gonads must be removed after bone growth. Hypogonadism, indicates unstimulated gonads. These patients must be evaluated for intracranial tumors by checking thyroid function and levels of growth hormone, prolactin, and cortisol. Pituitary stimulation tests may also be appropriate. Skull X-rays to detect calcifications and to evaluate the sella turcica, and a CT/MRI of the pituitary region is also recommended.

10. What is athletic amenorrhea? Should it be treated?

Amenorrhea in athletic women with no other etiology. The cause is not well-understood, although many of these patients have eating disorders as well as high stress levels. Many of these women are hypoestrogenic with significant loss of bone density that can lead to osteoporosis and stress fractures. These patients should be encouraged to improve their diet, decrease their stress levels, decrease the amount of strenuous exercise, if possible, and replace their estrogen and progesterone, if other chances do not increase estrogen levels.

11. What percentage of amenorrhea is due to hyperprolactinemia?

Ten to twenty percent.

12. How do stress and exercise cause amenorrhea?

Stress and exercise cause the level of catecholamine estrogens and beta-endorphins to increase; this influences the release of GnRH by acting on the neurotransmitters. Without appropriate release of gonadotropin-releasing hormone (GnRH), follicle-stimulating hormone (FSH) and luteinizing hormone (LH) are not released appropriately and anovulation occurs, which may lead to amenorrhea.

13. How does weight loss cause amenorrhea?

At less than 15% of ideal body weight, normal release of GnRH does not occur. At less than 25% of ideal body weight, not only GnRH release is abnormal, but pituitary release of LH and FSH is also abnormal. The pituitary gland cannot be induced to secrete LH and FSH normally, even if GnRH is supplied in the normal pulsatile function.

14. Which drugs cause amenorrhea?

- Any drug that stimulates prolactin secretion
- Antipsychotic, such as phenothiazine derivatives, haloperidol and droperidol (Inapsine)
- Tricyclic antidepressants
- Antihypertensive, such as reserpine and methyldopa
- Antianxiety agents, such as benzodiazepines
- Other drugs, such as metoclopromide (Reglan), opiates, barbiturates, and estrogens.

15. Which psychiatric disorder in adolescent is a major cause of amenorrhea?

Anorexia nervosa: The incidence of this disorder is 1/1,000 white adolescent females. Besides amenorrhea, these patients have severe weight loss, often have bradycardia, hypotension, and have low T3 levels from impaired peripheral conversion of T4 to T3. The mortality rate is 5–15%.

16. What are the pituitary causes of amenorrhea?

Damaged cells—lack of LH and FSH secretion caused by anoxia-thrombosis, or hemorrhage, as in Sheehan's syndrome (related to hypotension in pregnancy) or Simon's syndrome (unrelated to pregnancy).

Neoplasms—Most common of which secrete prolactin, but are not always associated with galactorrhea. Amenorrhea is also associated with acromegaly and Cushing's syndrome.

17. Which initial blood tests should be performed in the patient with amenorrhea?

Thyroid function tests are to rule out rare cases of asymptomatic hypothyroidism in patient with hypothyroidism, regular menses will resume with thyroid replacement. Prolactin levels should be measured to rule out hyperprolactinemia, which may occur even without galactorrhea. Patients with galactorrhea should also undergo skull X-ray with a coned-down view of the sella turcica or a CT scan or MRI to rule out a small pituitary adenoma, LH/FSH level.

18. What is post-pill amenorrhea?

Suppression of the hypothalamic–pituitary axis can persist for several months after discontinuing oral contraceptive

Flow chart 36.1: Diagnosis of amenorrhea

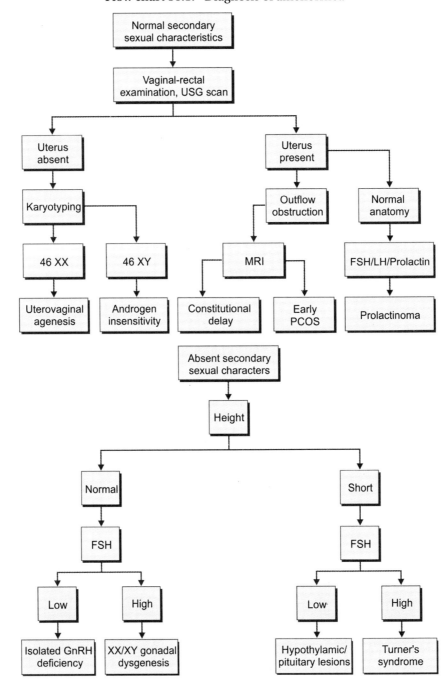

agents. The incidence of post-pill amenorrhea lasting greater than 6 months is equal to the incidence of secondary amenorrhea. It is no longer believed that oral contraceptives cause prolonged amenorrhea or infertility, and thus other etiologies must be considered.

19. What is premature ovarian failure?

Ovarian failure and, thus, amenorrhea before age of 40 years. These patients have symptoms of hypoestrogenism, increased levels of FSH and generalized sclerosis. Only primordial follicles with no progression past the antrum stage on ovarian biopsy is seen. Many patients have autoimmune diseases, such as Hashimoto's syndrome, Addison's disease, and hypoparathyroidism. If the patient is less than 25-year-old, a karyotype should be performed to determine if the patient is a 46 XX/46 XY mosaic pattern. If so, the gonads must be removed to prevent malignancy after age 20 years. Antithyroid antibodies, antinuclear antibodies, and 24 hours cortisol levels should also be checked. Ovarian failure may also result from irradiation or chemotherapy.

20. What is a progesterone challenge test?

10 mg of oral medroxyprogesterone acetate for 5 days or intramuscular injection of 100–200 mg of progesterone in oil. The test is positive if any bleeding (even spotting) occurs within 2 weeks of the test. A negative pregnancy test should be obtained first.

21. What does a positive progesterone challenge test indicate?

The patient has a serum estradiol level greater than 40 pg/mL, and thus, the anterior pituitary is producing LH and FSH and the endometrium and outflow tract are functioning. This indicates that, if thyroid function tests and prolactin levels are normal, the patient is anovulatory.

22. Which tests should be performed on a patient with amenorrhea after a progesterone challenge test reveals no bleeding?

A course of conjugated estrogen, 2.5 mg for 21 days prior to progesterone challenge, should be used to define a uterine defect as the cause of amenorrhea, such as complete destruction of the endometrial lining by Asherman's syndrome or fibrosis following severe endometritis. Next, the patient's FSH level should be determined. If FSH is elevated, the patient has premature ovarian failure. If FSH is normal, a CT scan of the hypothalamus–pituitary area should be done to rule out a central nervous system tumor, such as craniopharyngioma, or granulomatous diseases (tuberculosis, sarcoid). The patient's reserve of adrenocorticotropic hormone (ACTH) should be checked. If all of these tests are normal, the diagnosis of exclusion is hypothalamic–pituitary failure. All of these patients are hypoestrogenic and require hormone replacement therapy.

MUST REMEMBER

- Primary amenorrhea is defined as the absence of menstruation by age of 16 years. The absence of secondary sexual characteristics by age of 14 is an indication for further investigations. If secondary sexual characteristics are absent, then it indicates absent or unstimulated female gonad (ovaries). Presence of secondary sexual characteristics suggests investigating them further for the presence or absence of uterus. The absence of uterus indicates Müllerian agenesis.
- Secondary amenorrhea defined as the absence of menses for a period of 6 months in a previously menstruating woman. The common causes are pregnancy, menopause, lactational amenorrhea, polycystic ovary syndrome (PCOS), tuberculous endometritis, Asherman's and Sheehan's syndrome. Polycystic ovary syndrome (PCOS) is diagnosed when any two of the following criteria are present: (a) Oligo or anovulation, (b) Hyper-androgenism, and (c) Polycystic ovaries.

Endometriosis

Sudha Sharma, Vishal R Tandon, Sonali Deshpande

1. What is endometriosis and adenomyosis (endometriosis interna)?

The presence of functioning endometrium (glands and stroma) in sites other than uterine mucosa is called endometriosis. Ectopic endometrial tissue may be found in the myometrium then it is called adenomyosis. More commonly these tissues are found at sites other than uterus and are generally referred to as endometriosis.

2. What are the endometrial cells?

The endometrium is the mucus surface that lines the inside of the uterus. It contains several layers of cells (i.e. endometrial cells) that vary in appearance and number throughout the menstrual cycle, as the levels of estrogen and progesterone fluctuate. During the luteal phase (the two-week period just before a woman bleeds); for example, the endometrium is thick, its cells are enlarged, the glands bulge, and the arteries are swollen. At menstruation, the endometrium sheds. Following menstruation, new cells grow and the endometrium regenerates. The cells that make up the endometrium normally grow only inside the uterus and are called endometrial cells.

3. What is the epidemiological correlation?

- Endometriosis is a disease of the childbearing period. Women are usually 30–40 years old at the time of diagnosis. A familial tendency has been identified
- Its incidence appears to be on increase, partly due to improvements in diagnostic technique and partly due to changing social patterns like late marriage and limitation of family size. It is more common amongst the affluent class
- Evidence of the disease is present in 20% of women undergoing laparoscopic investigation for infertility. Approximately 24% of women who complain of pelvic pain are subsequently found to have endometriosis
- The overall prevalence, including symptomatic and asymptomatic women, is estimated to be 5–10%. Because surgical confirmation is necessary for the diagnosis, the true prevalence of the disease is unknown.

4. What is its pathogenesis?

Pathogenesis is not well-understood and is probably multifactorial in origin.

Retrograde menstruation (Sampson's theory)

The most widely embraced theory involves retrograde menstruation. This means retrograde flow of menstrual blood through tubes during menstruation, which enters the pelvis. While this theory can explain pelvic endometriosis, it fails to explain the endometriosis at distant sites.

Direct implantation occurs

According to this theory, the endometrial or decidual tissue starts to grow in susceptible individual when implanted in the new sites. Such sites are abdominal scar following hysterotomy, cesarean section, tubectomy and myomectomy. Endometriosis at the episiotomy scar, vaginal or cervical sites can also be explained by this theory.

Coelomic metaplasia (Meyer and Ivanoff theory)

Refers to cells that transform into endometrial cells, perhaps as a result of chronic inflammation or irritation from retrograde menstrual blood. This theory of coelomic metaplasia is based on the observation that coelomic epithelium is the common ancestor of endometrial and peritoneal cells, thus, allowing transformation of one type of cell into another.

Metastatic theory [lymphatic theory (Halban) and vascular theory]

It is very difficult to explain the occurrence of endometriosis at less accessible sites like the umbilicus, pelvic lymph nodes, ureter, rectovaginal septum, bowel wall, and remote sites like lung, pleura, endocardium, and extremities. Hence, this might be possible through embolization of menstrual fragments through vascular or lymphatic channels leading to launching of endometriosis at distal sites.

Congenital factors

Endometriosis may be a congenital condition (existed from birth). During fetal development, uterine tissue may remain in the pelvis and grow as a result of hormonal influence. Müllerian remnants can differentiate into endometrial tissue.

Hormonal theory

Ovarian steroid hormones probably play an important role in the induction and maintenance of the disease, as symptoms improve in cases of low hormone levels. Medical treatment that suspends cyclic ovarian function (oral contraceptives, medroxyprogesterone acetate, danazol, gonadotropin-releasing hormone agonist) or surgical removal of the ovaries will result in symptom improvement. Pregnancy causes atrophy of endometriosis mainly through high progesterone levels. Endometriosis is rarely seen before puberty, and it regresses after menopause.

5. What recent hypotheses are emerging explaining pathogenesis of endometriosis?

Role of oxidative stress in endometriosis

The presence of elevated concentrations of free radicals and lowered antioxidant potential leads to oxidative stress. The development of oxidative stress in the local peritoneal environment may be one of the links in the chain of events leading to endometriosis. Antioxidant supplementation, immunomodulators, and selective progesterone receptor modulators with antioxidant effects have been investigated as possible treatments for endometriosis, but compelling evidence on the benefits of the various modalities is lacking.

Genetic and immunological theory

Genetic basis of endometriosis probably accounts for less than 10% of patients. There is increased incidence in 1st degree relatives. Multifactorial inheritance is thought. Endometriosis is more frequently diagnosed in patients with infertility than in a normal population suspicion arises, is there immunological link between endometriosis, recurrent miscarriage and implantation failure. This can possibly be explained by alterations in humoral and cell-mediated immunity in women with endometriosis. Humoral immunological changes include increased formation of antibodies against endometrial antigens, antilaminin-1 autoantibodies, and other auto-immune antibodies (e.g. antiphospholipid). Cell-mediated immunological changes include alterations in peritoneal and follicular fluid immune cells and cytokines. The possible negative effect of these immunological changes on folliculogenesis, ovulation, oocyte quality, early embryonic development and implantation in women with endometriosis suggest that infertility in endometriosis patients may be related to alterations within the follicle or oocyte, resulting in embryos with decreased ability to implant.

6. How endometriosis is classified?

Stages of endometriosis

- *Stage I*—Minimal (Score 1-5): Few or superficial implants are evident in the early stages of endometriosis
- *Stage II*—Mild (Score 6-15): More implants, deeper involvement
- *Stage III*—Moderate (Score 16-40): More implants; ovaries affected, adhesions present
- *Stage IV*—Severe (Score >40): Similar to Stage III, but multiple and more dense adhesions present.

7. What are common sites of endometriosis?

It is seen widely spread throughout the lower pelvis usually below the level of umbilicus. Most often it is seen in the ovaries, posterior cul-de-sac, including uterosacral ligaments, in the adnexal region, Fallopian tubes, pelvis, peritoneum over bladder, sigmoid colon, back of the uterus, intestinal coils, pelvic lymph nodes, rectovaginal septum and appendix.

8. Which are less common sites?

Umbilicus, ureter, bowel wall and remote sites like lung, pleura, liver, endocardium and extremities. It is also reported to be seen over scar following hysterotomies, classical cesarean, myomectomy, amputated stumps of cervix, scar of vulva and episiotomy.

9. What is most common pathology of endometriosis?

Early implants look like small, flat dark patches or flecks of blue or black paint (gunpowder-burns) sprinkled on the pelvic surfaces. The small patches may remain unchanged, become scar tissue or spontaneously disappear over a period of months. Endometriosis may invade the ovary, producing blood filled cysts called endometriomas. With time, serum gets absorbed and the blood darkens to a deep, reddish brown or tarry color, giving rise to the description chocolate cyst. These may be smaller than a pea or larger than a grapefruit. In some cases, bands of fibrous tissue called adhesions may bind the uterus, tubes, ovaries, and nearby intestines together.

10. What are endometriomas/chocolate cysts?

This disease process is also known as endometriosis of the ovaries. Tiny implants of cells that line the uterine cavity become transplanted and form small cysts on the outside of the ovary. These cysts enlarge and produce endometriosis of the ovary. They respond to hormone stimulation during the menstrual cycle and produce many small cysts, which may then occupy and even replace the normal ovarian tissue. These endometriomas are filled with a thick chocolate-type material, which is the reason they are known as chocolate cysts. When this type of ovarian cyst ruptures, the material spills over into the pelvis and onto the surface of the uterus, bladder and bowel and the corresponding spaces between. Adhesions can develop because of this rupture and may lead to pelvic pain.

11. Can endometriosis be cancerous?

0.7–1% chances of endometroid adenocarcinoma. The endometrial tissue may invade neighboring tissue, but it is not a cancer. In rare instances, advanced endometriosis may be associated with ascites, pleural effusions, and large pelvic masses. Interestingly, in only 8% of the cases in one recent study recorded cancerous changes of the ovary diagnosed suggesting possible malignant transformation however, it still remains to be confirmed.

Symptoms

Pain

Endometriosis should be considered in any woman of reproductive age who has pelvic pain as it is the most common symptom that generally occurs just before and during menstruation and then decreases after menstruation. About 25–67% of women with endometriosis suffer congestive dysmenorrhea (painful menstruation). About 25% experience painful intercourse. Pelvic examinations can also be painful. Depending on the location of the implants, rectal pain and painful defecation may also occur. The diagnosis of endometriosis should be considered especially if a patient develops dysmenorrhea after years of pain-free menstrual cycles. Abdominal pain or low backache also can be chief complaints.

Infertility

Infertility is common. In fact, infertility is the most common symptom that prompts a visit to the doctor office for diagnosis. Endometriosis is diagnosed in up to 60% of infertile women.

12. What can be the possible reasons for infertility?

Extensive scarring interferes with tubal motility or entirely blocking the tubes. Ovarian dysfunction can also be one of the reasons. Increased or decreased secretion of various cytokines that regulate the immunologic processes has been shown to occur among women with endometriosis. These changes may affect sperm, egg function, or embryo development. Abnormal sperm motility has been shown in association with endometriosis. It has been also suggested that endometriotic implants may secrete substances that interfere with normal sperm motility and, thereby, impair the process of fertilization.

Menstrual symptoms

Menorrhagia is common with adenomyosis, and irregular bleeding may occur with cervical, and vaginal bleeding. Polymenorrhea is noted with ovarian involvement.

Other symptoms

Painful or difficult defecation, diarrhea, melena and bloody urine if sigmoid or rectum, and bladder are involved. If the lungs are involved, endometriosis may cause pleuritic pain or hemoptysis. If endometrial cells implant in the brain, the patient may experience seizures.

Medical history

About 90% of women with pelvic pain have endometriosis. Pelvic pain that is typical of endometriosis includes menstrual cramps, low back pain that worsens during menstruation, and pain in the pelvis that occurs during or after sexual intercourse. Depending on where the implants are located, a woman may feel pain in her rectum during defecation.

Physical examination

The expected positive findings are pelvic tenderness, nodules in the pouch of Douglas, nodular feel of the uterosacral ligaments, fixed retroverted uterus and unilateral or bilateral adnexal mass of varying sizes. Rectal or rectovaginal examination is often helpful to confirm the diagnosis.

Diagnosis

Pelvic ultrasonography, computed tomography and magnetic resonance imaging are occasionally used to identify individual lesions, but these modalities are not helpful in assessing the extent of endometriosis.

Laparoscopy

Most women with endometriosis have normal pelvic findings, and laparoscopy is necessary for definitive diagnosis. It permits to see inside the pelvic region to observe classic lesion of endometriosis.

13. Are there any biochemical markers for diagnosis of endometriosis?

a. Many patients with endometriosis have an elevated CA-125 blood level (CA-125 is an antigen).
b. Antiendometriosis antibodies.

Differential diagnosis of endometriosis by symptom

- Generalized pelvic pain
- Pelvic inflammatory disease
- Endometritis
- Pelvic adhesions
- Neoplasms, benign or malignant
- Ovarian torsion.

Lesions which mimic endometriosis

- Old sutures
- Epithelial inclusions
- Carbon deposits from electrosurgery or laser
- Reaction to oil-based contrast media
- Remnants of trophoblast, malignant deposits

Endometriosis with nonpigmented lesions
- Flat white opacification, red flame lesions
- Subovarian adhesions, yellow peritoneal patches, hypervascular areas.

Dysmenorrhea
- Primary → Spasmodic
- Secondary → Congestive.

Dyspareunia
- Musculoskeletal causes (pelvic relaxation, levator spasm)
- Gastrointestinal tract causes urinary tract (urethral syndrome, interstitial cystitis) infection
- Pelvic vascular congestion diminished lubrication or vaginal expansion because of insufficient arousal.

Infertility
- Male factor
- Tubal disease (infection)
- Anovulation
- Cervical factors
- Luteal phase deficiency.

14. What are the treatment modalities for endometriosis?

Following modalities are of use:
- Expectant—minimal endometriosis with no other pelvic findings like in unmarried or young married females.
- Hormones and others
- Surgery
- Conservative
- Radical
- Combination of surgery and hormones.

15. What is medical treatment of endometriosis?

Drug
- Combined estrogens and progestogens
- Progestogens (such as dydrogesterone, medroxyprogesterone acetate, norethisterone)
- Synthetic androgens (such as danazol, gestrinone)
- Gonadotropin-releasing hormone analogs (such as buserelin, goserelin, leuprorelin acetate, nafarelin, triptorelin)
- Nonsteroidal anti-inflammatory drugs (such as diclofenac, ibuprofen, mefenamic acid)
- Gonadotropin releasing hormone analogues and any combined hormone replacement therapy (continuous or sequential) or tibolone the combined oral contraceptive pill for endometriosis.

16. What are the main advantages of OC pills?

The main advantages of the pill are that it is inexpensive and is usually reasonably well-tolerated by women. It can also be taken safely for many years, if necessary, unlike most of the other hormonal drug treatments for endometriosis.

How it works?
Like all the other hormonal treatments, the pill does not cure endometriosis. Rather, it alleviates the pain of endometriosis by suppressing menstruation and inhibiting the growth of the endometrial implants.

Progestins as a treatment for endometriosis
The progestins are effective treatments for the symptoms of endometriosis. However, like all the hormonal drugs used for endometriosis, they have side effects, which some women find intolerable. They are safer and cheaper than the GnRH-agonists and danazol, which some gynecologists believe makes them appropriate for women who need prolonged or repeated treatments.

How it works?
It is not known precisely how progestins relieve the symptoms of endometriosis, but they probably work by suppressing the growth of endometrial implants in some way, causing them to gradually waste away. They may also reduce endometriosis-induced inflammation in the pelvic cavity. The progestins control pain symptoms in approximately 3 out of 4 women. However, they may not relieve symptoms completely.

Does its use after surgery has any role?
There is some evidence to justify using hormonal drug treatments following surgery to suppress the growth and development of any remaining or new endometrial implants.

Use in recurrent endometriosis (Pseudomenopausal treatment)
Repeat courses of progestins may be used for women with recurrent endometriosis.

Danazol as a treatment for endometriosis (Pseudomenopause treatment)
Danazol is a synthetic androgen. Danazol is an effective treatment for endometriosis, and has the same effectiveness as the other hormonal treatments. However, it has many androgenic (male-like) side effects, including weight gain, increased body hair and acne. Its unpleasant side effects and its tendency to adversely affect blood lipid (cholesterol) levels mean it is not usually the first choice of treatment for endometriosis.

How it helps?
It suppresses its growth and development temporarily, so the disease may recur following treatment. Danazol has a multitude of effects on the body. Some of these effects combine to produce high levels of androgen and low levels of estrogen in the body. This hormonal environment stops menstruation and suppresses the growth of endome-

trial implants, causing them to degenerate. The symptoms of endometriosis usually begin to diminish by the end of the second month. Most women will resume ovulating and menstruating within 4–6 weeks of stopping treatment. It relieves pain in approximately 90% of women.

GnRH-agonists as a treatment for endometriosis (Reversible medical oopherectomy).
They are modified versions of a naturally occurring hormone known as gonadotropin-releasing hormone, which helps to control the menstrual cycle.

How they work?
When used continuously for periods of longer than 2 weeks, they stop the production of estrogen by a series of mechanisms. This deprives the endometrial implants of estrogen, causing them to become inactive and degenerate. They appear to be at least as effective as progestins in relieving pain.

NSAIDs
These drugs can be effective in alleviating pain and inflammation but they do not reduce the size of the implants or treat the source.

How they help?
It is thought that much of the pain of endometriosis, especially menstrual pain, is due to inflammation that may be caused in part by high levels of prostaglandins. Women with endometriosis have been shown to produce an excess of a prostaglandin called PGE2, which causes inflammation, pain, and uterine contractions. Theoretically, NSAIDs would seem to be a good choice for relieving menstrual pain because most of them work by blocking the production of all prostaglandins.

17. What are the recent advances in the medical treatment?
- Gonadotropin-releasing hormone analogues and any combined hormone replacement therapy (continuous or sequential) or tibolone
- *Aromatase inhibitors as a treatment for endometriosis:* At the moment, the treatment of endometriosis with aromatase inhibitors is still experimental, because the research is still in its early days. Research has shown that aromatase is also found in high levels in the ectopic endometrial tissue of women with endometriosis, which contributes to the growth of their endometriosis. Aromatase inhibitor suppresses the growth of their endometriosis, and reduces the associated inflammation. This, in turn, significantly reduces their pelvic pain.
- GnRH agonist treatment combined with tibolone
- Tumor necrosis factor—(alpha) blockers
- Leflunomide, an immunomodulator induces regression of endometriosis.

Surgery
Surgery is used to treat moderate-to-severe cases of endometriosis.

Laparoscopy
A laparoscopy is usually the only surgical option for women who want to preserve fertility. A laparoscopy can be used to freeze the implants, burn them with a laser, or surgically remove them, depending on the type of lesion. In a laparascopy done for diagnostic purposes, the lesions are usually removed at the same time.

18. What is an endometrioma?
An endometrioma is a mass of tissue (noncancerous cyst or tumor) that contains shreds of endometrial tissue.

19. How are endometriomas treated?
Several surgical treatments are available for endometriomas:
- *Simple puncture:* Draining the fluid from the cyst
- *Ablation:* Drain the cyst and remove its base with laser or electrosurgery
- Cutting away of the cyst wall. This is the procedure of choice to decrease recurrence of disease
- *Draining, drug therapy and surgery:* Endometriomas can also be drained, treated with medication, and later removed by surgery.

Laparotomy
In severe cases, however, and in women who choose not to preserve fertility, a laparotomy may be necessary.

20. How is advanced endometriosis treated?
Laparoscopy or by laparotomy, traditional abdominal surgery, which requires a larger incision, is the management of advanced endometriosis.

21. Is laparoscopy more effective than laparotomy?
Laparoscopy and laparotomy are equally effective in relieving pain and improving fertility. Endometriosis recurs in about 20% of cases over 5 years in both procedures. Patients who undergo laparoscopy, however, experience a more rapid and less painful recovery.

22. What treatment algorithm should be followed?
Primary prevention of endometriosis (Flow chart 37.1)
- Going for pregnancy
- Correct cervical obstruction
- Oral contraceptives use
- Tubal patency test should be avoided just before the commencement of menstruation
- Operations on the genital tract should be scheduled in postmenstrual period

Flow chart 37.1: Treatment of endometriosis

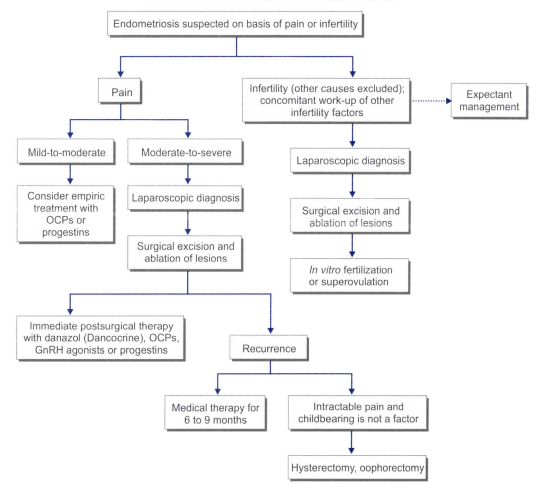

- Classical cesarean section and hysterotomy should be avoided to prevent scar endometriosis
- Avoid pelvic examination in menses.

23. What are risk factors for endometriosis?

Delayed childbearing, nulliparity, higher social class, family history of endometriosis, early menarchae, obstructive Müllerian anomalies.

24. What are the causes of pain in endometriosis?

Peritoneal inflammation, nerve irritation with deep infiltration, tissue damage, local production of prostaglandins, collection of blood in endometriotic implants.

25. Name the investigations.

USG, MRI, Doppler, CA-125.

MUST REMEMBER

- Endometriosis is the presence of gland and stroma outside the uterus.
- Risk factors for endometriosis include early menarche, delayed child-bearing low parity, high social class, Müllerian anomalies.
- Symptoms of endometriosis includes severe dysmenorrhea, dyspareunia, chronic pelvic pain, menstrual abnormalities, infertility and bowel/bladder symptoms. Pain is most predominant symptom.
- Visual inspection of pelvis at laparoscopy is gold standard for diagnosis of endometriosis.
- Infertile women with endometriosis may require ART (assisted reproductive technique).
- Management may be medical or surgical.

Menopause

Girija Wagh, Sanjay Gupte

1. What is menopause? What is climacteric?

Menopause is defined as cessation of menses for a period of 12 months or more. It is that point in time when permanent cessation of menstruation occurs following the loss of ovarian activity (men: month, pause: cessation).

The years prior to menopause marked by irregularity of cycle which encompass the change from normal ovulatory cycles to cessation of menses is called premenopausal transition.

Climacteric (ladder)—more general term which indicates the period of time when a woman passes from the reproductive stage of life through perimenopausal transition and the menopause to the postmenopausal years.

2. What is menopausal syndrome?

Menopausal transition usually begins in women's forties. During this time, women report of varied physical and psychological symptoms which together comprise the menopause.

3. What are the symptoms of menopause?

Immediate:
- Menstrual irregularity
- *Vasomotor symptoms:* Flushes and night sweats (75%)
- *Psychological:* Irritability (92%), lethargy (88%), depression (78%), forgetfulness (62%), crying spells (42%), and insomnia (51%)
- Urinary complaints such as dysuria (20%), incontinence, etc.
- Local symptoms such as dryness.

Intermediate:
- Genital atrophy
- Skin and hair changes
- Musculoskeletal
- Joint and muscle spasm (48%)
- Sexual disturbances (decreased libido (20%))
- Ocular changes
- Weight gain (61%).

Late (hidden):
- Osteoporosis
- CVS—palpitations (44%).
- Dementia.

4. What are the changes in the gonadotropins at menopause?

Shortly after menopause, there are no ovarian follicles. There is 10–20 fold increase in FSH and approximately 3 fold increase in LH. These hormones reach maximum levels in 1–3 years after menopause. Then they gradually decline. High levels of FSH confirm ovarian failure.

5. Why are the FSH levels higher than LH levels?

Luteinizing hormone (LH) is cleared from blood faster. Half-life for LH is 20 minutes and for FSH, it is 3–4 hours. Also there is no specific negative feedback peptide for LH-like inhibin.

6. How is the fertility potential reduced at menopause? How can one assess the ovarian reserve?

Ten to fifteen years before menopause, there is significant decline in fertility. There is subtle increase in FSH during this period. The increase is due to the quality and quantity of aging follicles. Once the oocyte pool reduces to approximately a 1000 follicles, menopause starts. For optimum ovarian function, a cohort is essential which only will help in successful ovulation. Decreased fertility may occur without any obvious changes in the menstrual cycle. Despite of decreased fertility, pregnancy is possible.

The functional ovarian reserve can be directly measured by a basal day-3 serum FSH level.

There also is a lot of advocacy about anti-Müllerian hormone (AMH) levels which can be tested any time during the cycle (women with low AMH levels in the first test <1 ng/mL on average yielded only about six eggs, while women who had more than three times as much AMH provided about 20 eggs on average) but this needs more validation. Also the sonographic evaluation of the ovary for antral follicle count too can be of help (at least four follicles, 4 mm in size).

7. How to differentiate between menopausal irregular uterine bleeding and abnormal uterine bleeding?

No unusual presentation or definition of irregular periods is approved. On an average 4–8 years prior to menopause, irregularity in cycle is observed in majority of women.

Most common 3 parameters are seen:
1. Oligomenorrhea (70%)
2. Menorrhagia, metrorrhagia (18%)
3. Sudden amenorrhea.

8. What type of abnormal uterine bleeding requires investigation?

- Heavier than usual bleeding (blood loss > 80 mL, clots +, associated anemia)
- Prolonged bleeding (>7 days)
- Frequent menstrual period (cycles <21 days)
- Metrorrhagia (intermenstrual bleeding)
- Postcoital bleeding.

9. What are hot flashes, hot flushes or night sweats? What is their etiopathogenesis and cause?

The symptoms of vasomotor instability are called hot flashes. Some distinguish the hot flash from hot flush. However, the terms are interchangeable.

A hot flash is a sudden transient sensation that ranges from warmth to intense heat. A sudden wave of hot sensation spreads over the body, especially the upper body and face (causes flushing). The skin temperature rises as the blood flow to the skin increases, especially in the fingers and toes, where skin temperature can rise by 1–7 degrees. This can follow by an experience of a chill because of reduction of the core temperature.

Hot flashes that occur with drenching diaphoresis (perspiration) during sleep are termed as night sweats. They can occur frequently, i.e. hourly or in close succession (monthly or weekly). Some women experience them during the premenopausal transient phase especially in association with menses. The precise cause is not known. Thermoregulatory center situated in the hypothalamus is under the control of catecholamines and catechol-estrogens. There are estrogen receptors present in these centers. The estrogen present in blood combines with catecholamines to produce catecholestrogen. When there is lack of estrogen, there is an imbalance between catecholamine and catecholestrogen, which results in hot flashes.

It is doubtful whether it is estrogen-dependent but it has shown a dose-dependent response to estrogen supplementation.

10. What is the presentation and cause of urinary and fecal symptoms in menopause?

Urinary complaints like urinary incontinence, recurrent UTI, the urethral syndrome are common in postmenopausal women. Some women can also have fecal incontinence as a result of menopausal changes. Persistent involuntary leaking of urine, i.e. urinary incontinence of all forms affects 10–30% women between the age group of 50 and 64 years. The prevalence of urge incontinence increases with number of postmenopausal years while stress incontinence is more common during perimenopause.

The female urethra and trigone of bladder share the same embryonic origins as the vagina. Therefore, they contain estrogen receptors which are affected by the reduced level of estrogen. So urinary incontinence occurs as a result of reduced bladder and urethral tissue tone.

Various other types of urinary presentation like frequency, urgency, nocturia are also seen to be associated after middle-age.

Urethral syndrome is characterized by recurrent episodes of urinary frequency, dysuria and urgency. Urethral mucous membrane atrophy leads to urge incontinence which is characterized as sudden, strong desire to void, can be many a times misdiagnosed and treated as UTI.

About 15–26% of women with urinary incontinence also have fecal incontinence. This is due to lowered estrogen level giving rise to neuromuscular dysfunction of the pelvic floor. The anorectum is found to be abundant with estrogen receptors.

11. Why are menopausal women susceptible to urinary tract infection?

Lack of estrogen results in shortening and shrinking of the distal portion of the urethra. This reduces the defense against offending pathogens and increases the risk of UTI.

Reduced endogenous estrogen levels lead to reduction in the epithelial cell glycogen production. This increases the alkalinity of the vaginal, urethral, and bladder environment.

12. Enumerate the factors leading to urinary incontinence during menopause.

- Reduced endogenous estrogen levels
- Urethritis and cystitis
- Neuromuscular dysfunction of the pelvic floor
- Previous childbirth injuries or perineal floor damages
- Substance abuse like smoking, alcohol and caffeine
- Obesity
- Pelvic organ prolapse
- Medications like diuretics and tranquilizers
- Neurological disorders like multiple sclerosis and Parkinson's disease
- Diabetes mellitus.

13. Describe the androgen levels at menopause.

The two sources of androgen secretion are: Ovaries and the adrenal glands.

The ovary secretes androstenedione and testosterone, and after menopause, predominantly androstenedione.

The androstenedione levels in the blood reduce to half of that seen before menopause. The source of this is mainly from the adrenal gland. The levels of DHEA and its sulfate, DHEA-S, which originate in the adrenal gland, decline markedly with aging, and about 70–74% less respectively after about 10 years of menopause.

Testosterone production decreases by approximately 25% after menopause, but in most women, the ovary secretes more testosterone after menopause. With the disappearance of follicles and estrogen, the elevated gonadotropins stimulate the ovarian stroma to secrete more testosterone. The total level of testosterone after menopause, however, is reduced because there is no peripheral conversion of androstenedione. Compared with young women, the overall androgen exposure of perimenopausal women is less.

14. Describe the estrogens levels at menopause.

Postmenopausal women have serum estradiol levels below 15 pg/mL, and mean estrone levels of 30 pg/mL. Although estradiol levels are negligible, it has been observed that estrone levels are higher in older men and women. Older women convert androstenedione to estrone. The circulating estradiol levels after menopause are derived from the peripheral conversion of estrone, which in turn, is derived from the peripheral conversion of androstenedione. This is because the adipose tissue aromatase mRNA expression increases and is the highest in the hip fat, and the lowest in the abdomen. The average postmenopausal production rate of estrogen is approx 45 mg/24 hour. The percent conversion of androstenedione to estrogen correlates with body weight. This probably is due to the ability of fat to aromatize androgens and reduce levels of SHBG. These low levels of estrogen are insufficient to sustain secondary sex tissues.

	Premenopausal	Postmenopausal
Estradiol	40–400 pg/mL	10–20 pg/mL
Estrone	30–200 pg/mL	30–70 pg/mL
Testosterone	20–80 ng/dL	15–70 ng/dL
Androstenedione	60–300 ng/dL	30–150 ng/dL

15. Why is there hirsutism at menopause?

The androgen to estrogen ratio changes drastically after menopause, because of the more marked decline in estrogen. With increasing age, a decrease can be measured in circulating levels of DHEA and DHEA-S, whereas androstenedione, testosterone and estrogen remain constant. Mild hirsutism is a reflection of this marked shift in the sex hormone ratio.

16. What is the impact of menopause on the CVS?

Menopause worsens serum lipid and plasma fibrinogen profiles. Estrogen deficiency adversely affects circulating lipid levels, leading to increase in low density lipoproteins, cholesterol, total serum cholesterol and triglyceride levels.

Menopausal estrogen deprivation leads to reduction in HDLP. This positively correlates with adiposity at the trunk and central fat deposition.

Atherosclerosis develops rapidly after menopause. Triglycerides increase in these women and if at levels of 400 mg/dL or higher are a strong risk factor for CHD.

As women grow older, their rates of myocardial infarction and stroke approach and then exceed that of men.

In younger women throughout adulthood, the HDL cholesterol levels are about 10 mg/dL higher and total and LDL cholesterol levels lower, thus being cardioprotective. In addition, estrogen is known to have a direct inotropic effect on the myometrium which can probably contribute.

17. How should one evaluate a menopausal woman?

Medical evaluation includes a complete history and physical examination with a focus on the target areas affected by menopause, namely, the CVS, the skeleton, the genitourinary system and the neuroendocrine system.

The questionnaire should include information with respect to hot flashes, sleep disturbances, mood and memory changes and urinary symptoms.

The medical, gynecological, and sexual history along with exercise habits will help assess the health status of these women.

A dietary history should include a specific enquiry into fat and calcium intake.

Physical examination should include blood pressure measurement, examination of thyroid, breast and the CVS. The abdominal and pelvic examinations will also be part of this routine.

Following laboratory investigations should be performed:
- Total cholesterol levels and HDL cholesterol levels—if they are deranged, 12 hour fasting lipid profile including triglycerides should be evaluated. Marked hypertriglyceridemia is an independent risk factor for coronary artery disease in women.
- FSH and estradiol levels are usually not needed to diagnose menopause.
- FSH level of >20 IU/L and estradiol levels of 20–40 pg/mL confirm primary gonadal failure.
- A Pap smear and a screening mammogram, or at least a thorough breast examination should be performed on menopausal women.

18. What is the effect of exogeneous hormones on CVS?

Several observational and epidemiological studies have strongly suggested that ERT could reduce cardiovascular deaths significantly. These studies inspired confidence that estrogen therapy would reverse the negative impact of menopause on the lipid profiles. The angiographic studies have suggested that estrogen could reverse atherosclerosis and improve tone and resilience of the vascular system.

Examples are:
- Leisure World Study, a prospective longitudinal study, documented, reduced risk of death due to myocardial infarction.
- The Lipid Research Clinics Follow-up Study (LRCFS) demonstrated 63% reduction in the relative risk of cardiovascular disease.
- A population based case-control study in Minnesota concluded 45% reduction in risk of MI in estrogen users.
- The Nurses Health Study (NHS) found decreased risk of CVD in current users, suggesting that estrogen should be used indefinitely for cardioprotection.
- The Postmenopausal Estrogen Progesterone Intervention trial (PEPI) suggested beneficial effects of estrogen on lipid profile, except it was associated with elevated triglycerides. But, it concluded that other beneficial-vascular effects like endothelium dependent vasodilatation, relaxation of smooth muscles, inhibition of lipoprotein oxidation, inhibition of foam formation, decreased fibrinogen levels and direct inotropic effect on the heart were beneficial, and it recommended conventional HT.

But all these positive effects of HT were counter-proved by many studies, where it was in fact now accepted that estrogen is not actually cardioprotective. In fact it is associated with risk of CVD's.
- Finnish study of pooled data from 22 small short term randomized studies found 39% increase in cardiovascular events in estrogen users. This was the first break in the pattern of support for estrogen.
- The large and respected Framingham Heart study reported 50% increased risk of CVD's in estrogen users.
- The Heart Estrogen/Progestin Replacement study (HERS): A carefully designed large scale prospective multicentered placebo-controlled trial of combined therapy for secondary prevention of CHD in postmenopausal women had 2783 postmenopausal non-hysterectomized women with established CHD or at least 50% occlusion of a major coronary artery as subjects. Their mean age is 66.7 years and were randomized to placebo or the most commonly used HT, i.e. 0.625 mg of oral Conjugated Equine Estrogen + 2.5 mg of Medroxy Progesterone Acetate daily. The primary endpoints of this study were non-fatal MI or CHD deaths. The trial began in 1993 and ended after 4.1 years with 179 primary CHD events in the hormone group. The study concluded that CEE and MPA were not to be used for secondary prevention of CHD, and received endorsement to this effect by the FDA. The subset HERS II trial, which completed the stipulated time frame also failed to show any cardiovascular benefit.
- The Women's Health Initiative (WHI) trial, the largest study of menopausal women in which 16608 women were randomized to receive HT (0.625 mg CEE + 2.5 mg MPA C.C. HT) or placebo. The trial was scheduled for 10 years, but altered prematurely in July 2002 (5.2 years) when it was discovered that the risk of invasive breast cancer exceeded in HT group. It also showed increased rates of coronary events, stroke and pulmonary embolism with two-fold increase in risk of venous thromboembolism with HT group.
- Estrogen replacement and atherosclerosis (ERA) trial and women's estrogen for stroke trial (WEST) also did not find cardioprotective benefits for estrogen.

19. What is the role of estrogen with respect to memory and cognition?

Estrogens play an important role in memory and learning which involves acquisition, encoding and consolidation of new information.

Recently, using sophisticated functional neuro-imaging techniques include MRI, SPECT (positron emission tomography), etc. Estrogens have been shown to modulate cerebral blood flow, neurotransmitter function and glucose utilization in postmenopausal women. Increase in cerebral blood flow was particularly noticed in the hippocampus, para-hippocampus, gyrus and temporal regions which are a part of the memory circuit. But, the very recent component study of WHI, named WHIM, has indicated absence of estrogen-induced neuroprotective role with respect to memory and cognition. The HT increased the risk of probable dementia in postmenopausal women aged 65 years and older.

20. What is postmenopausal osteoporosis? How serious is the problem?

Osteoporosis is a systemic skeletal disorder characterized by low bone mass, and a deterioration of micro-architecture of bone fragility as a result of which there is increased fracture rate with little or no trauma. Osteoporosis commonly affects the site of cancellous bone earlier and more severely than cortical bone, resulting in increased incidence of osteoporotic fractures in areas with predominance of cancellous bone, namely, vertebral bodies, proximal femur and distal forearm. It is the most prevalent bone problem in the elderly.

21. What is BMD? How do you assess it correctly?

Bone mineral density (BMD) is bone mass. It increases throughout the growth period and is completely achieved in young women by late adolescence. Therefore, normal diet and normal hormonal environment during adolescence is important to achieve higher peak bone mass. After 30 years, the bone loss occurs at the rate of 0.7% per year. After menopause, due to estrogen deficiency, the bone loss is accelerated up to 2% per year for 10 years (postmenopausal osteoporosis type 1). The bone loss continues at a much slower rate of 1% per year as the aging related loss (senile osteoporosis type 2).

The BMD can be correctly assessed by DEXA-scanning (Dual energy X-ray Absorptiometry). It is fast and simple, non-invasive method with minimal radiation exposure and can measure BMD at all sites. It has a precision of 1 to 2% with the pencil-beam machine and 0.5–1% with fan-beam machine. At least 2 major osteoporotic sites are scanned. The report gives us total BMD in g/cm sq as well as T-score and Z-score along with a graph with the fracture threshold.

T-score is defined as the patient's BMD as compared to the peak bone mass in normal young adults. While, Z-score is the patient's BMD compared to the peak bone mass in age-to-sex matched adults.

When T-score is less, it indicates bone loss over number of years, probably due to postmenopausal or senile changes. If Z-scores are less than 2, the bone loss is due to some pathological cause and needs to be investigated.
- –1 to –2.5 → osteopenia
- Less than –2.5 → osteoporosis
- + 2.5 to –1 normal.

22. Describe the effects of estrogen on bone.

Estrogens in women are essential for formation and maintenance of sufficient bone mass. Both the osteoclasts and the osteoblasts have estrogen receptors. Estrogens act directly on the osteoclasts by inhibiting lysosomal enzyme production and prevent bone resorption. Estrogenic action on osteoblasts directly is, however, not known but it acts indirectly through osteoblasts on osteoclasts. The estrogen promotes production of interleukins from the osteoblasts which inhibit the osteoclast activity.

23. Describe the effects of calcium on bone.

Ninety percent of the calcium in the body is in bones. A normal woman stores about 1000 g of calcium. The 1% of calcium is in circulation and in soft tissue and is necessary for muscle contraction and transmission of nerve impulse. A decrease in calcium intake and/or absorption lowers the serum level of ionized calcium. This stimulates PTH secretion to mobilize calcium from bone by direct stimulation of osteoclastic activity. A deficiency in estrogen is associated with greater responsiveness of bone to PTH. Thus, for any given level of PTH, there is more calcium removed from bone, raising the serum calcium.

24. What are the risk factors for osteoporosis?
- Unmodifiable risk factors:
  – Female sex
  – Premature menopause <40
  – Late menarche
  – Short stature
  – Slender built
  – Ethnic origin (Asian, Caucasian)
  – Nulliparity
  – Family history of osteoporosis
  – Fair skin.
- Potentially modifiable risk factors:
  – Smoking
  – Physical inactivity (burkha)
  – Low dietary calcium
  – Low vitamin D
  – Alcohol, caffeine and nicotine abuse
  – Estrogen deficiency (as in menopause)
  – Hyperthyroidism
  – Hyperparathyroidism
  – Hyperadrenalism
  – Anticoagulant therapy
  – Glucocorticoid use.

25. Describe the clinical features of established osteoporosis.

Most of the osteoporotic postmenopausal women are asymptomatic till fractures occur.
- Back pain is a major clinical symptom of vertebral compression fractures. The pain with a fracture is acute, then subsides over 2–3 months and lingers as chronic low back pain due to increased lumbar lordosis. There is loss of height and postural deformities called the "kyphotic Dowager's hump". Fifty percent women more than 65 years of age have spinal compression fractures (2/3rd are unrecognized). Each complete compression fracture causes loss of approximately 1 cm in height. The most common sites for vertebral fractures are T12, L1, L2, L3 vertebrae.
- Colles' fracture—a ten-fold increase is seen from age 35 to 60 years.

- Hip fracture—0.3 to 20% incidence is observed with increasing age from 45 to 85 years. Eight percent of all hip fractures are associated with osteoporosis.
- Tooth loss—oral annular bone loss is strongly associated with osteoporosis.

26. How do you diagnose osteoporosis? What are the WHO criteria?

Osteoporosis can be easily diagnosed on plain X-ray spine by prominent horizontal trabeculae and wedging or compression of dorsolumbar vertebrae due to gross demineralization. But by this time, 40% bone loss has already occurred and patient is in advanced stage of osteoporosis. Early diagnosis should be done in the stage of osteopenia where X-ray is subjective. DEXA scanning is a gold standard to diagnose osteoporosis.

The WHO defines osteoporosis in terms of BMD T-score:

Bone density	T-score
Normal	> –1.0
Osteopenic	–1.0 to –2.5
Osteoporotic	< –2.5
Severely osteoporotic	< –2.5 + 1/>1 fragility fractures

27. What are the NOF guidelines for prevention and treatment of osteoporosis?

National Osteoporosis Foundation 2000 Guidelines suggest initial screening for following group of postmenopausal women:
- All women over 65 years of age
- Women more than 50 years with one or more clinical risk factors
- Any fracture after age 40
- Osteoporotic fracture in a first-degree relative
- Current smoking
- Weight less than 127 lbs
- Postmenopausal women presenting with fractures.

Prevention
- *Primary prevention*: Should start at menarche and adolescent years with a combination of adequate nutrition, physical exercise and healthy lifestyle to achieve optimal peak bone mass.
- *Secondary prevention*: To diagnose osteoporosis and to prevent osteoporotic fractures and further deterioration.
- *Tertiary prevention*: To prevent further osteoporotic fractures where they have already occurred in the past.

Treatment
- HT is recommended after menopause but not generally so. But HT is necessary when osteoporosis or its risk factors already exist.
- Weightbearing exercises
- Smoking and alcohol discouraged
- Nonhormonal treatment includes:
  - Biphosphonates
  - Calcitonin
  - Fluoride
  - Calcium (1500 mg elemental Ca/day) and vitamin D (20 mg/day) supplementation.

28. What is conventional HRT?

Conventional hormone replacement therapy (HRT) is replacement of the predominant circulating hormones in the premenopausal woman namely, estrogens, progestogens and to some extent androgens after the decline of ovarian function.

Conventional hormone therapy includes:
- Estrogen replacement therapy (ERT)
- Estrogen progestogen therapy (EPRT)
- Sequential EPRT (SEPRT)
- Continuous combined HT (CCHT)
- Continuous combined EPRT (CCEPRT)
- Continuous sequential HT (CSHT)
- If androgens are given, it is known as AT.

29. What are tibolone and SERM?

Tibolone is a widely acting gonadomimetic hormone with a combination of all estrogenic, progestogenic and androgenic actions. It is a uni compound with tissue-specific mode of action and is described as STEAR, i.e. Selective Tissue Estrogen Activity Regulator. It has estrogenic effects on the bone and vaginal tissue, functions as progesterone in endometrial tissue, and has androgenic effects on the brain and liver. It is administered orally as once daily dose of 2.5 mg. It may not be effective against severe vasomotor symptoms in this dose. Its long-term effects are still under research. It is not a conventional HT as it does not contain estrogen or progesterone.

Side effects include breast tenderness, acne, hirsutism, visual disturbances, headache and weight gain.

Selective estrogen receptor modulator (SERM) is a compound that produces estrogen agonism in desired target tissues such as bone, liver, vascular system, etc. together with estrogen antagonism and/or minimal agonism in reproductive tissues such as breast and uterus. They are a group of anti-estrogens, eR ligands which activate transcriptional activational functions in estrogen receptors TAF 1 (agonistic) and TAF 2 (antagonistic).

There are 3 generations of SERM's:
1st: Tamoxifene
2nd: Raloxifene
3rd: Iodoxifene.

30. What is the MORE study?

The multiple outcomes of raloxifene evaluation (MORE) study, which involved 7705 postmenopausal women over 4 years. It showed raloxifene had beneficial effects on osteoporosis after 36 months, it reduced the incidence of breast cancer but had no effect on endometrial cancer, 10% alteration in lipid profile.

31. What are biphosphonates?

Biphosphonates are enzyme resistant analogues of pyrophosphates which inhibit mineralization in bone. They reduce the resorption of bone in a dose dependent manner mainly by inhibiting recruitment and promoting apoptosis of osteoclasts. They also indirectly stimulate osteoblast activity. There are three generations of biphosphonates:

1st: Etidronate
2nd: Tiludronate
3rd: Risedronate.

Absorption is impaired by food and, therefore, have to be taken on empty stomach.
Dose: 5 mg/day for prevention and 10 mg/day for treatment.

Forty-eight percent reduction in new vertebral fractures was observed over a period of three years of Alendronate therapy.

32. What are phytoestrogens?

Phytoestrogens are plant compounds that are structurally or functionally similar to steroidal estrogens produced by the body. These compounds are weaker than natural estrogens and are found in herbs, seasoning, vegetables, fruits and drinks. Oats, fennel, liquorice, barley, yeast, etc. contain phytoestrogens.

Flavonoids are the dominant phytoestrogen in the human diet with 4000 different flavonoids having been identified.

They are divided into 7 subfamilies:
i. Flavons
ii. Isoflavons
iii. Flavanones
iv. Flavonols
v. Coumestans
vi. Lignans
vii. Chalcones.

Phytoestrogens are selective estrogen enzyme modulators functioning as proestrogens when estrogen deficiency is present and as antiestrogens when excess estrogen is present. Thus, they selectively balance the estrogen metabolism in the body. They are antioxidants, bone protective, cancer preventive, anti-atherogenic, and delay aging. It is a good alternative to women in whom conventional HT is contraindicated.

Table 38.1: Stages of menopause

Stages	Stage I		Stage IIA	Stage IIB	Stage III
Years	Roughly 3-5 years before the menopause		One year	Up to five years after the menopause	From five years after menopause up to her lifetime
Events	*IA:* Menstrual irregularity *IB:* Vasomotor instability *IC:* Early psychosomatic symptoms	MENOPAUSE	CONFIRMATION	• Local atrophic changes • Late psychosomatic symptoms	*IIIA:* Late atrophic changes *IIIB:* Ischemic heart disease *IIIC:* Osteoporosis *IIID:* Very late complications: e.g. cerebrovascular accidents, Alzheimer's disease, etc.
Action	Establish communications			Treats	Prevent I

33. Can menopause be staged?

The menopausal transition is a period and it is a good practice to stage this transition in relevance to the clinical presentation. This also helps us to rationalize the correct HT options and its utility. Such a classification was proposed by Prof Behram Anklesaria (IMS staging) way back in 1997 following which the STRAW classification for reproductive ageing was proposed. The IMS staging now has been found to be useful and is cited by the Jeffcott's textbook of gynecology and is a helpful tool to guide menopause management in the clinical setting.

34. What is the IMS staging and its advantage?

IMS staging is depicted in Table 38.1.

The advantages are that offers the correct guidelines in the use of different modalities of menopause management and also helps in identifying the correct window of opportunity for treatment.

35. What are the factors responsible for age of menopause?

Genetic, ethnicity, socioeconomic status, parity, smoking, prior surgery—hysterectomy, ovarian surgery, prior chemotherapy, prior radiotherapy.

MUST REMEMBER

- Menopause is normal cessation of menses.
- Climacteric is the symptomatic perimenopausal years.
- Diagnosis is by amenorrhea, FSH level >20 mIU/mL.
- Premature menopause is spontaneous cessation of menses before the age of 40 years.
- Investigations—Pap smear and mammography, blood sugar and lipid profile, bone densitometry.
- Management options—lifestyle modification, HRT, SERMS, bisphosphonate, calcium, weightbearing exercise.
- HRT is the best known treatment for vasomotor symptoms, mood changes, vaginal symptoms and prevention of osteoporosis.
- Contraindications to HRT—family history—breast cancer, hyperlipidemia. Past history—breast cancer, CHD, venous thromboembolism, hypertriglyceridemia.

Hormones and Allied Medications in Gynecology

39

Shirish Daftary, Pralhad Kushtagi

1. Name the clinical situations where hormones are required to be prescribed in gynecological practice.

The broad indications of use of hormones in gynecological practice are:
- Management of infertility
- Menstrual disorders
- Contraception
- Menopause
- Substitution therapy in deficiency states
- Cancer.

2. Which are the common hormonal drugs used in clinical practice?

The commonly used hormonal drugs used in gynecological practice are:
- Estrogens
- Progestogens
- Androgens
- Antiestrogens
- Antiprogesterone
- Antiandrogens
- Pituitary gonadotropins
- Gonadotropin releasing hormones (GnRH) and analogs.

ESTROGENS

3. What is the basic chemical structure and source of estrogen? What are its different types?

Estrogen is a naturally occurring C-18 steroid hormone. Its common sources are ovaries, adrenal glands and during pregnancy, the placenta. The natural estrogens belong to one of three types: Estriol, estradiol and estrone.

4. Outline the actions of estrogens on an individual.

The tissue actions of estrogens are as follows:
- Contributing to growth and maturation of female genital tract
- Initiation and maintenance of secondary sexual characteristics
- Provide negative feedback to the pituitary and hypothalamus
- Causing proliferative phase of the endometrium
- Cervical mucus favorably to sperm ascent
- Preparing the endometrium for progesterone action prior to nidation.

5. What are the indications for their use in clinical practice?

The various therapeutic indications of estrogens are:
- Ethinyl estradiol (EE) as a common component of oral contraceptive pills (OCP)
- In the treatment of dysfunctional uterine bleeding
- Conjugated estrogens in the management of menopause
- Local application as dienestrol cream for senile vaginitis
- HRT in perimenopausal and menopausal women
  - To control symptoms
  - For cardioprotective effect
  - To prevent osteoporosis
- Estrogen patches
  - HRT for controlling menopausal symptoms
  - Intersex cases to promote female sexual development
  - Prostate cancer.

6. What are the contraindications for use of estrogens?

The contraindications for use of estrogens are:
- Suspected genital tract malignancy
- Breast cancer
- History of thromboembolism
- Liver and gallbladder disease
- Cardiac, hypertensive or diabetic women
- Suspected pregnancy and during lactation
- Sickle cell anemia.

7. Which are the drugs that interact and affect the potency of estrogens?

Drugs that interact with estrogens include:
- Rifampicin
- Barbiturates
- Phenytoin
- Anticoagulants.

8. What are the side effects/complications due to the use of estrogens?

The side effects of estrogen use are:
- Nausea and vomiting
- Water retention and weight gain
- Mastalgia
- Thromboembolism
- Cerebrovascular accidents
- Endometrial cancer/breast cancer
- Gallbladder disease
- Hepatoma.

PROGESTOGENS

9. What is the basic chemical structure and source of progesterones?

Progesterone, a natural steroid hormone is with C-21 ring. It is not orally absorbed. They are elaborated by theca cells of the corpus luteum of the ovary.

10. What are the different types of progesterones?

Basically progesterones are considered as:
- Pure progesterone
- Progestogens—synthetic compounds with progestational effects.

11. Which are the progesterone preparations in common clinical use?

The common progesterones used are:
- Pure progesterone
  - Micronized progesterone
- Esters of progesterone
  - 17 alpha-OH progesterone caproate (proluton)
  - Medroxyprogesterone acetate (MPA)
- Retroprogesterone (dydrogesterone, duphaston)
- Alkyl derivatives of testosterone
  - Ethisterone
- Alkyl derivatives of nortestosterone
  - Norethisterone
  - Lynestrenol
  - Norgestrel
  - Desogestrel
  - Norgestimate
  - Gestodene.

12. What are the different routes of administration for contraceptive use of progestogens?

Routes of administration of progestogens for contraception are:
- Oral
  - Singly
  - Along with estrogen
- Intramuscular
  - Proluton depot—Injectable DMPA; as long-acting contraceptive
- Implants
  - Norplant
- Intrauterine device
  - Mirena coil progestasert
- Vaginal ring.

13. How are micronized progesterone administered?

The routes of administration of micronized progesterone are:
- Oral use
- Intravaginal.

14. What are the indications for the use of progesterone in clinical practice?

The clinical conditions where progesterone/progestagen are used:
- Luteal phase defect
- Threatened abortion
- Recurrent abortions
- Advanced endometrial cancer—in high doses; used for palliation
- Endometriosis
- Prior to TCRE to thin down the endometrium
- Amenorrhea—progesterone challenge test
- Hormone replacement therapy
- Postponement of menses (social/cultural reasons).

15. What are the contraindications for use of estrogens?

The contraindications for use of progestagens are:
- Undiagnosed vaginal bleeding
- Breast cancer/tumor
- Thromboembolism.

16. What are the side effects due to the use of progestogens?

The side effects commonly noted due to use of progestogens are:
- Nausea and vomiting
- Headache
- Mastalgia
- Water retention
- Bloating
- Weight gain
- Cramps
- Hirsutism
- Depression
- Increase in low density lipoprotein and cardiovascular accidents.

ANDROGENS

17. What are the different androgens used in gynecological practice?

The androgens in clinical use for gynecological conditions are:
- Testosterone
- Danazol
- Gestrinone.

TESTOSTERONE

18. What is the basic chemical structure and source of testosterone?

Testosterone is the naturally occurring steroid hormone. It is produced in women from ovarian stroma and adrenal glands. The physiological level in the normal individual is 1 ng/mL.

19. What are the therapeutic uses of testosterone?

Therapeutic use of testosterone is limited because of fear of hirsutism. It is used in the treatment of:
- Heavy menstrual bleeding in women
- Infertility for male
  - Oligospermia
  - Decreased libido.

20. What are the side effects due to use of testosterone?

The side effects are:
- Hirsutism
- Virilization.

DANAZOL

21. What is danazol?

Danazol is isoxazole derivative of 17-alpha ethinyl testosterone.

22. What are the actions of danazol?

Danazol acts directly on the endometrium causing atrophy.

23. What are the clinical uses of danazol?

Danazol is used to treat the following conditions:
- Endometriosis
- Cyclic mastalgia
- Diminished libido
- To shrink fibroids
- To thin down endometrium prior to ablation (TCRE)
- Fibrocystic disease of the breast
- Gynecomastia.

24. What are the side effects due to use of danazol?

The side effects due to danazol use are:
- Weight gain
- Hirsutism, acne, muscle cramps
- Breast atrophy
- Voice change
- Increased low density lipoproteins can cause cardiovascular disturbance.

25. What are the significant complications due to use of danazol?

The complications due to use of danazol are:
- Liver damage
- Teratogenic to the female fetus, if administered during pregnancy.

GESTRINONE

26. What is gestrinone?

Gestrinone is a trienic 19-norsteroid derivative.

27. What are the actions of gestrinone?

Gestrinone has an androgenic, antiestrogenic, antiprogesterone and antipituitary actions similar to danazol.

28. What are the clinical uses and side effects of gestrinone?

Gestrinone is used for similar indications. It is milder and better tolerated.

ANTIESTROGENS

29. Name the antiestrogens in common clinical use.

The antiestrogens in clinical use are clomiphene citrate, tamoxifen and letrozole.

CLOMIPHENE CITRATE (CC)

30. What is the chemical structure of clomiphene citrate?

CC is a nonsteroidal compound related to diethylstilbestrol (DES). It is a mixture of 2 isomers (cis and trans). The cis fraction is responsible for ovulation induction.

31. What is the mechanism of action of CC?

CC blocks the negative feedback of estrogen to the hypothalamus and thus stimulates gonadotropin secretions FSH and LH, thereby, inducing ovulation. This action is optimal in presence of some estrogen in the body.

32. Name the clinical situations where CC is prescribed.

The indications for use of CC are:
- Anovulatory infertility
  - PCOD
  - Assisted reproduction
- Male infertility.

33. What are the contraindications for the use of CC?

The contraindications for prescribing CC are:
- Ovarian cyst
- Liver disease
- Scotoma.

34. What are the known side effects due to use of CC?

The various side effects due to the ingestion of CC are:
- Ovarian enlargement
- Hot flushes
- Nausea and vomiting
- Visual disturbances
- Headache and dizziness
- Hair loss
- Antiestrogen effects on cervical mucus
- Ovarian hyperstimulation
- Multiple pregnancy
- Higher abortion rate
- Neural tube defects in offspring
- Premature ovarian failure.

TAMOXIFEN

35. What is the chemical structure of tamoxifen and how does it produce its clinical effects?

Tamoxifen is a nonsteroidal antiestrogenic drug. Its pharmacological and clinical actions are due to binding and reducing the available estrogen receptors.

36. In which clinical condition is tamoxifen indicated?

It is used in the treatment of advanced breast cancer in the dose of 10–20 mg twice daily for not more than 5 years.

37. Name the side effects due to use of tamoxifen.

The side effects of tamoxifen use are:
- Gastrointestinal upsets, dizziness, pruritus
- Thrombocytopenia, leukopenia, thromboembolism
- Hot flashes
- Vaginal bleeding.

38. What are the risks associated with use of tamoxifen?

Use of tamoxifen is significantly associated with the occurrence of endometrial hyperplasia and endometrial cancer. Hence, monitoring endometrial thickness on USG and endometrial sampling periodically is an important safeguard.

LETROZOLE

39. What is letrozole?

Letrozole is a nonsteroidal aromatase inhibitor which suppresses estrogen effects.

40. What is the indication for the use of letrozole?

Letrozole is used for induction of ovulation for anovulatory infertility.

41. Is it advantageous to use letrozole for ovulation induction?

Letrozole scores over clomiphene because it does not have adverse effects on cervical mucus or endometrium.

42. What is the dose prescribed for ovulation induction?

The recommended dosage is 2.5 mg daily for 5 days in every cycle (just like clomiphene citrate).

ANTIPROGESTERONES

43. Name the antiprogestin.

The antiprogestin in clinical use is mifepristone (RU 486).

44. What is the structure of mifepristone and what is its mechanism of action?

Mifepristone is a 19-norsteroid derivative of synthetic progestogen, norethindrone. It binds to the receptors in the cell nucleus and blocks progesterone action on the target organ.

45. When is the peak action of mifepristone after administration?

About 85% of the drug is absorbed after oral intake. Peak levels are reached in 1–2 hours; the half-life of the drug is 24 hours. It is excreted in bile and feces.

46. Which are the conditions where mifepristone is useful?

The indications for use of mifepristone are:
- Therapeutic abortion for medical termination of pregnancy within 49 days of amenorrhea (with misoprostol)
- Postcoital pill for prevention of pregnancy
- Cervical ripening prior to induction of midtrimester MTP
- Induction of labor in case of intrauterine fetal death
- Missed abortion.

47. What are the side effects due to mifepristone?

The side effects in patient on mifepristone are:
- Headache
- Gastrointestinal upsets
- Rash

- Faintness
- Adrenal failure
- Teratogenicity, if MTP fails.

ANTIANDROGENS

The different antiandrogens used in gynecological practice are cyproterone acetate, spironolactone, flutamide and finasteride. These drugs are used in the treatment of hirsutism.

CYPROTERONE ACETATE
(Diane 35, Krimson 35, Ginette 35)

48. What is the chemical structure of cyproterone acetate and what are its actions on ingestion?

Cyproterone acetate is chemically related to progesterone. It is a potent anti-androgen, it competes with dihydrotestosterone for intracellular androgen receptor sites and inhibits its binding. It has a weak corticosteroid effect. In small doses, it does not affect the pituitary gland, but large doses cause amenorrhea, loss of libido. In males, it causes loss of libido and suppression of spermatogenesis.

49. What are indications for the use of cyproterone acetate?

Cyproterone acetate is used mainly in the management of PCOD. Various aspects of PCOD where the drug could be useful are:
- Hirsutism—prescribed along with ethinyl estradiol (EE) cyclically for 3 weeks in every cycle for 6–12 months; beneficial effects are seen only after 3 months when hirsutism and acne show reasonable clinical improvement
- Abnormal uterine bleeding—diane 35 regularizes menstruation
- Contraceptive effect
- Treat acne
- Prior to induction of ovulation to improve treatment results.

SPIRONOLACTONE

50. What is the structure and mechanism of action of spironolactone?

Spironolactone is an aldosterone antagonist having antiandrogenic and diuretic effects. It blocks androgen action at receptor level in hair follicles. It reduces 17 alpha-hydroxylase activity, lowers plasma levels of testosterone and androstenedione.

51. In which condition is spironolactone used and how is it prescribed?

Spironolactone is used in the treatment of hirsutism. The suggested dose is 150 mg daily along with cyclic EE. Treatment for 6–12 months provides adequate relief in most cases. This is followed with maintenance dose of 50 mg/day.

PITUITARY GONADOTROPINS

The hormones secreted by anterior pituitary and that are used in clinical gynecological practice are gonadotropins (FSH, LH) and prolactin (PRL).

52. Name the sources of pituitary gonadotropins utilized in clinical practice.

Follicular stimulating and luteinizing hormones are the important gonadotropins used in gynecological practice. FSH is derived from menopausal urine; LH resembles hCG and is extracted from the urine of pregnant women.

53. What are the clinical indications for use of gonadotropins in gynecology?

The indications/purpose for use of gonadotropins in gynecological practice are:
- Induction of ovulation in anovulatory infertility
- Induction of multiple ovulation prior to ART
- Hypogonadotropic hypogonadism
- Cryptorchidism
- Amenorrhea—secondary to pituitary failure
- Luteal phase defect—hCG is used.

54. What are the likely side effects due to use of gonadotropins for ovulation induction?

The side effects resulting from use of gonadotropins for inducing ovulation are:
- Hyperstimulation syndrome
- Multiple pregnancy.

GnRH AND ANALOGS

55. What is the chemical structure and biological action of GnRH/analogs?

GnRH is a decapeptide. It is released by hypothalamus in a pulsatile manner. The pulse rate and intensity determine pituitary release of glycoprotein hormone FSH or LH. Continuous administration, however, suppresses the pituitary gonadotropins.

56. What are the clinical uses of GnRH/analogs?

The clinical uses of GnRH and analogs are:
- Hypothalamic amenorrhea
  - Pulsatile GnRH analogs
  - 5-10 mcg IV every 90-120 minutes or
  - 15-20 mcg subcutaneous or
  - Intranasal 200 mcg every 2 hourly or
  - Induce cyclic menstruation
- Hypothalamic infertility—Pulsatile GnRH
- PCOS—in infertile women on ART for ovulation induction with down-regulation protocol before commencing FSH/LH regime
- Endometriosis
- Fibroid uterus—to shrink the size prior to surgery
- AUB—to thin down the endometrium prior to ablation (TCRE)
- Cryptorchidism in males
- Precocious puberty—continuous administration (zoladex, leupride); to buy time until normal age of puberty is reached.
- Contraception—expensive
- Dysfunctional bleeding—when other measures have failed.

57. What are the side effects due to use of GnRH and analogs?

The side effects in the patient on GnRH and analogs are:
- Hyperstimulation syndrome
- Multiple pregnancy incidence same as in general population
- Higher abortion rate
- Menopausal symptoms including osteoporosis on prolonged use
- Decrease in breast size
- Decreased libido
- Nausea, insomnia, dizziness and myalgia.

BROMOCRIPTINE

58. What is bromocriptine?

Bromocriptine is a synthetic ergot alkaloid—derivative of lysergic acid and ergoline.

59. What is the mechanism of action of bromocriptine?

Bromocriptine is a dopamine agonist, it suppresses prolactin while promoting the secretion of gonadotropins. It induces menstruation, ovulation and pregnancy.

60. What is the role of administration of bromocriptine preparations?

Bromocriptine can be administered:
- Orally—Parlodel, serocrip, proctinal
- Vaginally—Pergolide
- Parenterally—Parlodel-LAR (glycolipid microspheres).

61. What are the therapeutic uses of bromocriptine?

Indications for use of bromocriptine are:
- Hyperprolactinemia causing/oligomenorrhea/anovulation and infertility with/without galactorrhea
- Suppression of lactation
- Prolactinomas.

62. If the woman on bromocriptine conceives, which are the specific issues that should be covered in counseling?

Woman on bromocriptine:
- She can continue bromocriptine during pregnancy
- It does not cause teratogenic effects
- May grow during pregnancy
  - Needs to be monitored for growth of prolactinomas with MRI scan and assessment of visual fields.

63. How is the treatment with bromocriptine initiated?

Bromocriptine treatment is initiated with a low dose of 1.25 mg at bedtime; the dose is then gradually built up to 2.5 mg twice daily or more as required to normalize prolactin levels.

64. What are the side effects with the use of bromocriptine?

The common side effects associated with use of bromocriptine are:
- Nausea and vomiting
- Dizziness and hypotension
- Postural hypotension.

Pelvic Organ Prolapse

CN Purandare, Jayam Kannan, Madhuri A Patel, Manjusha Yetalkar, Nikhil Purandare

HISTORY

Age

Parity

Symptoms: Fullness in vagina, mass descending per vaginum—on straining, at rest, urinary symptoms, urinary complaints, bowel complaints, sexual dissatisfaction, backache, discharge/bleeding.

Past History

Connective tissue disorder, myopathy/neuropathy.

Obstetric History

Number of pregnancies, vaginal deliveries, duration of second stage, size of the baby, instrumental delivery.

Menopausal Status

- Occupation
- Chronic cough/constipation
- Smoking
- Previous surgery—for prolapse, hysterectomy
- Physical examination
- Bone mass index (BMI)
- Joint hypermobility
- Other signs of myopathy/neuropathy
- *RS:* For features of COPD
- *PA:* Abdominal mass
- *LA:* Vulval atrophy, perineal body, introitus gaping, vaginal rugae
- *Prolapse:* POP-Q classification staging, tone of levator ani, lateral vaginal sulcus, stress incontinence, decubitus ulcer
- *Pelvic examination:* Uterine size, mobility
- *Rectal examination:* Rectocele, enterocele, tone of anal sphincter.

1. What is POP?

A prolapse is the protrusion of an organ or structure beyond its normal anatomical position (Procidentia, word, Latin *Procidese* = to fall).

2. Why genital prolapse occurs?

Genital prolapse occurs due to relaxation and weakening of pelvic supports which result in displacement of either uterus or vagina or both from its anatomical position.

3. What is the anatomical classification of POP?

Normal—cervix at the level of ischial spine.
I°—cervix below the ischial spine but above introitus
II°—cervix at the level of introitus
III°—cervix outside introitus
Procidentia—uterine fundus outside introitus.

4. Can you tell us about grading of POP?

Grading of POP either via the Baden–Walker system or the pelvic organ prolapse quantification (POP-Q) system is presently being followed in many centers, especially in academic and research centers (Fig. 40.1).

Baden–Walker system for the evaluation of pelvic organ prolapse on physical examination	
Grade	Posterior urethral descent, lowest part other sites
0	Normal position for each respective site
1	Descent halfway to the hymen
2	Descent to the hymen
3	Descent halfway past the hymen
4	Maximum possible descent for each site

Pelvic organ prolapse quantification (POP-Q) system	
Stage	Description
0	No prolapse anterior and posterior points are all –3 cm, and C or D is between -TVL and -(TVL-2 cm)
1	The criteria for stage 0 are not met, and the most distal prolapse is more than 1 cm above the level of the hymen (less than 1 cm)
2	The most distal prolapse if between 1 cm above and 1 cm below the hymen (at least one point is -1, 0, or +1)
3	The most distal prolapse is more than 1 cm below the hymen but no further than 2 cm less than TVL
4	Represents complete procidentia or vault eversion; the most distal prolapse protrudes to at least (TVL-2 cm)

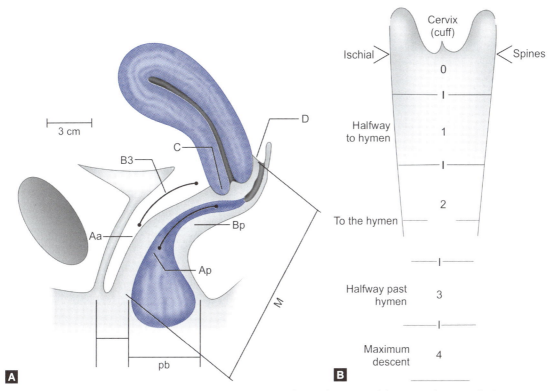

Figs 40.1A and B: Diagrammatic representation for explanation of the quantification of POP

	Grades of Cystocele
1+	Bulge inside vagina on straining
2+	Bulge up to to vulval outlet on straining
3+	Bulge seen outside vulval outlet on straining
4+	Bulge seen outside vulval outlet at all times

5. What is II° degree cystocele?

It is prolapse of the upper 2/3rd of anterior vaginal wall and underlying bladder up to the introitus.

6. What is II° degree rectocele?

It is prolapse of lower 2/3rd of the posterior vaginal wall underlying rectum up to the introitus.

7. What is an enterocele?

Enterocele is herniation of pouch of Douglas which contains loops of small bowel or omentum.

Types of enterocele

- *Pulsion:* In this type, the vaginal vault is pushed outwards by conditions which increase the intra-abdominal pressure, e.g. chronic respiratory problems, lifting heavy weights, etc.
- *Traction:* There is a pre-existing weakness in the anterior compartment, uterine does not pull down the vault.
- *Congenital:* Results from the failure of fusion or reopening of the previous fusion of the peritoneum so that the bowel filled cul-de-sac can extend by dissection all the way to the perineal body.
- *Iatrogenic:* This follows a vault suspension procedure like Burch/Marshall-Marchetti-Krantz, which produces a change in the vaginal axis and subject the vault to abnormal procedures.

Types of enterocele according to site
- Anterior—anterior to vagina
- Posterior—located between vagina and rectum
- Lateral (pudendal enterocele)—located lateral to vagina.

8. Why there is chronic backache in a case of genital prolapse?

Chronic backache in a case of genital prolapse occurs due to stretching of pelvic ligaments, i.e. uterosacral and Mackenrodt's ligament.

9. Why there is leukorrhea in a case of genital prolapse?

Leukorrhea in a case of genital prolapse occurs due to vaginitis or due to decubitus ulcer or due to increased cervical glandular activity associated with congestion.

10. Why there is dyspareunia in a case of POP?

Dyspareunia in a case of genital prolapse occurs due to:
- Prolapse of ovaries in POD,
- Associated with PID/endometriosis, etc.

11. Why there is bearing-down sensation in a case of POP?

Bearing-down sensation in a case of genital prolapse occurs due to stretching of mesentery of the enterocele.

12. Why in severe degree of cystocele incomplete evacuation of urine occurs and more the patient strains she has more difficulty to pass urine?

When the intra-abdominal pressure is raised during straining, the urine is pushed down into the cystocele below the level of the external meatus. She can only empty the bladder by reducing the cystocele into the vagina with her fingers.

13. What are the supports of the uterus?

Supports of the uterus:
- *Muscular levator ani:* Coccygeus
- *Urogenital diaphragm:* Sphincter urethrae
- *Ligamentous:* Transverse cervical, pubocervical, uterosacral, and uterocervical. Except the round ligament, the others are robust and contain smooth muscles along with fibrous tissue to offer good support
- Perineal body
- Anteverted position of uterus.

14. What are the etiological factors in POP?

Developmental weakness of the supports (congenital prolapse), spina bifida, myelodysplasia.

Menopausal atrophy predisposes to prolapse.

In this case, home delivery probably unattended by an expert has resulted into POP.

During vaginal delivery, there may be:
- Excessive stretching of pelvic floor muscle and ligaments
- Bearing down before full dilatation
- Prolonged 1st and 2nd stages of labor
- Application of ventouse before full dilatation
- Pudendal nerve injury
- Delivery of big baby
- Resuming heavy work soon after delivery, without pelvic floor exercises.

15. What are the aggravating factors for POP?

Increased intra-abdominal pressure:
- Chronic cough
- Chronic constipation
- Ascites
- Tumor in the abdomen especially in the lower abdomen
- Lifting heavy weights
- Straining at stools.

Increased weight of the uterus:
- Subinvolution
- Myohyperplasias
- Traction on uterus
- Vaginal traction
- Large cervical polyp
- Pulling strongly on the cervix during operation.

16. What are the differential diagnoses of POP?
- Congenital elongation of the cervix
- Cervical polyp
- Vulvar tumor
- Urethral caruncle
- Chronic inversion of uterus
- Vaginal/periurethral cysts
- Diverticulae/prolapse of the urethra.

17. What is the mode of treatment in young patient?

If patient is young and interested in further childbearing function, hence conservative surgical management in form of sling operation is advised.

18. How will you investigate patient with POP?
- CBC X-ray/chest PA view
- RFTs and ECG
- LFTs/USG
- Blood group, clotting time, bleeding time
- Urine analysis, Pap smear.

19. What are the aims of surgery in young patient?
- To relieve symptoms
- To restore anatomy
- To restore sexual function
- To restore reproductive function.

20. What are the different types of sling operation?
- *Shirodkar's abdominal sling:* It is closed loop, posterior sling and static type of sling.
- *Purandare's cervicopexy:* It is closed loop but anterior and dynamic type of sling.
- *Khanna's sling:* It is open and neutral type of sling.
- *Virkud's composite sling:* It is a combination of static and dynamic support open type and anterior plus posterior type of sling.

21. What is an ideal prosthetic material?
- Biologically nonirritating to tissues
- Inorganic in nature
- Easily sterilized
- Chemically inert in tissue fluids
- Unaltered by sterilization
- Nonelectrolytic, nonhygroscopic
- Inexpensive and readily available

- Pliable, nonrigid so as to adjust to tissue movement
- Strong enough to withstand local stress and intra-abdominal pressures
- Not subjected to fragmentation
- Non opaque to X-ray
- Should be usable in potentially infected area.

22. What are the selection criteria for sling operation?

- Young women with II/III degree cervical descent want to preserve the reproductive function
- Absent or minimal cystocele/rectocele
- Uterocervical length of less than five inches
- If moderate to large cysto/rectocele is present, it should be repaired from below at the same sitting before performing the sling
- Not suitable for hypertrophic, lacerated and infected cervix.

23. Describe Shirodkar's sling operation for genital prolapse and its advantages and disadvantages.

- This is conservative type of surgery for genital prolapse where the Mersilene tape is fixed to the posterior aspect of isthmus and sacral promontory
- It is an alternative to Purandare's cervicopexy, especially if cervicopexy in past has failed.

Advantages
- It maintains the uterus in its correct anatomical position
- It provides a strong static bony support
- No tendency to enterocele formation
- No difficulty in subsequent LSCS.

Disadvantages
- Technically difficult to perform especially on left side where the sling has to pass blindly under the sigmoid mesentery
- Risk of injuring the colon, ureter, iliac vessels and genitofemoral nerve on left side
- Injury to presacral veins and hematoma formation
- Being a closed loop sling, if it becomes tight, there is a risk of bowel obstruction.

24. What is Purandare's cervicopexy?

In this type of sling anterior rectus sheath or mersilene tape when anterior rectus sheath is defective is anchored to the anterior aspect of isthmus and anterior abdominal wall. It is indicated in II/III degree prolapse with minimal or no cystocele and/or rectocele and no supravaginal elongation of cervix.

Advantages
Technically easy to perform, every time the patient strains the recti contract and uterus is pulled up instead of being pushed down as in the natural effect of straining.

Disadvantages
- Injury to the inferior epigastric vessels
- Not correct anatomically, being anterior sling, uterus becomes retroverted.

To prevent this on right side, round ligament plication is done
- Deepens POD, so tendency to develop enterocele
- As the tape is anchored anteriorly, it may get damaged at subsequent LSCS surgery.

25. What is Khanna's sling operation?

In this, Mersilene tape is anchored to posterior aspect of isthmus and anterior superior iliac spine. It is fairly easy to perform. There is no risk of bowel obstruction. Being neutral, it does not cause anterversion or retroversion of uterus.

Disadvantages
- Tape is easily felt by the patient as it is being superficial
- If skin wound gets infected, periostitis will occur which is a very painful condition and the tape may get detached
- The tape will be uncomfortable for Indian traditional dress wearers.

26. What is Virkud's composite sling operation?

In this surgery, the Mersilene tape is anchored from the posterior aspect of isthmus to sacral promontory on right side and anterior abdominal walls on left side and left uterosacral ligament is plicated.

Advantages
- Easy to perform
- Provides double support
- Uterus remains anteverted
- No tendency to enterocele formation
- No risk of injury to sigmoid colon, iliac vessels, ureter or genitofemoral nerve
- Being open type of sling, no risk of bowel obstruction.

Disadvantages
Tendency towards dextrorotation which can be compensated by left uterosacral ligament plication.

27. What are the advantages and disadvantages of endoscopic approach to sling operation?

Advantages
- All the benefits of minimally invasive surgery
- Magnification and better exposure of tissue.

Disadvantages
Expert and trained hands are required.

28. What are the other conservative surgical procedures that can be done in this age group?

Other conservative surgical procedures can be done in this age group are:

- Fothergill's operation
- Shirodkar's modification of Fothergill's operation
- Nadkarni's operation.

29. What are the principles of Fothergill's operation and disadvantages of it?

Principles of Fothergill's operation are
- Dilatation and curettage
- Shortening of cardinal ligament
- Partial amputation of cervix
- Sturmdorf suture
- Anterior colporrhaphy
- Posterior colpoperineorrhaphy.

Disadvantages
- Cervical stenosis
- Infertility
- Incompetent os
- Cervical dystocia
- Recurrence after vaginal delivery.

30. What is Shirodkar's modification of Fothergill's operation?

- Shirodkar's modification of Fothergill's operation is same operation as Fothergill's operation except partial amputation of cervix and Sturmdorf's suture are not taken, as there is no supravaginal elongation of cervix.

31. What is the use of mesh in POP?

The aim of surgery in POP is to provide support for vagina or uterus. 70% women undergoing conventional vaginal prolapse surgery have a successful outcome. Mesh reinforcement is used with the aim of reducing the risk of recurrence of the prolapse. It may provide a longer lasting repair and has been shown to be successful in 80% of people.

Additional use of a vaginal support device (VSD), along with the mesh, is a new approach to surgery. The purpose of the VSD, which remains in the vagina for four weeks following surgery, is to provide extra support for the vagina during the healing period. The VSD also simplifies surgery when mesh is used, and this may have additional benefits, such as shorter operating time and less complications from surgery. The VSD is made of a soft comfortable material, which is well-tolerated by most patients. The VSD may cause a discharge from the vagina approximately 2 weeks after surgery. VSD may move down slightly after 3 weeks. About 10–15% may have difficulties.

32. In patient of genital prolapse of advanced age who is not interested in childbearing and menstrual functions, what type of surgery will be advised?

Patient of genital prolapse with advanced age who is not interested in childbearing and menstrual functions, vaginal hysterectomy with anterior colporrhaphy and posterior colpoperineorrhaphy is advised.

33. What are the different operations done for enterocele repair?

The different operations done for enterocele repair are:

Abdominal route
Moschcowitz operation is done in a patient of enterocele associated with condition that requires exploratory laparotomy or along with Burch procedure, Purandare's cervicopexy, ventral suspension to prevent development of enterocele in future.

Vaginal route : Halban culdoplasty
During vaginal hysterectomy, high vaginal peritonization is done or during vaginal hysterectomy before peritonization, the peritoneum of the posterior cul-de-sac is sharply mobilized of the anterior surface of the rectum and lower sigmoid and excised. One to three internal McCall sutures are taken depending upon the size of the enterocele. In internal McCall suture, the monofilament zero suture is placed deeply into left pararectal fascia, after which the suture is continued across the front of the sigmoid colon and placed deeply into right pararectal fascia. Similarly, one or two external McCall sutures are taken, where suture is taken from posterior vaginal wall to the peritoneum to the same left pararectal fascia across the front of the sigmoid to the right pararectal fascia and brought through vagina. These sutures are tied after completion of anterior colporrhaphy.

34. What are the different operations done to correct posthysterectomy vault prolapse?

Operation to correct posthysterctomy vault prolapse can be done by
- Vaginal route.
- Abdominal route, if vagina is narrow or if laparotomy is required for other reasons.

Different operations are
- Complete colpocleisis
- Sacrospinal vaginal fixation
- Williams—Richardson operation
- Ventral suspension of vaginal wall
- Abdominal sacropexy: The posterior cul-de-sac is obliterated by Moschcowitz culdoplasty where Mersilene tape, Teflon tape or Marlex mesh is used to suspend vault.

35. What are the indications and methods of conservative nonsurgical management?

Indications
- Unfit for surgery
- Denies for surgery
- Waiting for surgery
- Prolapse during 1st trimester of pregnancy
- Puerperal prolapse
- Planning for pregnancy in near future.

Methods of conservative nonsurgical management pelvic floor exercises: Pelvic floor exercise also known as Kegel's exercises.

Principles

A sustained program of voluntary isometric contractions of pelvic floor muscles.

Technique

Patient is taught these exercises by asking her to contract her pelvic floor muscles around the examining vaginal finger as she would do so in order to interrupt her flowing stream of urine. Patient is asked to do these exercises at home at least three times a day gradually increasing in duration.

Patient should be counseled that is a very important nonsurgical modality of treatment, and it is patient-dependent. Patient is also advised to avoid strenuous work or factor to prevent recurrence. Patient has to be explained that it is a very time consuming therapy and result will be seen after at least 6 months of continuous and regular exercises.

Vaginal support devices

 i. Pessaries
 ii. Cube
 iii. Gehrung.

Principles: It stretches the levator muscle which cause reflex contraction of it over the pessary which prevents it from falling down. It is a ring-shaped device made of polyethylene, which is used as pelvic support device. It is most commonly and simplest to use. It causes less inflammation as it is made up of polyethylene. It is available in different diameters, according to outer circumferences.

Indications

- Prolapse uterus during pregnancy up to first 4 months
- Immediate postpartum lactation
- Patient unfit for surgery or not willing for surgery
- Patient waiting for surgery, e.g. healing decubitus ulcer.

Contraindications

- Complete procedentia
- Very patulous vaginal orifice
- Stress incontinence
- Local infection/ulceration
- Correct size of pessary is chosen by trial and error methods, so that the largest sized pessary is comfortably retained during walking, standing, exercising, etc. It should not be expelled even partially/completely by Valsalva maneuver
- It should be sterilized before used
- Counseling, regular removal and cleaning should be done. Initially, remove overnight, clean with soap and water, lubricate and reinsert in the morning. Later weekly overnight removal to be done

- Regular follow-up is asked
- Explain hazards of leaving the pessary inside for prolonged period like impaction, ulceration, infection, malignancy, SUI, vesicovaginal fistula.

36. What are the complications of genital prolapse?

Local complications

- Keratinization
- Decubitus ulceration
- Hypertrophy of cervix because of congestion, edema, hyperplasia of cervical glands and supravaginal elongation of cervix
- Incarcerated prolapse
- Malignancy
- Remote complications
- *Infection:* UTI, cystitis, pyelitis, pyelonephritis
- Calculus formation
- *Obstructive complications:* Because of hypertrophy of bladder wall and trabeculation, constriction of ureters, hydroureter, hydronephrosis and renal failure.

37. What are the preventive measures for genital prolapse?

- Antenatal physiotherapy
- Prevention of anemia
- Promote delivery under supervision of a trained attendant
- Avoid bearing-down before full dilatation of cervix
- Avoid prolonged first and second stages of labor
- Generous episiotomy in primigravida and when required low forceps if delay in II stage of labor
- Perineal tears immediately and accurately sutured after delivery
- Postnatal exercises and physiotherapy
- Early postnatal ambulation
- Adequate rest for 6 month after delivery
- Adequate interval between pregnancies
- Family planning
- *Other strategies*
  – Cessation of smoking
  – Maintaining ideal body weight
  – Avoid constipation
  – Prevent diabetic complications
  – No role of elective LSCS for protection of pelvic floor.

38. Describe genital prolapse in pregnancy.

Symptoms

- Severe backache
- Excessive vaginal discharge
- Spotting per vagina
- Constipation
- Urinary retention and increased SUI.

Complications
- Abortion, retention of urine
- UTI, decubitus ulcers
- PROM, cervical dystocia
- Cervical tears, PPH
- Subinvolution of uterus
- Puerperal infection.

Management
- Bed rest
- Pessary
- Introital tightening.

39. What is the cause of decubitus ulcer in case of prolapse?

It is a trophic ulcer formed due to dependent part of the prolapsed mass outside the introitus. There is an initial surface keratinization, "cracks", "Infection sloughing" ulceration.

MUST REMEMBER
- The latest addition to the group of staging systems is the POP-Q system, which is becoming increasingly popular with specialists all over the world, because, although is not very simple as a concept, it helps defining the features of a prolapse at a level of completeness not reached by any other system to date. In this vision, the POP-Q system may reach the importance and recognition of the TNM system use in oncology.
- Two-dimensional translabial scanning is now a standard technique and has been reported for assessing position and mobility of the bladder neck and proximal urethra, stress incontinence, bladder wall thickness (with transvaginal scanning as well), levator ani activity (with perineal scanning), and prolapse quantification. Multiple two-dimensional images can be combined, like slices of bread, to yield a three-dimensional image. Three-dimensional ultrasound has been used to image the urethra, levator ani complex, paravaginal supports, prolapse, and synthetic implant materials. Ultrasound is not recommended in the primary evaluation of women with incontinence and prolapse and is an optional test for complex problems.
- MRI may be helpful in patients with complex organ prolapse to supplement the physical examination, the dynamic MRI of the pelvic floor proved itself as an excellent tool for assessing functional disorders of the pelvic floor, including organ prolapse and incontinence. Recent studies suggest that dynamic MRI correlates very well with clinical examination in detection of the prolapse but may offer superior results when it comes to staging. This investigation seems to be also useful in assessing the results of surgery for pelvic organ prolapse, even when the patient has no clinical symptoms. Dynamic MR imaging underestimates the extent of cystoceles and enteroceles, it has the advantage of revealing all pelvic organs and the pelvic floor musculature.
- Surgery should be tailored to suit the patient's need.
- Vaginal hysterectomy with vaginal repair should be done with patient's consent, knowing that there are alternatives to hysterectomy. Perineorrhaphy is recommended, vault suspension is an essential step.
- Laparoscopic sacrocolpopexy as an alternative to open surgery is considered. Further studies are required on the long-term efficiency in laparoscopic paravaginal repair and vaginal wall prolapse. Computational models have been demonstrated to be an effective tool to investigate the effects of vaginal delivery and PF dysfunctions interdisciplinary and multidisciplinary collaborative research, involving bioengineers and clinicians, is crucial to improve clinical outcomes in patients with PF dysfunctions.
- Sacrospinous hysteropexy is done, if interested in uterine preservation and should be considered by surgeons well-versed in transvaginal surgery.
- LeFort colpocleisis technique was associated with a good patients' satisfaction and functional results in a population aged over 75.
- Ischiospinous ligament fixation is a safe and efficacious management.
- Incidence of posthysterectomy vault prolapse correlated with the degree of preoperative rectocele.
- Multifilament sutures result in higher levels of postoperative morbidity when compared with 2/0 monofilament sutures.
- While theoretically appealing, the implantation of synthetic mesh in the pelvis may be associated with inherent adverse consequences, such as erosion, extrusion, and infection that further complicates the decision to use synthetic mesh.
- Levator avulsion injury is main etiological and risk factor associated with uterine and vaginal prolapse as the sequel of delivery trauma. This injury also increases significantly the risk of prolapse recurrence after native tissue vaginal repair.

Uterine Fibroids

Suchitra N Pandit, Prachi S Koranne, Vaman B Ghodake, Shashikant M Umbardand

1. What is incidence of fibroid?

Incidence: It occurs in 20–40% of women in the reproductive age group. These are more common in nulliparous. The prevalence is highest between 35 and 45 years of age.

2. What is etiology of fibroid?

Exact etiology is not known. Each individual myoma is unicellular in origin. It appears to be that the growth of fibroid depends on ovarian steroids, since fibroids are not seen prior to menarche and usually there is regression in size after menopause and no new growth.

Estrogen: Though there is no evidence that it is a causative factor, it has been implicated in growth of myomas. Myomas contain estrogen receptors in higher concentration than surrounding myometrium.

Progesterone: Increases mitotic activity and reduces apoptosis which results in increase in size.

There may be a genetic predisposition for fibroid formation.

3. What are the risk factors for fibroid?

Risk factors

Increased risk:
- Age
- Nulliparous woman
- Obesity
- Family history
- Early menarche
- Diabetes
- Black women.

These factors mainly influence the hormonal mileu. There is an association between the prevalence of *symptomatic endometriosis* and *symptomatic uterine fibroids.* Both of these diseases seem to be related to increased subfertility independently of each other. In a recently published study a majority of symptomatic uterine fibroid patients were also diagnosed with endometriosis. There is a hypothesis that a hyperestrogenic state might have a role in the development of both fibroids and endometriosis. It seems that uterine fibroid cells significantly express aromatase, resulting in elevated tissue concentrations of estrogens in fibroid nodules compared to the surrounding myometrium. Similar to uterine fibroids, endometriotic tissue has been demonstrated to express aromatase and to produce estrogen independently of the ovaries. In addition, the role of estrogens is supported by the fact that neither fibroids nor endometriosis appear before the age of onset of fertility, and during the menopause, the symptoms of both diseases diminish.

4. What is Rein's hypothesis?

Rein and coworkers have proposed a hypothesis to explain the pathogenesis of myomata. This hypothesis suggests a critical role for progesterone in their growth.

They state: The initiation and growth of myomas likely involves a multistep cascade of separate tumor initiators and promotors. The initial neoplastic transformation of the normal myocyte involves somatic mutations. Although the initiators of the somatic mutations remain unclear, the mitogenic effect of progesterone may enhance the propagation of somatic mutations. Myoma proliferation is the result of clonal expansion and likely involves the complex interactions of estrogen, progesterone, and local growth factors. Estrogen and progesterone appear equally important as promotors of myoma growth.

5. How will you classify fibroid?

Classification: Fibroids can be classified on the basis of either location or the uterine layer affected.

Corporal fibroids (91.2%):
- *Submucus fibroids* are—located beneath the endometrium. These are sessile or pedunculated. Submucous fibroids are often associated with a disturbed bleeding pattern. The pedunculated fibroids can protrude into or through cervical canal, and are called pseudocervical fibroid, this makes them more susceptible for infection or intermenstrual bleeding.
- *Intramural or interstitial:* These are the most common sites occurring within the uterine wall.
- *Subserous*: Located just beneath the serosal surface. They grow out towards the peritoneal cavity, and can be sessile or pedunculated. These fibroids are either partially or completely covered by peritoneum. When

completely covered by peritoneum, it usually attains a pedicle—called *pedunculated subserous fibroid*. On rare occasions, the pedicle may get torn and gets its nourishment from the omental or mesenteric attachment. It is called a *parasitic or wondering fibroid*.

Sometime intramural fibroid may be pushed out between the layers of broad ligament and is called as *psuedobroad ligament fibroid*.

Cervical (2.6%):

These are rare and further subclassified as:
- *Interstitial:* These often displace the cervix or expand so much that the external os is difficult to identify.
- *Subperitoneal*
- *Polypoidal:* According to the position, they are classified as:
  - Anterior
  - Posterior
  - Lateral
  - Central.

6. What are the clinical features of fibroid?

Clinical features
- Symptomatic in only 35–50% of women
- Symptoms depend on location, size, changes and pregnancy status.

Menorrhagia:
- The most common symptom present in 30% of patients
- Heavy/prolonged bleeding can lead to anemia
- Submucous myoma produces the most pronounced symptoms of menorrhagia, or pre- and postmenstrual spotting.

It is seen due to:
- Increased total surface area of the endometrium
- Mechanical distortion of the endometrial cavity
- Interference with uterine contractility
- Dilatation and congestion of the endometrial venous plexuses
- Endometrial hyperplasia due to high estrogen
- Pelvic congestion
- Ulceration of endometrium over the submucous fibroid.

Dysmenorrhea:
- Congestive as well as spasmodic dysmenorrhea
- Pedunculated submucous fibroids have areas of venouses thrombosis and necrosis on the surface which can cause intermenstrual bleeding.

Subfertility in these cases is due to:
- Distortion and elongation of uterine cavity—difficult sperm ascent
- Impaired uterine contractility—difficult sperm ascent
- Congestion of endometrium—defective implantation
- Corneal block due to fibroid
- Elongation and stretching of tube over large fibroid
- Anovulation associated with hyperestrogenism.

Fibroids that change the shape of the uterine cavity (submucous) or are within the cavity (intracavitary) decrease fertility by about 70% and removal of these fibroids increases fertility by 70%. Other types of fibroids, those that are within the wall (intramural) but do not change the shape of the cavity, or those that bulge outside the wall (subserosal), do not decrease fertility.

Pressure effects are:
- Pelvic pain or backache
- Bladder—frequency or retention, seen more commonly with isthmic fibroid
- Ureter—hydroureter, hydronephrosis
- Bowel—constipation, tenesmus.

Rarely a posterior fundal tumor causes extreme retroflexion of the uterus distorting the bladder base leading to urinary retention. Parasitic tumor may cause bowel obstruction.

Pain:

It can be due to vascular occlusion leading to necrosis or infection. Torsion of a pedunculated fibroid causes acute pain. Other main reasons for pain are:
- Myometrial contractions to expel the myoma
- Red degeneration → acute pain
- Heaviness/fullness in the pelvic area
- Feeling a mass
- If the tumor gets impacted in the pelvis → pressure on nerves → back pain radiating to the lower extremities.

Dyspareunia if it is protruding into the vagina

Cervical tumors can cause *serosanguinous vaginal discharge, bleeding, dyspareunia* or *infertility*.

7. What is the relationship between pregnancy and fibroid?

Effects of fibroids on pregnancy can lead to:
- Repeated abortions
- Antepartum hemorrhage
- Malpresentations
- Postpartum hemorrhage
- Inversion of uterus
- Puerperal sepsis
- Defective implantation of placenta
- Obstructed labor.

Effects of pregnancy on fibroid:
- Increased size in 20–30% cases
- Torsion
- Infection

- Red degeneration
- Expulsion
- Necrosis.

Fibroids are seen in 1–2% of pregnant women. Interestingly, studies that report changes in growth of existing leiomyoma during pregnancy are not consistent. Some leiomyomas grow, others shrink, but many show little change. Depending upon the *size, number* and *location* of the fibroids, they may give rise to problems in pregnancy. If the placenta implants over or in close proximity to a fibroid, there may be an increased risk of miscarriage, abruption, preterm labor, PROM and IUGR. Fibroids located in the lower segment can produce malpresentation and PPH. A large retrospective review of ultrasound and medical records of 12,708 cases of pregnancy with fibroids showed that the fetal growth, PROM and the mode of delivery was generally unaffected by the presence of fibroids. Concern of possible complications related to fibroids in pregnancy is not an indication for myomectomy, except in women who have experienced a previous pregnancy with complication related to these fibroids. Only indication for cesarean myomectomy is if the presence of the fibroid makes hindrance to baby delivery or adequate closure of the uterine incision impossible as there is increased incidence of PPH and increased operative morbidity.

8. What are the clinical signs of fibroid?

Signs:
- G/E—anemia due to heavy and prolonged bleeding
- P/A—palpable lump if more than 12 weeks size. Firm, nodular, well-differentiated mass arising from pelvis and mobile from side-to-side
- P/S—cervix pulled up in large fibroids
- P/V—transmitted movements present
  - Uterus not felt separately from the mass
  - No groove felt between mass and uterus
  - Uterus is enlarged and nodular.

9. What are the different diagnostic modalities for fibroid?

Diagnosis:

Apart from clinical examination, various radiological modalities can be used for diagnosis of fibroids.

a. *Ultrasonography (USG):* USG is the modality of choice for diagnosis and evaluation of uterine fibroids. On USG, fibroid appears as hypoechoic lesions.

b. *Transvaginal sonography (TVS)* is the most accurate modality for diagnosis of fibroid. TVS would differentiate the subserous leiomyoma from other adnexal masses quite easily. Transvaginal ultrasonography is as efficient as magnetic resonance imaging in detecting myoma presence, but its capacity for exact myoma mapping falls short of that of magnetic resonance imaging, especially in large (>375 mL) multiple-myoma (>4) uteri. Distortion of endometrial echoes is seen in the cases of submucous fibroids whereas a bulging contour is seen in cases of subserosal or large intramural leiomyomas. In a few cases, cleavage plane surrounding the fibroid may also be visible. However, patients with massive uterine enlargement caused by leiomyomata are better evaluated with a TAS.

c. *Sonohysterography (SHG)* is a newer diagnostic modality wherein, saline is injected into the uterine cavity with the help of a pediatric infant feeding tube of 5F diameter. The anechoic interface provided by the saline allows the examiner to determine whether the abnormality visualized on TVS is intracavitary, endometrial or submucosal, without using ionizing radiations or contrast agents.

d. *Duplex Doppler and color flow imaging:* These play an important role in the assessment of vascular leiomyomata and intravenous leiomyomatosis. A high peak systolic velocity with mild diastolic elevation has been noted in the periphery of leiomyosarcomas. Thus, Doppler studies help to suggest the possibility of malignancy by increased vascularity in a case of fibroid uterus especially leiomyosarcoma. Evidence of vascular invasion also suggests sarcoma or intravenous leiomyomatosis (explained later).

e. *Three-dimensional ultrasound (3D-USG)* allows the display of anatomy and pathologic conditions usually not possible with 2D-USG. Three-dimensional saline infusion sonography is valid and reliable in women suspected of having intrauterine abnormalities and has relevant clinical value in addition to conventional saline infusion sonography. Three-dimensional sonohysterography allows precise recognition and localization of lesions. If 2D and 3D SHG are normal, invasive diagnostic procedures such as hysteroscopy could be avoided. 3D power Doppler imaging can detect structural abnormalities of the malignant tumor vessels, such as arteriovenous shunts, microaneurysms, tumoral lakes, disproportional calibration, coiling, and dichotomous branching. Therefore, it enhances and facilitates the morphologic and functional evaluation of both benign and malignant pelvic tumors.

f. *Magnetic resonance imaging (MRI)* has an important role in defining the anatomy of the uterus and ovaries in patients in whom USG findings are confusing or in case of large fibroids. This is expensive though. MRI has a potential of distinguishing each type of secondary changes that occur in leiomyomata. Speckled pattern was associated with a mild degree of hyaline or myxoid degeneration or focal necrosis. Nodular pattern was caused by necrosis or cellular leiomyomata, and cystic pattern was related to severe hyaline or myxoid degeneration or necrosis. Each type of secondary changes within leiomyomata showed distinctive MR findings, if they were severely involved. However, because various other uterine tumors can also have similar signal intensity on MRI, further evaluation for the heterogeneous leiomyomata appears to be necessary.

g. MRI is also helpful in fibroid, mapping before planning myonectomy.
h. *CT scan* has limited role in diagnosis of fibroids. On CT scan, fibroids are indistinguishable from healthy myometrium unless they are calcified or necrotic.
i. *X-ray* has a limited role in diagnosis of fibroids. Unless heavily calcified, fibroids are not detected on radiographs.
j. *Hysteroscopy*, submucous fibroids or fibroid polyp can be diagnosed on hysteroscopy. It can help us to know the exact origin, size and vascularity of the fibroids.

10. What are differential diagnosis of fibroid?

Differential Diagnosis:
a. *Pregnancy:* History of missed periods can give a clue.
b. Full bladder.
c. *Adenomyosis:* In adenomyosis, the lining of the uterus infiltrates the wall of the uterus, causing the wall to thicken and the uterus to enlarge. On ultrasound examination, this will often appear as diffused thickening of the wall, while fibroids are seen as well-defined hypoechoic areas with a discrete border. Adenomyosis is usually a diffused process, and rarely can be removed without taking out the uterus.
d. *Ovarian tumor*
e. *Endometriosis*
f. *Tubo-ovarian mass.*

11. What is cervical fibroid?

Cervical fibroids:
- *Anterior cervical fibroids:* These burrow beneath the bladder base, elevating the bladder above it and causing hesitancy and urinary retention. Occasionally while incising the uterovesical fold, an accidental cystotomy may occur unless surgeon is aware of the elevated upper most limits of the bladder.
- *Posterior cervical fibroids:* These fibroids may grow in pouch of Douglas and may compress the rectum and cause constipation and tenesmus.
- *Central cervical fibroids:* They protrude in to the cervical canal. This may result in ureteric obstruction, hydronephrosis and hydroureter.
- *Lateral cervical fibroids:* These fibroids bury between the leaves of the broad ligaments. Uterine artery always runs on its lateral aspect. Identification of this structure is essential step during hysterectomy.

12. What is broad ligament fibroid?

Broad ligament fibroids: Broad ligament fibroids are of two types: (a) True (b) False. True: Broad ligament fibroids arise from smooth cells. These fibroids grow into the layers of broad ligament. The important differentiating feature is that the uterine vessels are always medial to true broad ligament fibroids. Each of above mentioned fibroids require modifications in the steps during surgical management.

13. What are the management options for asymptomatic fibroids?

Incidental detection in an asymptomatic woman causes certain concerns:
- The psychological impact of the diagnosis on the woman
- The possible risks due to intervention.

Once diagnosed to have fibroids, the woman though asymptomatic at the time of detection is likely to be disturbed by its presence and may attribute several symptoms to its presence. Counseling plays a major role in creating awareness about the innocuous nature of the fibroids and allaying her fears. Apart from inherent risks of drug therapy, medical therapy produces an anovulatory state that inhibits fertility. Myomectomy can cause infertility due to adhesions and increased risk of rupture uterus during pregnancy. One also needs to consider the morbidity and mortality associated with the various interventional procedures.

Under its evidence-based practice program, the Agency for Healthcare Research and Quality (AHRQ) has produced an evidence report on the Management of Fibroids. Guidelines for management asymptomatic fibroids have changed.

Recent guidelines (Guidelines for the management of Fibroid, Te-Linde's 10th edition):
- Asymptomatic women with fibroids where the uterine size is less than 12 weeks in size (and where other causes of pelvic mass have been excluded) do not need further investigations but should be advised to seek medical advice only if symptoms occur.
- Regular follow-up of patient is mandatory.
- Asymptomatic women with fibroids >12 weeks should have specialist referral to discuss options including observation.
- Silent, stable fibroids may be observed.

- Removal of fibroids that distort the uterine cavity may be indicated in infertile women, where no other factors have been identified, and in women about to undergo *in vitro* fertilization treatment.
- Concern of possible complications related to fibroids in pregnancy is not an indication for myomectomy, except in women who have experienced a previous pregnancy with complication related to these fibroids.
- Women who have fibroids detected in pregnancy may require additional fetal surveillance when the placenta is implanted over or in close proximity to a fibroid.
- Size of the fibroids by itself does not warrant removal.
- Possibility of malignant change is not an indication for intervention.

14. What are principles of medical management in fibroid?

The objectives of medical management:
- To improve menorrhagia
- To minimize size and vascularity
- To correct anemia before surgery
- As an alternative to surgery in perimenopausal women or women with high-risk factors for surgery
- Where postponement of surgery is planned temporarily.

Drugs used:
a. *Progesterones*: They are not very effective. They mainly correct menorrhagia and hormonal disturbances associated with fibroids. Norethisterone acetate or Medroxyprogesterone acetate 5–10 mg is administered cyclically from day 5th of the cycle for 20 days.
b. *Antiprogesterones*: Mifepristone (RU486) has been found to be more effective in treatment of menorrhagia. It reduces size of the fibroid. A daily dose of 25–30 mg is recommended for three months. 5 mg dose for 3 months is also effective but long-term treatment is not recommended due to the risk of endometrial hyperplasia
c. *Androgens*: Danazol 200–400 mg can be given daily for three months. This minimizes blood loss significantly or it can produce amenorrhea. It also reduces size of the fibroid.
d. *GnRH agonists:* For example, goserelin, buserelin, leuprorelin acetate are commonly used. These cause pituitary down regulation and suppression of the ovarian function. They are considered first line medical therapy.
e. *GnRH antagonists*: For example, cetrorelix or ganirelix causes immediate suppression of the pituitary gland and ovaries.

15. What are different surgical options available for the management of fibroid?

Surgical management: Different modalities of surgical management are as follows:

Myomectomy
It is a conservative surgical modality. It includes enucleation of myoma from the uterus leaving behind potentially functioning uterus, capable of further reproduction. It is a more risky operation when fibroid is too big or there is a chance of recurrence.

Indications: The patient is in reproductive age group:

Current indications in infertility
- Deformity of endometrial cavity
- Distortion of Fallopian tubes
- Fibroid associated with unexplained infertility
- Before ART (artificial reproductive techniques)
- Prophylactic to prevent future complications—though evidence for this is limited.

Contraindications: Other factors for infertility should be ruled out.
- If the husband is proved infertile and does not want to make use of donor sperms
- Infected fibroid
- Associated pelvic pathology
- Suspected malignancy in fibroid
- Perimenopausal women >48–50 years of age having complete family (controversial).

Hysterectomy
It is the operation of choice in symptomatic fibroids in patients over the age of 40 years and in those not desirous of future fertility. If there is an adnexal pathology, it is also dealt with. If the ovaries are healthy and there is no family history of ovarian cancer, they can be left behind in women over 40 years of age. Removal of healthy ovaries can lead to sudden menopausal syndrome and long-term problems of osteoporosis. Though, these women can be offered hormone replacement therapy but compliance is poor. Whenever possible vaginal route preferred. The contraindications for vaginal route are:
- Uterus >16 weeks size
- No UV descent
- Fibroid >7–9 cm/multiple fibroids making parametrial access difficult
- Associated pelvic pathology, malignancy
- Abdominal route preferred where C/I to vaginal route.

16. What are principles of myomectomy?
- Planned in postmenstrual period
- Remove as many fibroids through least number of incisions

- Main incision on largest fibroid (Tunneling of smaller fibroids)
- No incision impinging on cornu or kinking the Fallopian tube
- Adequate hemostasis
- Minimize adhesion formation
- Use of adhesion barrier, may reduce adhesion formation
- Incisions on anterior and posterior wall: Vertical
- Incision for fundal fibroid: Transverse called as Bonney's hood incision.

17. What is role of laparoscopy in the management of fibroid?

This requires specialized expensive equipment and training in endoscopic surgery. It is suitable for subserous and intramural fibroids.

Advantages are:
- Shorter hospital stay
- Faster postoperative recovery
- Decreased postoperative pain
- Decreased incidence of ileus and thromboembolic phenomenon
- Lesser incidence of pyrexia
- Comparable pregnancy rates with abdominal myomectomy.

Contraindications (Relative):
- Size of fibroid >15 cm
- Multiple fibroids
- Unfavorable location (intraligamentary, in POD, posterior wall)
- Submucosal myoma amenable to hysteroscopic removal)
- Medical C/I for abdominal distension
- Diffuse leiomyomata
- More than 3 myomas >5 cm.

Limitations:
- Special equipment and special skill required
- *Difficulty in:* Broad ligament/cervical fibroid
- Size >8 cm
- Number >3 fibroids
- Separate incisions needed
- Closure of dead space and hemostasis difficult
- Weaker scar
- Increased operating time and blood loss
- Inherent complications of laparoscopic surgery.

18. What is a hysteroscopic myomectomy?

Hysteroscopic myomectomy is a technique that can be performed only if fibroids are within or bulging into the uterine cavity (submucosal). This procedure is performed as outpatient surgery without any incisions and virtually no postoperative discomfort. Anesthesia is needed because the surgery may take one to two hours and would otherwise be uncomfortable. A small telescope, the hysteroscope, is passed through the cervix and the inside of the uterine cavity can be seen. Electricity passes through the thin wire attachment at the end of the hysteroscope, allowing the instrument to cut through the fibroid like a hot knife cutting through butter. As the fibroid is shaved out, the heat from the instrument sears blood vessels and the blood loss is usually minimal. Women go home the same day, and recovery is remarkably fast, with most patients able to go back to normal activity, work and exercise in one or two days (Fig. 41.1).

When fibroids are the cause of infertility, pregnancy rates following hysteroscopic myomectomy have been about 50% and when performed for heavy bleeding, nearly 90% of women have a return of normal menstrual f low.

Only a few years ago, treatment for fibroids in the cavity of the uterus involved major surgery—an abdominal incision and either cutting open the entire uterus to remove the fibroid or performing a hysterectomy. Hysteroscopic myomectomy has been a major advance in the treatment of women who have submucous fibroids.

19. Can new fibroids grow after myomectomy?

Once fibroids are removed, they do not grow back. Therefore, the term "recurrence" is technically incorrect. Although new fibroids may grow after a myomectomy, most women will not require any additional treatment. If the first surgery is performed for a single fibroid, only 11% of women will have another surgery within the next 10 years. If multiple fibroids are removed, about 26% will have subsequent surgery and the risks are lower for women as they get close to menopause, when new fibroids do not form. It would be extremely unusual for a woman to need another operation or procedure if she had a myomectomy after age 40 years.

Treatment with GnRHa before surgery makes the fibroids smaller and may make them harder to identify and remove during surgery. One study found that after surgery 63% of the women treated with GnRHa had small fibroids found with ultrasound, but only 13% of women who did not get GnRHa had similar fibroids.

20. What is robotic myomectomy?

The da Vinci surgical robot is a major advance in the ability to precisely operate through small incisions. As shown in Figure 41.2, the surgeon sits at a console and looks through a three-dimensional video camera.

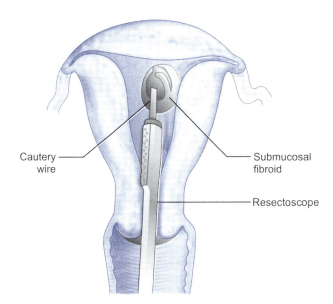

Fig. 41.1: Myoma resection

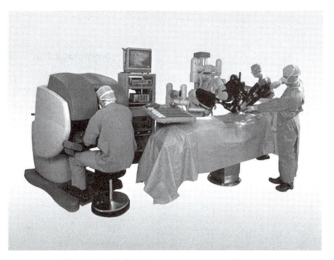

Fig. 41.2: Robotic surgery team and setup
(For color version, see Plate 1)

The hand movements in the surgeon are duplicated in the patient by the robot. Most importantly, the instruments duplicate the wrist movements of the surgeon, allowing the instruments to change angles to allow precise suturing.

The da Vinci does not always eliminate the need for abdominal myomectomy. When there are very large myomas and/or many myomas an abdominal myomectomy may be preferable.

21. What are the secondary changes in fibroid?

a. *Benign degenerations:*
- Atrophic
- Hyaline → yellow, soft gelatinous areas, most common
- Cystic → liquefaction follows extreme hyalinization
- Calcific → circulatory deprivation → precipitation of calcium carbonate and phosphate usually starts in the periphery
- Septic → circulatory deprivation → necrosis → infection
- Myxomatous (fatty) → uncommon, follows hyaline or cystic degeneration
- *Red (carneous) degeneration:*
  - Commonly occurs during pregnancy, usually in 3rd trimester
  - Edema and hypertrophy → impede blood supply → aseptic degeneration and infarction with venous thrombosis and hemorrhage
  - Painful but self-limiting
  - May result in preterm labor and rarely DIC

b. *Malignant transformation:* Leiomyosarcomatous changes.

22. What is leiomyosarcoma?

When a fibroid undergoes malignant degeneration, it becomes a leiomyosarcoma. It is difficult to know the actual incidence of malignant transformation as fibroids are common whereas malignant leiomyosarcomas are rare and can also arise *de novo*. The incidence of malignant degeneration is less than 1.0% and has been estimated to be as low as 0.2%. Moreover, preoperative diagnosis of a leiyomyosarcoma is infrequent. Cervical cytology, endometrial sampling, ultrasound (including color Doppler) are not reliable in diagnosing leiomyosarcoma. MRI is promising in distinguishing between benign and malignant fibroid. Earlier, a rapidly growing fibroid in a premenopausal woman was thought to indicate a possible malignant change. However, in a study of uterine sarcoma in patients operated for presumed leiomyoma and rapidly growing leiomyoma, Parker WH et al. have shown that this is not true. They concluded that the clinical diagnosis of a rapidly growing leiomyoma in a premenopausal woman did not predict uterine leiomyosarcoma in the absence of any other symptoms and thus, should not be used as the sole indication for myomectomy or hysterectomy.

23. What are the complications of fibroid?

Complication:
- Red degeneration
- Sarcomatous change (0.5%)
- Torsion (pedunculated subserous fibroid)
- Inversion of uterus
- Capsular hemorrhage
- Infection
- Atrophy
- Necrosis

- Vacuolar changes
- Hemorrhage.

24. Why polycythemia is common with fibroid?
- Altered erythropoietic functions of kidney through ureteric pressure
- Erythropoietic functions by tumor itself.

25. What is intravenous leiomyomatosis?
This is tumor with extension into vascular space outside leiomyoma. It is benign in nature and can extend into IVC pelvic vein, etc.

26. What are the modifications in the surgical techniques with different locations?
a. *Posterior cervical fibroid*: Grows in POD and presents as mass in posterior vaginal wall. Surgical technique: May need bisection of uterus more on posterior wall.
b. *Central cervical fibroid*: Protrudes into cervical canal, elevates the uterus and cervix becomes globular and close to ureters causing ureteric obstruction and hydronephrosis.
    Surgical technique: Transverse incision and hemisection of uterus to deliver fibroid.
c. *Anterior cervical fibroid*: Elevates the urinary bladder. Patient complaints of hesitancy and frequency of urination.
    Surgical technique: Transverse incision and enucleation prior to hysterectomy allows easy access to uterine vessels and avoids ureteric injury.

27. What are newer modalities of management of fibroid?
Newer therapies for fibroids are as follows:
a. *Uterine artery embolization:* It is a minimally invasive procedure, which can be used as an alternative to major surgical procedures for fibroids and failure of medical treatment.
    The blockage of the blood supply caused degeneration of the fibroids and this resulted in resolution of their symptoms. This has led to the use of this technique as a stand-alone treatment for symptomatic fibroids.
    Uterine artery embolization effectively reduces bleeding, pain, and fibroid size. Under local anesthesia, a catheter is advanced from the femoral artery to the uterine arteries to allow direct injection of polyvinyl particles. The procedure is not recommended for large fibroids. The failure rate is about 10–15%. Most patients experience pain, nausea, and low-grade fever with a very high white blood count for 1–2 days following the procedure. The long-term impact of the radiation absorbed during the procedure is unknown. In addition, serious complications occur, including complication-related hysterectomy, amenorrhea, premature menopause, septicemia, bowel obstruction, and pulmonary embolus. *Embolization should not be performed in women who desire to retain their fertility.*
b. *Mirena (levonorgesterol IUD):* It is third generation IUD, containing 52 mg of progesterone and licensed for five years use. It releases 20 mcg of levonorgestrel daily, which acts directly on the endometrium. This is followed by a decrease in uterine size and a dramatic reduction in menstrual blood loss, with 40% of patients achieving amenorrhea. This method of treatment is not recommended when distortion of the uterine cavity is evident on examination with ultrasonography.

If side effects do occur, they are transient and include:
- Spotting per vagina
- Headache
- Breast tenderness
- Water retention.

However this can be inserted only if the cavity is regular and size of uterus is less than 12 weeks.

The beneficial effect of locally applied levonorgestrel is unexplained, contrasting with the studies that indicate growth promotion of myomas by progestins.

28. What is new in the medical management of fibroid?
Multidisciplinary teams continue to develop innovative ways to treat fibroids. Medical therapies to date have primarily focused on estrogen's role in fibroid formation and growth. Progesterone, however, is clearly important in fibroid tumor cell proliferation and growth, and fibroid tissue has been found to express both estrogen receptors and progesterone receptors.
a. *Selective progesterone receptor modulators (SPRMs):* Based on this knowledge, a new class of progesterone ligands are under development, although they are not yet approved for clinical use. These selective progesterone receptor modulators (SPRMs) have both progestogenic and antiprogestogenic activities, depending on dose and the presence or absence of progesterone. Selective progesterone receptor modulators could potentially decrease fibroid size and blood flow to the myomas without systemic hypoestrogenism. In addition, SPRMs affect the spiral arteries, inhibiting proliferation of the endometrium, which could potentially control abnormal uterine bleeding. These are an exciting set of compounds that have potential in

multiple aspects of female reproductive health. Large clinical trials will be necessary to evaluate their future role in fibroid treatment.

b. *Aromatase inhibitors*: Another class of compounds, which is under investigation for fibroid therapy, is *aromatase inhibitors*. They directly inhibit estrogen synthesis in the ovary, which results in a rapid decrease in estrogen without the initial flare-up period that can occur with GnRH-a.

c. *Use of low dose mifepristone*: Mifepristone in doses of 5 mg or 10 mg results in comparable leiomyoma regression, improvement in symptoms, and few side effects. Further study is needed to assess the long-term safety and efficacy of low-dose mifepristone.

d. *Pirfenidone* is a new, not yet available, medication that blocks the growth of existing fibroids and may stop the formation of new fibroids. Although the exact mechanism of action is not known, pirfenidone affects the production of collagen, a major component of fibroids. Other effects of pirfenidone on cell growth factors may also be important. Studies are now under way to evaluate how fibroids respond to this new drug and to evaluate its side effects. In the future, women with small fibroids may be able to take pirfenidone, or a medication like it, to prevent fibroid growth and avoid any other need for treatment.

e. *Asoprisnil* is a novel selective steroid receptor modulator that shows unique pharmacodynamic effects in animal models and humans. Asoprisnil, its major metabolite (J912), and structurally related compounds represent a new class of progesterone receptor (PR) ligands that exhibit partial agonist and antagonist activities *in vivo*. Asoprisnil demonstrates a high degree of receptor and tissue selectivity, with high-binding affinity for PR, moderate affinity for glucocorticoid receptor (GR), low affinity for androgen receptor (AR), and no binding affinity for estrogen or mineralocorticoid receptors. Early clinical studies of asoprisnil in normal volunteers demonstrated a dose-dependent suppression of menstruation irrespective of the effects on ovulation, with no change in basal estrogen concentrations and no antiglucocorticoid effects. Unlike progestins, asoprisnil does not induce breakthrough bleeding. With favorable safety and tolerability profiles, thus far, asoprisnil appears promising as a novel treatment of gynecological disorders, such as uterine fibroids and endometriosis.

29. What are the contraceptive options for women with fibroid?

Proper selection of contraception is prudent. OC pills are not contraindicated in fibroid. Progesterone containing contraceptives are beneficial in menorrhagia. Copper containing IUCDs used with caution after USG to ruleout distortion of cavity. LNG IUCD is also a good option if there is no distortion of uterine cavity, helps to decrease menorrhagia.

30. What is HIFU?

High-intensity focused ultrasound (HIFU, or sometimes FUS) is a highly precise medical procedure using high-intensity focused ultrasound to heat and destroy pathogenic tissue rapidly through ablation. HIFU treatment for uterine fibroids was approved by the Food and Drug Administration (FDA) in October 2004.

This is a noninvasive treatment option for patients suffering from symptomatic fibroids. Most patients benefit from HIFU and symptomatic relief is sustained for two plus years. Up to 16–20% of patient will require an additional treatment.

When MRI is used for guidance, the technique is sometimes called "magnetic resonance-guided focused ultrasound", often shortened to MRgHIFU or MRgFUS. When ultrasonography is used, the technique is sometimes called ultrasound-guided focused ultrasound, often shortened to USgFUS.

Ultrasound can be focused, either via a lens (for example, a polystyrene lens), a curved transducer, or a phased array (or any combination of the three) into a small focal zone, in a similar way to focusing light through a magnifying glass focusing light rays to a point. As an acoustic wave propagates through the tissue, part of it is absorbed and converted to heat. Tissue damage occurs as a function of both the temperature to which the tissue is heated and how long the tissue is exposed to this heat level in a metric referred to as "thermal dose". By focusing at more than one place or by scanning the focus, a volume can be thermally ablated.

This technology can achieve precise ablation of diseased tissue, therefore is sometimes called HIFU surgery. Because, it destroys the diseased tissue noninvasively, it is also known as "non-invasive HIFU surgery". Anesthesia is not required, but should be recommended.

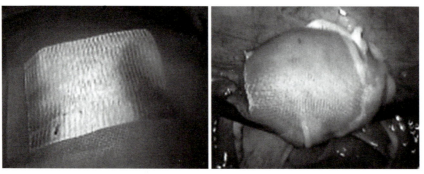

Fig. 41.3: Cloth like material being wrapped around the raw areas from surgery
(For color version, see Plate 1)

31. Can adhesion barriers prevent postmyomectomy adhesions?

Another new advance in surgery has been the use of special substances, called adhesion barriers, which help prevent the formation of scar tissue after surgery. Small sheets of cloth-like material can be wrapped around the raw areas from surgery and the material prevents nearby tissue, such as the intestines from sticking to the surgery sites. After a few weeks, the material dissolves, leaving the newly healed surgery sites fairly free of adhesions. While the barriers are not perfect, they have been shown to help reduce the formation of adhesions (Fig. 41.3). (e.g. interceed (oxidized regenerated cellulose).

32. Is there any relationship between fibroids and food or exercise?

Some of the dietary factors have shown following effects on fibroid cells in laboratory:

Vitamin D—decreases fibroid cell size and disrupts the formation of fibroid muscle cells.

Resveratrol (found in grapes)—decreases growth and increases death of fibroid cells in a test tube.

Curcumin (spice)—decreases growth and increases death of fibroid cells in a test tube.

Licorice (isoliquiritigenin)—decreases growth and increases death of fibroid cells in a test tube.

Green tea (epigallocatechin gallate)—decreases growth of fibroid cells in a test tube.

Also theoretically regular exercise may help in reducing size or restrict growth of fibroid as it reduces the fat and ultimately the conversion into estrogen by aromatase. But evidence for this effect is poor.

MUST REMEMBER

- Fibroids are mainly benign tumors of uterine myometrium with monoclonal origin.
- In many women, these are asymptomatic and diagnosed incidentally.
- Asymptomatic fibroids can be left alone provided other pathologies and malignancies are ruled out and patient is available for periodic follow-up.
- Women with symptomatic or problematic uterine leiomyomas should be considered candidates for surgical or radiologic intervention.
- Management options, including medical, radiologic, and surgical should be discussed with patients, emphasizing risks and benefits of each option.
- Careful preoperative evaluation for women who undergo surgical treatment of leiomyoma should include radiographic evaluation to determine the extent, location, and size of leiomyomata.
- In patients with infertility, myomectomy is performed by either an abdominal or laparoscopic approach and should only be performed after complete evaluation of other potential causes of infertility.
- Pregnancy rates and outcomes after laparoscopic myomectomy compare favorably with those after abdominal myomectomy.
- Meticulous repair of the uterine myometrium is essential for patients desiring pregnancy after a myomectomy.
- Hysteroscopic myomectomy is an effective surgical alternative to relieve symptoms associated with submucous myomas.
- Current information regarding uterine artery embolization (UAE) is promising, but patients should be made aware that limited long-term data are available regarding outcomes, especially relating to fertility and pregnancy.

Infertile Couple

Late Mandakini Parihar, Ashish R Kale

HISTORY

Female Partner

Age, number of married years, contraceptives used, sexual history—frequency/week, dyspareunia. Menstrual history—previous cycles, dysmenorrhea, midcycle bleeding/pain. Obstetric history—previous pregnancies, postabortal/puerperal sepsis, history of curettage. Medical history—PCOS, diabetes, hypertension, TB, STIs, medications, galactorrhea, previous surgery—vaginal, pelvic surgery, substance abuse, smoking, alcohol.

Male Partner

Age, occupation, substance abuse, smoking, alcohol. Sexual history—erectile dysfunction, premature ejaculation, anosmia, hyposmia. Past history—surgery- herniorrhaphy, surgery for undescended testis, injury. Infections—mumps orchitis, epididymitis, STIs.

EXAMINATION

Female Partner

General examination: BMI, BP, acne, hirsutism, acanthosis nigricans, breast examination—galactorrhea, signs of thyroid dysfunction
P/A: Mass arising from pelvis, surgical scar
P/S: Circumflex stenosis, scarring of circumflex
P/V and P/R: Uterus size, adnexal mass, nodularity in POD, induration of uterosacral ligament.

Male Partner

General examination: BMI, gynecomastia, genital examination.

1. When will you label a couple infertile?

When the couple has been trying for conception and have been unable to conceive after 1 year of regular unprotected sexual intercourse, we will call these couples as infertile and investigate them for the same.

2. What are the basic investigations advised to the couple?

- Clinical evaluation for both partners
- Semen profile
- Ovulatory status by history and natural cycle follicular monitoring
- Tubal patency and tuboperitoneal evaluation.

3. What are the common causes of infertility?

The causes can be divided into:
- Male factor
- Female factor
  - Ovulatory dysfunction
  - Tubal factor infertility
  - Uterine factor
  - Cervical factor
  - Peritoneal factor
- Unexplained infertility.

4. What is the percentage of male infertility?

Approximately 30% have causal or associated male factor as the cause of infertility.

5. What are the different investigations when a couple comes for evaluation of infertility?

Investigations done for a couple with infertility:

For males:

- *Semen analysis:* Most of the time, this is the only investigation asked for. However, if the initial semen analysis is abnormal, then additional investigations are needed and these are as follows:
  - Endocrine investigation for FSH, LH, prolactin and testosterone
  - Evaluation of sperm function.
    For example: Sperm migration test
    Sperm survival test
    Hypo-osmotic swelling test
  - Immunological investigation, e.g. antisperm antibody by ELISA

- Microbiological investigation, e.g. semen culture
- Testicular biopsy
- Varicocele assessment using Doppler blood flow
- Genetic investigation by karyotyping to look for translocations and microdeletions.
- Tests of ovulation.

For females:
- Basl body temperature (BBT)
- *Hormonal assay:* These are baseline hormone evaluations done on the second or third day of the cycle to check for normal HPO axis. These include, FSH, LH, estradiol, TSH and prolactin levels
- Cervical mucus study
- Baseline ultrasonography along with natural cycle follicular monitoring for evidence of ovulation
- Hysterosalpingography (tubal patency)
  If these are abnormal then additional tests may be needed and these include:
  - Laparoscopy with hysteroscopy
  - Immunological test (cervical factor), e.g. antisperm antibody, antiphospholipid antibody
  - Endometrial biopsy or curettage.

6. What are the different types of infertility?
These can be divided as:
- Primary and secondary infertility, or
- Male factor, female factor, and unexplained infertility.

7. What are the different ways for detecting ovulation?
- Basal body temperature
- Cervical mucus study
- Endometrial biopsy
- Urinary LH monitoring
- Ultrasound follicular study is the most accurate way and is today the gold standard for ovulation detection
- Serum progesterone level day 8/9 after ovulation (approximately day 21/22 of a 30 day cycle) >15 ng/mL.

8. What are the criteria taken into account for normal semen count?
There are wide variations in normal semen counts and hence WHO has defined common minimum criteria for normal semen. Lower limit within perenthesis.

WHO parameters as per 2010 for normal semen count are:
- Volume >1.5 mL
- Concentration >15 million/mL
- Motility >32% forward progressive motility (combination of rapid and slow forward progressive motility)
- Morphology >40% normal
- Vitality >75% live
- WBC <1 million/mL
- Immunobead <20% adherent
- MAR <10% adherent.
- Total sperm count >40 million/ejaculate

9. What are the common causes of infertility in women?
- Ovulatory disorder—(40%)
- Tubal diseases—(20-25%)
- Endometriosis—(10-15%)
- Uterine factor—(5%)
- Cervical factor—(5%)
- Unexplained—(10-15%).

10. What is meant by follicular studies?
Follicular study is monitoring of growing follicles in the ovary by sonography. Earlier it was done abdominally, but with the advent of vaginal probes, follicular studies are mostly done by the transvaginal sonography as it gives better resolution and information about the pelvic organs than abdominal sonography.

Baseline sonography is done to know the ovarian volume and antral follicle count on day 2/day 3 of the menstrual period. There after serial sonography done to evaluate the follicular growth and to see endometrial growth (thickness and pattern) from day 7/8 onwards. The growing follicle is identified and monitored till the day it ruptures.

11. What are the different types of anovulatory infertility?
Broadly anovulation can be divided into four categories based on the levels of pituitary gonadotropin hormones:

i. *Hypogonadotropic anovulation:* Here the levels of gonadotropin hormones are very low and hence there is no ovarian response, e.g. Kallman's syndrome, anorexia nervosa, exercise-induced amenorrhea. Isolated gonadotropin deficiency, pituitary deficiency, etc. Here the gonadotropin levels are low and hence there is anovulation.

ii. *Normogonadotropic anovulation:* Here the levels of gonadotropin hormones are normal range but ratio is altered and hence there is no or inappropriate ovarian response, e.g. PCOS. Here the levels of gonadotropin hormones are normal but there is chronic anovulation due to metabolic disturbance.

iii. *Hypergonadotropic anovulation:* Here the gonadotropin hormones are markedly elevated due to resistant ovaries and this signifies absent or nonfunctional ovaries, e.g. premature ovarian failure, absent ovaries, etc.

iv. *Hyperprolactinemic anovulation:* Raised prolactin levels cause anovulation by affecting the pituitary secretion of the gonadotropins and this leads to anovulation, e.g. idiopathic hyperprolactinemia, micro- and macroadenomas of the pituitary, lactational anovulation, etc.

12. What is meant by PCOS? Who discovered it and when?

Polycystic ovarian syndrome (PCOS) was first described by Irvin F Stein and Michael L Leventhal in 1939 and hence the earlier name was Stein–Leventhal syndrome.

It is the most common endocrine abnormality affecting female reproductive performance. It leads to infertility, menstrual disturbances and is associated with hyperandrogenism, obesity, insulin resistance. It is a metabolic dysfunction and needs active management to avoid long-term complications of hyperestrogenism.

13. What are the clinical features of PCOS?

- Obesity
- Hirsutism
- Oligomenorrhea/amenorrhea
- Infertility.

14. What is the pathophysiology behind PCOS and in the recommendation for it?

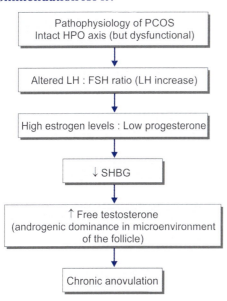

It is also been established that PCOS is associated with profound insulin resistance as well as with defects in insulin secretions. Insulin affects ovarian function in multiple ways, causing anovulation and hyperandrogenism.

15. What are the baseline hormonal evaluations done and what do they signify?

Basal level of FSH and LH is done between 2nd and 4th day of menstrual cycle. Along with FSH and LH, it is customary to check the levels of estradiol, TSH and prolactin. Based on the levels of FSH and LH, we can determine the type of anovulation that the patient suffers from and institute the appropriate treatment.

16. Why does hyperprolactinemia cause anovulation?

Hyperprolactinemia has a negative feedback effect on hypothalamic pulsatile secretion of GnRH, resulting in gonadotropin deficiency and secondary ovarian failure. Patient may have amenorrhea and galactorrhea sometimes.

17. What are the different effects of tuberculosis on the genital tract?

- Fallopian tubes are the most common site of initial involvement
- Infection can lead to adhesion formation, tubal blockage or tubo-ovarian masses
- Most common presenting symptom is infertility (75%)
- Other may present with abdominal or pelvic pain, abnormal vaginal bleeding or peritonitis. The tubes may be beaded, rigid lead pipe appearance or develop a hydrosalpinx
- If the uterine endometrium is affected, it results in destruction of the basal layer and subsequent intrauterine adhesions—Asherman's syndrome.

18. What are the clinical manifestations of Asherman's syndrome?

Most common clinical manifestation of Asherman's syndrome is secondary amenorrhea. Patients may also present with infertility and hypoamenorrhea or amenorrhea. Hysteroscopy is the gold standard in diagnosis, but it can also be aided by USG and HSG.

19. What are the treatment options advised to manage Asherman's syndrome?

Hysteroscopic resection is the primary treatment for Asherman's syndrome. Efficacious treatment also requires prevention of repeat adhesions and IUCD or Foley's catheter have been used in the past to prevent readhesions along with exogenous estrogen to promote endometrial growth.

20. What are the common infective organisms affecting the Fallopian tubes?

Common infective organism affecting Fallopian tubes are:
- *Chlamydia trachomatis*
- *Neisseria gonorrhea*
- *Mycobacterium tuberculosis*
- *Mycoplasma hominis*
- Endogeneous aerobic and anaerobic bacteria.

21. What is meant by Fitz–Hugh–Curtis syndrome?

Women with PID complaining of acute right-sided upper abdominal pain. It is due to fibrosis band extending from under surface of diaphragm to the surface of the liver. The most common organisms causing these in PID are gonococcal and chlamydial infection.

22. What is the relevance of hydrosalpinx in infertility management?

Hydrosalpinx represents the end-result of a previous acute salpingitis and is often bilateral. The fimbrial end is closed and tubal fluid collects and causes dilatation of the tube. In patients who are undergoing IVF, prior removal of hydrosalpinx is warranted, as fluid contained in it can be embryotoxic and significantly decreases the pregnancy rate.

23. What is endometriosis and what are the different ways in which it causes infertility?

Occurrence of ectopic endometrial tissue outside the cavity of uterus is called endometriosis. It has a unique pathology of a benign proliferative growth process having the propensity to invade the normal surrounding tissue. About 15% of infertile women suffer from endometriosis.

It interferes with tubal motility and function due to biochemical as well as physical alterations in the tubo-ovarian anatomy. It may inhibit ovulation and cause luteinized unruptured follicular syndrome, hyperprolactinemia, and short luteal phase cycle. Due to the altered tubo-ovarian anatomy, there is dyspareunia and hence the frequency of sexual intercourse is reduced.

24. What is meant by planned relations?

Planned relation means sexual intercourse done at and around the time of ovulation, signs of ovulation can be monitored either by sonography, urinary LH kit or basal body temperature charting.

25. What is meant by intrauterine insemination? And how is it done?

Intrauterine insemination (IUI) is a process by which semen which is processed in culture media is introduced into the uterine cavity under aseptic conditions. Processing is done so that all the debris, dead sperms and seminal secretions are separated out from motile sperms and a good harvest of actively motile sperms can be introduced in the uterine cavity using a small disposable plastic cannula. The dead sperms and debris need to be removed so as to prevent painful uterine contractions. At the time of ovulation or in the periovulatory period, about 0.5–0.7 mL of motile sperms suspended in culture medium are inserted in the uterus, so as to place it in close proximity with the egg in the Fallopian tube.

26. What is IVF? Describe process in brief.

In vitro fertilization (IVF) means fertilization of oocyte by sperm gamete in the laboratory. The mainstay of the program consists of stimulation of the ovary using gonadotropins and the giving the trigger for oocyte maturation. About 34–35 hours later, aspiration of mature oocytes from both ovaries under ultrasound guidance is done. These oocytes are kept in specific culture for a few hours to complete oocyte maturation. Especially processed sperm are kept with these oocytes in culture media under specific temperature and CO_2 environment so that oocytes are fertilized by sperm. Evidence of fertilization is seen in 18 hours and formation of an embryo occurs in the next 24 hours. These embryos when formed are then transferred into uterine cavity after 2–3 days of oocyte retrieval (cell division). With extended culture media available, we can now culture the embryos up to the blastocyst stage and transfer on day 5/6 after oocyte retrieval.

27. Name the world's first IVF baby and the scientists who were responsible for her birth.

First child born, as a result of IVF was Louise Brown in 1978, in Bourne-Hall clinic in London by the efforts of two great scientists, Robert Edwards and Patrick Steptoe.

28. What is general success rate with IVF procedure?

As the process of implantation is still a mystery, the overall pregnancy rate with IVF is 35–38%. There will be a 20–25% pregnancy loss due to abortions and hence take home baby rate is usually 22–25%.

29. What is meant by ICSI and how does it differ from IVF?

ICSI stands for intracytoplasmic sperm injection. It is a micromanipulation technique in which a single spermatozoan is injected directly into cytoplasm of mature oocyte using a micropipette. This technique increases the likelihood of fertilization when there are abnormalities in the number, quality or function of sperm. While in IVF, motile sperms are put with mature oocyte in culture media in incubator for 16–18 hours and fertilization takes place naturally.

30. What is varicocele and how does it affect fertility?

Varicocele is elongated, dilated and tortuous spermatic vein within the scrotum. The increased vascularity causes the temperature in the scrotum to be raised and hence affects normal spermatogenesis and maturation. It is found in 20–25% of infertile men with oligo/astheno/teratospermia and can be the cause of low sperm counts and or motility.

31. What are the different types of azoospermia? What are the differentiating features?

Azoospermia is the absence of sperm in the semen and this can be obstructive and nonobstructive in nature. The differentiating features between the two types are absence of fructose in obstructive azoospermia. Though, there is absence of sperm in semen in both cases but in patients with obstructive azoospermic sperms can be retrieved by various microsurgical technique from testes/epididymis for IVF and ICSI. Obstructive azoospermia as the name suggests is absence of sperm due to a physical block and there is presence of mature spermatozoa in the testes and/or epididymis.

Nonobstructive azoospermia is total absence of sperm in the semen and in the testes too. This is usually due to absence of one of the germ cells or testicular destruction beyond repair, e.g. fibrosis and atrophy, post mumps orchitis, cryptorchidism, etc. As there is no sperm, the only option for pregnancy is using donor sperm or adoption.

32. What constitutes the semen?

Normal semen contains seminal plasma and cellular elements: Spermatozoa, sperm precursors and other cells from genital tract and few leukocytes. The seminal plasma consists of seminal proteins, prostatic secretions, fructose and secretions from bulbourethral glands.

33. Write the full form of PESA, MESA, TESA, TESE.

PESA: Percutaneous epididymal sperm aspiration.
MESA: Microsurgical sperm aspiration.
TESA: Testicular sperm aspiration.
TESE: Testicular sperm extraction.

And when are the procedures done?

When there is absence of sperm in semen but the cause is obstructive azoospermia, sperms can be retrieved by various microsurgical technique from testes/epididymis for IVF and ICSI and achieve pregnancy.

34. Define unexplained infertility and options for treatment.

Unexplained infertility means failure to establish a pregnancy despite an evaluation uncovering no obvious reason for infertility, or after correction of factor identified as probably responsible for infertility. It is seen 10–15% couples.

It is recommended to try using an ovulation induction agent like clomiphene citrate (CC) for 3–4 cycles. If there is no pregnancy then it is reasonable to CC+ HMG or only HMG cycles with IUI for 3–4 cycles. If this too fails then IVF with ICSI is the recommended treatment.

35. What are the treatment options in a patient with endometriosis and infertility?

Endometriosis is divided into minimal mild moderate and severe disease and the treatment will depend on the degree of the disease. However, the most important point to remember is that start treatment for infertility as a primary treatment and there is no place for suppression of endometriosis to improve outcome. For minimal and mild endometriosis, controlled ovarian stimulation with IUI is the recommended treatment. They should be treated as unexplained infertility. Surgery is the mainstay in patients with moderate to severe endometriosis with infertility. Depending on the degree of spread, GnRH agonists may be used for a short-term. Goals of surgery are to remove all implants, resect adhesions, relieve pain, reduce the risk of recurrence and adhesion formation and restore the normal anatomy and physiology to whatever extent possible. If endometriosis is of severe type when surgery cannot restore the normal tubo-ovarian relationship or if tubes are blocked then assisted-reproductive techniques are the only option.

36. What is meant by donor insemination?

When the sperm is obtained from the sperm bank and inseminated in the female partner for achieving pregnancy, the process is called as donor insemination. The donor is always unknown donor and the process is carried out with consent from both the partners and is legally valid. The sperm used is cryopreserved semen for insemination for the patients with sterility due to diseases or vasectomy, orchidectomy, chemicals or radiation exposure or because of genetic consideration, e.g. hemophilia, Huntington's diseases.

37. Where does one get sperm for donor insemination and what precautions should be followed prior to donor insemination?

Sperm for donor insemination should be used from cryopreserved semen from certified sperm banks. Each sample of semen is tested for common viral markers, viability of the sample after thawing the sample and is stored in liquid nitrogen for at least 3 months. The donor is tested for viral markers again and when proven negative, the sample is released for clinical use. This ensures storage of properly checked sample for various infective organisms, including HIV and HbsAg and HbC. Adequate counseling prior to starting the donor cycle treatment is vital. Couple should be assured of complete confidentiality and the method by which the donors are selected, matched and the possibility of success should be informed. It is necessary to match the blood group of the donor with that of the husband and basic physical characteristics. Confidentiality is the key issue and must be strictly adhered to.

38. What is meant by ART and what does it include?

ART stands for assisted-reproductive technologies. These mean any procedure involving manipulation of gametes *in vitro* and include *in vitro* fertilization (IVF), intracytoplasmic sperm injection (ICSI), gamete intra-Fallopian transfer (GIFT), zygote intra-Fallopian transfer (ZIFT).

39. What is the most common drug used for ovulation induction and how it is used?

Clomiphene citrate is the most common drug used for anovulatory infertility. It is nonsteroidal compound with weak estrogenic effect.

When it binds to estrogen receptors, central perception of circulating estrogen level is prevented, dampening or abolishing the usual negative feedback response. So, GnRH pulsatility and gonadotropin secretions are enhanced which further result in stimulation of follicular growth and development. Treatment is usually following spontaneous menses or progestin withdrawal bleed. Clomiphene is prescribed for 5 days beginning with cycle days 2–5. Starting dose is typically 50 mg while a dose of 100 mg is more appropriate for obese patient.

If no response is noted in that cycle, dose should be increased by 50 mg in next cycle until ovulation is noted till maximal dose of 150 mg is reached. It should be reasonable to limit patient to six consecutive cycle.

40. What is the role of gonadotropin therapy in infertility? Name the different types of gonadotropins available.

For the patients who do not respond to clomiphene therapy or is not a candidate for clomiphene will need administration of exogeneous gonadotropins.

Various gonadotropin preparations available are:
- Urinary human menopausal gonadotropins (hMG) (LH: FSH 1: 1)
- Urinary FSH (u FSH)
- Highly purified urinary FSH (Uhp-FSH)
- Recombinant FSH (r-FSH)
- Recombinant LH.

41. What is bromocriptine and what are common side effects?

Bromocriptine is an ergot derivative that stimulates dopaminergic receptors in the brain and anterior pituitary. It is used for treatment of hyperprolactinemia. It is usually started at dose of 1.25 mg each evening for first 7–14 days to decrease possible side effects. Dose can be increased by 1.25 mg every 2–3 weeks until normoprolactinemia is achieved. Common side effects are GI disturbances like nausea and vomiting, orthostatic hypotension, nasal congestion and headache.

42. What is cabergoline and where is it used?

It is a dopamine agonist. It is used in cases of hyperprolactinemia. It has advantages over bromocriptine as it has longer half-life and a higher binding capacity for D_2 receptors. This allows a biweekly dose and hence a significant decrease in the side effects seen with bromocriptine.

43. What is the role of GnRH analogues in assisted reproduction? Name the types of GnRH analogues.

GnRH analogues are used in assisted reproduction for down regulation of the pituitary and hence achieving an appropriate cycle control by preventing premature LH surge. This prevention of LH surge allows further maturation of follicles which has been shown to increase clinical success rate. They can be classified into agonists and antagonists.

The agonists are further divided into:
- Nonapeptides.
  - Buserelin
  - Leuprolide
  - Histrelin
  - Goserelin.
- Decapeptides.
  - Nafarelin
  - Triptorelin.

The antagonists are:
- Cetrorelix
- Ganirelix.

44. What is the drug used to trigger ovulation? When? What dose?

Human chorionic gonadotropin is used as an LH surrogate to trigger ovulation. Injection hCG is usually administered, in doses of 5000–10,000 IU, when there is at least one follicle measuring 18 mm in diameter. Ideally, the estradiol levels should be at least 200–300 pg/mL per mature follicle and endometrial thickness of at least 8 mm.

45. What is meaning of surrogacy?

Gestational surrogacy: Women who have an embryo transferred to their uterus. This embryo genetically belongs to the intended parents, but is implanted in the surrogates womb. At the end of the gestational period, the surrogate will deliver and then the child is given to the genetic/biological parents. As per the Indian law, the biological parents must officially and legally adopt the child.

46. By what means can we achieve pregnancy in postmenopausal women?

In postmenopausal patient, pregnancy can be achieved either by means of ovum donation or embryo donation. This is because her own ovaries cannot produce any eggs and hence ova from a younger woman are fertilized with the husband's sperm and then transferred in the menopausal woman's uterus. In embryo donation, the ready embryo from unknown donors is implanted in the uterus.

Three main principles for donor oocyte program are:
i. Preparation of recipient's endometrium
ii. Window for embryo transfer
iii. Early pregnancy management with exogenous hormones.

47. What are complications of use of gonadotropins in ART?

By and large, the gonadotropins are quite safe but there can be some immediate side effects with the use of gonadotropins.

These are:
- Retention cyst
- Mild injection site reaction
- Headache
- Ovarian hyperstimulation syndrome (mild-to- moderate)
- Abdominal pain and gastrointestinal symptoms, e.g. nausea, vomiting, diarrhea, abdominal cramps and bloating
- Multiple pregnancy.

Uncommon:
- Severe OHSS
- Ovarian torsion, a complication of OHSS.

48. What is postcoital test?

It is to evaluate the semen, cervical mucus and the immunological cause of infertility.

The couple is asked to have coitus around periovulatory period. The posterior pool from the vagina is aspirated within 2 hours of coitus. Normal 10–50 motile sperms/HFP is considered as normal. <10 sperms or absent sperms or dead sperms are cases for extensive evaluation of the male partner.

49. What is sperm penetration test?

Capability of a live sperm to penetrate, zona free hamster egg *in vitro* is called as sperm penetration.

50. What is Kurzrok–Miller test?

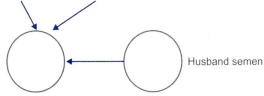

Normal cervical mucus permits invasion of motile sperm.

51. What are markers of ovarian reserve?

Day 3 serum FSH >15 mIU/mL, serum inhibin <400 pg/mL, serum AMH < 8.1 pmol/L, TVS-antral follicle count, mean ovarian volume, clomiphene citrate challange test.

52. What is WHO classification for disorders of ovulation?

Type I: Hypogonadotropic hypogonadism—low FSH, LH, low estradiol
Type II: Normogonadotropic hypogonadism—normal FSH, normal estradiol
Type III: Hypergonadotropic—high FSH, LH, low estradiol.

53. Explain about postcoital test.
- It is done to assess cervical mucus, sperm mucus interaction.
- Performed 1–2 days prior to ovulation
- Within few hours of intercourse
- Five motile sperms/HPF–normal
- Poor reproducibility and sensitivity
- Does not alter management.

54. What are the complications of ovulation induction?
- Ovarian hyperstimulation syndrome
  - Ovarian enlargement, ascites, hemoconcentration
  - Occurs with gonadotropin therapy
  - Managed conservatively
  - Replace fluid/ albumin
- Multifetal pregnancy.

55. What are different terminologies in relation with semen analysis?
- *Aspermia:* Absence of semen
- *Azoospermia:* Absence of sperms in semen
- *Oligozoospermia:* < 20 million sperms/mL of semen
- *Asthenospermia:* Decreased sperm motility
- *Hypospermia:* Low semen volume.
- *Teratospermia:* Sperm with abnormal morphology

56. Explain about intrauterine insemination (IUI).
- *Indication:* Male factor, cervical factor, unexplained infertility, minimal—mild endometriosis
- Requires semen processing
- Superovulation with chlomiphene citrate/gonadotropins
- Timing of ovulation—follicular monitoring, hCG to trigger ovulation.

MUST REMEMBER
- Infertility may be primary, which is the inability to conceive in a couple when no prior pregnancy has occurred or secondary which is the inability to conceive after at least one conception has occurred.
- Infertility may be due to male factors or combined male and female factors.
- Female factors may be anovulation, tubal, uterine, combined male and female factors.
- Male factor infertility is due to pretesticular, testicular, post-testicular factors.
- Midluteal serum progesterone measurement is used for documentation of ovulation. Basal body temperature can be used when progesterone assay is not available.
- HSG/laparoscopy—for evaluation of tubal infertility.
- IUI—for cervical factor infertility.
- If semen analysis is abnormal, further evaluation is by hormonal assay, karyotyping and ultrasound.
- Management of unexplained infertility is by ovulation induction/IUI or ART, when traditional treatment is unsuccessful, IVF is used.

Ovarian Tumors

Swati S Shiradkar

Ovarian malignancy is a persistent challenge to gynecologist, because the symptoms are very nonspecific and its anatomical position makes access difficult, they are usually diagnosed late.

As ovary develops from three structures, namely celomic epithelium, specialized mesoderm called as sex cords and germ cells, the origin of neoplasms is also from three structures. So one tumor marker is not diagnostic.

Underdiagnosis or overdiagnosis further affect morbidity and mortality.

Ovarian tumors is group of neoplasms, classified in five categories according to WHO.

- Epithelial tumors—75% of all ovarian tumors and 90-95% of ovarian malignancies
- Sex cord tumors—5-10% of all ovarian tumors
- Germ cell tumors—15-20% of all ovarian tumors
- Metastatic—5% of all ovarian tumors, secondary to breast, colon, endometrial and cervical malignancy
- Non-neoplastic/neoplasm from soft tissue.

Different subtypes are common in different age groups, germ cell tumors in younger age, sex cord tumors in 4th/5th decade and epithelial tumors in postmenopausal age.

Predisposing factors are also different according to tumor types.
1. *Germ cell tumors:*
   a. Genetic causes
   b. Constitutional chromosomal abnormalities
   c. Dysgenetic gonads.
2. *Sex cord tumors:*
   a. Peutz-Jeghers syndrome
   b. Cushing's syndrome
   c. Meigs' syndrome
   d. Gorlin syndrome.
3. *Epithelial ovarian cancers:*
   a. Hereditary breast ovarian cancer syndrome
   b. Hereditary nonpolyposis colon cancer
   c. Site specific ovarian cancer syndrome
   d. Increased number of ovulation cycles
   e. Pelvic irradiation
   f. Viral infection
   g. High fat diet
   h. Lactose consumption
   i. Racial predisposition in caucasians.

Mode of spread is different according to the type of tumor.
1. Epithelial—Direct spread.
2. Germ cell tumors—Intraperitoneal and hematogenous. Only dysgerminoma spreads by lymphatic route.
3. Sex cord tumor metastasis is rare, they remain localized.

There are different tumor markers for different types of ovarian tumors as:
1. *Epithelial tumors:*
   a. CA-125—nonmucinous
   b. Carcinoembryonic antigen (CEA)—mucinous.
2. *Germ cell tumors:*
   a. AFP—endodermal sinus tumor
   b. hCG—choriocarcinoma
   c. LDH—dysgerminoma.
3. *Sex cord tumors:*
   a. Inhibin
   b. Activin
   c. Estrogen
   d. Androgen.

TYPES

Non-neoplastic and neoplastic (benign/malignant)
- Retention cyst—Epithelial tumors
- Functional cyst—Stromal cell tumors
- Chocolate cyst—Germ cell tumors
- TO mass.

POINTS TO BE NOTED IN HISTORY

- Benign tumors are comparatively asymptomatic unless complication of torsion or rupture occurs. Malignant tumors produce vague symptoms. Functioning ovarian tumors produce menstrual disorders.
- Type of ovarian tumor is different in different age groups, e.g. dermoid in young girls.

- Nulliparity, induction of ovulation increases the risk while multiparity, use of OC pills, tubal ligation, breastfeeding is protective.
- Family history of ovarian, lung, colonic malignancy increases the risk.

GENERAL EXAMINATION

- Evidence of weight loss points towards malignancy
- Evidence of hirsutism, obesity points towards functioning ovarian tumors
- Tachycardia associated with pain and tenderness points towards torsion
- Left supraclavicular lymphadenopathy.

PER ABDOMEN EXAMINATION

Characters of benign tumors:
- Usually free fluid is absent
- Regular, cystic, mobile, nontender tumors
- Size variable.

Characters of twisted ovarian tumors:
- Regular, cystic, tender mass, mobility restricted
- Guarding rigidity present, signs of acute abdomen.

Characters of malignant ovarian tumors:
- Free fluid usually present/ascites present
- Irregular, variable consistency and mobility, nontender (unless bleeding or rupture of capsule), fixed mass
- Rapidly growing tumor.

PER SPECULUM EXAMINATION

Position of cervix may be shifted to same side of mass as uterus is deviated to opposite side.

PER VAGINUM EXAMINATION

- Confirmation of findings on abdominal examination
- Cervical movements will not be transmitted to mass as mass is separate from uterus (unless there are dense adhesions with uterus).

Differential diagnosis of pedunculated fibroid
- A notch will be felt between mass and uterus, differential diagnosis of pedunculated fibroid, pelvic TB, TO mass
- Tumor felt in anterior fornix with tenderness—more chances of torsion
- Fixed tumor in posterior fornix—more chances of malignancy.

PER RECTAL EXAMINATION

Nodularity felt in posterior fornix goes in favor of malignancy.

CONFIRMATION OF DIAGNOSIS

- USG + color Doppler. Morphological index score
- CT scan: To know about involvement of surrounding structures, nodes
- Markers, mainly CA 125 for epithelial ovarian tumors
  - <35 IU/mL is normal
  - >96 IU/mL in postmenopausal, high-risk of malignancy
- Risk of malignancy index.

1. What are the differential diagnosis of an ovarian mass?

- Full bladder
- Pregnant uterus
- Myoma
- Ascites.

2. What is unique feature of ovarian malignancy?

Because of multicentric origin, there can be epithelial tumor, stromal cell tumors and germ cell tumors present simultaneously. It makes diagnosis critical.

3. What are the features indicating malignancy on USG?

- Size/volume (>8 cm in premenopausal)
- Papillary projections from inner wall
- Bilaterality
- Solid tumors
- Multiloculations.
- Presence of ascites
- Involvement of other organs
  Each point carries 1 score.

4. What is role of color Doppler in diagnosis of ovarian malignancy?

Neoangiogenesis characterized by:
- AV shunts
- Microaneurysms
- Coiling
- Complex irregular branching
- Central vessels.

Most useful in postmenopausal women.

5. What is risk of malignancy index?

- It is index to predict risk of malignancy in given patient.
- Factors considered are:
  a. Menopausal status (M)
     - Premenopausal score 1
     - Postmenopausal score 3
  b. Ultrasound morphology scoring (U)
  c. Actual serum CA-125 level.
     - RMI = M × U × S. CA-125 level
     - If >300, chances of tumor being malignant are high.

6. How to decide line of management in premenopausal ovarian tumor?

- Cyst <6 cm, no symptoms, no evidence of malignancy with unilocular cyst
- Treatment of choice is observation with hormonal suppression of HPO axis
- Cyst >8 cm, increasing size, symptoms suggesting complications, suspicion of malignancy, exploration is must
- Extent of surgery depends on age, parity and findings at laparotomy

Treatment may range from:
- Removal of cyst only
- Or removal of cyst along with that sided ovary and tube
- Or total abdominal hysterectomy with bilateral salphingoopherectomy
- Or total staging laparotomy with radical surgery.

7. What is line of management in postmenopausal ovarian tumor?

- Exploration is must
- Extent of surgery depends on RMI and findings at laparotomy
- In case of suspected benign, total abdominal hysterectomy with bilateral salphingo-oophorectomy
- In case of suspected malignant, staging laparotomy with maximum possible debulking.

8. What are the steps of staging laparotomy?

- Adequate vertical incision
- Collection of ascetic fluid or peritoneal wash for cytology
- Examination of liver capsule, undersurface of diaphragm, parietal peritoneum, mesentery, omentum, intestinal surface, palpation of lymph nodes, biopsy from omentum and other suspected sites
- Examination of tumor itself noting bilaterality, morphology, surface, evidence of local infiltration
- Decision of extent of surgery, maximum possible debulking, aiming at <5 mm residual disease.

9. What are the advantages of cytoreduction?

- Reduction in ascites
- Removal of omental cake will reduce nausea
- Removal of intestinal metastasis will improve intestinal function, nutrition and tolerance to CT and RT
- Minimal cells in GO phase so better response to CT
- According to fractional cell kill hypothesis, less number of cells at end
- Requires less duration/dose of CT, so better patient compliance.

10. What is plan of treatment in stage Ia, Ib?

- TAH with BSO with omentectomy, follow-up, no need of adjuvant therapy
- If desirous of childbearing, in case of Ia, conservative surgery with careful follow-up and radical surgery as soon as childbearing is complete
- Role of fertility preserving/sparing surgery in young patients with stage Ia, (low grade), unilateral oophorectomy with follow-up can be considered. Hysterectomy with contralateral oophorectomy after completion of family.

11. What is plan of treatment in stage Ic onwards?

- TAH with BSO with omentectomy
- Adjuvant therapy, either chemotherapy or in selected cases radiotherapy
- Second look-laparotomy/scopy to confirm response
- Follow-up with SCA-125.

12. What should be the plan of treatment if radical surgery is not possible on exploration?

- Maximum feasible cytoreduction at first exploration
- Three cycles of combination chemotherapy
- Interval cytoreduction
- Remaining three cycles of chemotherapy
- Second-look surgery.

13. What is second-look surgery?

It is a laparotomy/scopy aiming to:
- Confirm response of therapy after completion of cycles, where there is no residual disease on CT scan, CA-125 levels normal
- To complete cytoreduction if evidence of residual disease
- To take decision to change combinations of drugs.

14. What are the prognostic factors in ovarian malignancy?

- Pathological—Histological grade and differentiation
- Biological—Nuclear characters (ploidy)
- Clinical—Stage, extent of residual disease, presence of ascites, age overall prognosis is 25% with 5-years survival.

15. What is secondary laparotomy?

After giving chemotherapy, patients with persistent or recurrent pelvic and abdominal tumors are candidates for secondary cytoreduction (usually within 9 to 12 months).

16. What are the treatment options available for treatment of malignant ovarian tumor?

- Surgery
- Chemotherapy
- Radiotherapy

- Immunotherapy
- Combined approach.

17. How do you stage Ca ovary?

FIGO staging:
Stage-I : Growth limited to ovaries
Stage-II : Growth involving one or both ovaries with pelvic extension
Stage-III : Tumor involving one or both ovaries with peritoneal implant outside the pelvis
State-IV : Distant metastasis.

18. What is the significance of staging ovarian tumor at laparotomy?

It is done to confirm the diagnosis, nature of disease and to assess extent of disease.

19. Why prognosis is bad?

- Early diagnosis is difficult as condition causes vague symptoms and lack of appropriate markers makes mass screening difficult
- Suboptimal surgery either because malignancy is not suspected or surgeon is not experienced to handle such case
- Requirement of radical surgery and side effects of adjuvant therapy increase morbidity.

20. What is advantage of combination of chemotherapeutic drugs?

- Less dose of each drug, decreasing individual toxicity
- Less chances of development of resistance
- Combination of drugs acting at different cell phases increases response in the form of cell kill.

21. What are the complication of benign ovarian cyst?

- Torsion/axial rotation
- Rupture
- Pseudomyxoma peritonei
- Infection
- Extraperitoneal development.

22. What is the classification of ovarian tumor?

- *Common epithelial tumors:*
  - Serous tumors
  - Mucinous tumors
  - Endometrioid tumors
  - Clear cell
  - Brenner tumors
  - Mixed epithelial tumors
  - Undifferentiated carcinoma
  - Unclassified epithelial tumors.
- *Sex cord tumors:*
  - Granulosa, stromal cell tumors, theca cell tumors.
  - Androblastomas: Sertoli-Leydig cell tumors.
  - Gynandroblastoma
  - Unclassified.
- *Lipid (lipoid) cell tumors.*
  - Dysgerminoma
  - Endodermal sinus tumor
  - Embryonal carcinoma
  - Polyembryoma
  - Choriocarcinoma
  - Teratoma
  - Mixed forms.
- *Gonadoblastoma:*
  - Pure
  - Mixed with dysgerminoma or other germ cell tumors
- *Soft tissue tumors not specific to ovary*
- *Unclassified tumors*
- *Tumor-like conditions.*

23. What is Meigs' syndrome?

It consists of:
- Fibroma of ovary
- Hydrothorax
- Ascites.

24. State differential diagnosis of ovarian cyst.

- Full bladder
- Pregnant uterus
- Myoma
- Ascites
- Other tumors.

25. What is paraovarian cyst?

Extraperitoneal cyst lying in the broad ligament adjacent to the ovary, below the Fallopian tube.

26. What are non-neoplastic causes of ovarian cyst?

- Follicular cyst
- Corpus luteum cyst
- Theca lutein and granulosa lutein cyst
- Polycystic ovarian syndrome
- Endometrial cyst.

27. What is Krukenberg's tumor?

Type of secondary ovarian carcinoma. They are:
- Bilateral
- Have smooth surfaces which may be slightly bossed
- Are freely movable in the pelvis

- Tumors are secondary growth in ovary and most often arise from primary carcinoma of stomach (70%), large bowel (15%) and breast (6%). They arise by retrograde lymphatic spread.

28. What are the contents of ovarian pedicle?
- *Laterally:* Infundibulopelvic ligament containing structures therein, i.e. ovarian vessels, nerves and lymphatics.
- *Medially:*
  - Ovarian ligament
  - Medial end of the Fallopian tube
  - Mesosalpinx containing utero-ovarian anastomotic vessels.
- *Middle:* Broad ligament.

29. What is pseudomyxoma peritonea?
It is caused due to rupture of mucinous tumors. There is spillage of mucinous material in the peritoneal cavity which leads to adhesion formation. It is recurrent.

New developments in diagnosis and treatment of ovarian malignancies:
i. BRCA I and II genetic testing to identify individuals for further investigations.
ii. Cytogenetic studies
   - Trisomy 12 is most commonly found in germ cell tumor, trisomies 3, 8 and 14 are also found.
   - Trisomy 12, 14 and monosomy 22 have some relation with sex cord tumors.
   - There is no pathognomic rearrangement for epithelial tumors.
iii. At present platinum based drugs are used as mainstay of combination chemotherapy. The efforts are made to make blue prints of individual tumors so that specific drug can be given in chemotherapy.
iv. The finding that levels of folate receptors is increased, indicates some hope in immunotherapy.

MUST REMEMBER
- Unique feature of ovarian malignancy is multicentric origin giving rise to varied histopathological types.
- Nonspecific but persistent dyspeptic symptoms point towards malignant epithelial tumors.
- Acute abdomen in presence of pelvic mass, torsion of ovarian tumour should be suspected.
- Papillary excrescence on USG and low impedance flow on color Doppler are pathognomonic of malignancy.
- Apart from imaging, menopausal status and CA125 levels help to know risk of malignancy index (RMI).
- Careful assessment of patient before operative procedure is must to avoid undertreatment or overtreatment.
- Staging laparotomy is must for opt diagnosis.
- Maximum possible cytoreduction improves prognosis.
- Any palpable pelvic mass at any age should be evaluated with care as ovarian malignancy can occur at any age.
- Every effort must be made to diagnose ovarian malignancy at early stage to improve prognosis.

Cancer of Cervix

SR Wakode, Vidhya Choudhary

HISTORY

Patients with age between 35 and 65 years, multipara may be having abnormal uterine bleeding, postcoital bleeding, vaginal discharge, pain, loss of appetite, loss of weight. Past history of early age at first intercourse, multiple sexual partners, STIs.

SYMPTOMS

Intermenstrual/postcoital/postmenstrual bleeding, vaginal discharge, pain, urinary and bowel complaints.

SIGNS

- Cachexia, lymphadenopathy
- Physical examination
- Pallor, cachexia, lymphadenopathy
- PS—Cervical lesion—exophytic/endophytic/ulcerative lesion bleeds on touch, friability, fixity
- PR—Parametrial involvement, rectal mucosal involvement.

1. What is the most common cancer in female next to breast?

Cancer cervix—80% of genital cancers in India.

2. What are etiological factors for cervical cancer?

Factors predisposing cervical cancer are:
- Early coital activity and childbearing
- More frequency of intercourse
- Multiplicity of sexual partners
- Low socioeconomic status
- Viral infections—Human papilloma virus (16, 18, 31, 33) (70% cases), herpes virus type
- Prostitutes with HIV and STD, smoking (second most common).

3. How invasive cervical cancer develops in cervical epithelium?

Invasive cervical cancer is preceded by dysplastic changes in the cervical epithelium.

4. What is cervical intraepithelial neoplasia (CIN)?

Histopathological description where part or whole of the thickness of the cervical epithelium is replaced by cells showing varying degree of dysplasia.

5. What is meant by dysplasia?

Dysplasia means a change causing an alteration and disorderly arrangement of the cells of the stratified squamous epithelium.

6. What are the characteristics of dysplastic cells?

The cells are:
- Variable in size and shape
- Large, irregular, and hyperchromatic nuclei
- Mitotic figures found in cells.

Dysplastic cells have four characteristics:
- Anisocytosis (cells of unequal size)
- Poikilocytosis (abnormally shaped cells)
- Hyperchromatism (excessive pigmentation)
- Presence of mitotic figures (an unusual number of cells which are currently dividing).

7. What are types of cervical dysplasia?

- Mild dysplasia (CIN-I)—Undifferentiated cells are confined to the lower third of the epithelial layer
- Moderate dysplasia (CIN-II)—The lower 50–75% of the epithelial layer is undifferentiated
- Severe dysplasia—The entire thickness of the epithelium undifferentiated
- Carcinoma *in situ* (CIN-III)—This is replaced by anaplastic cells.

8. What type of vaginal infection shows changes of mild cervical dysplasia?

Trichomoniasis.

9. How many years period is required for progression of severe dysplasia to invasive cervical cancer?

5–10 years period is required.

10. How much percentage of mild and severe dysplasia progress to cervical cancer?

0.5% of mild and 9.6 percent of severe dysplasia can progress to cervical cancer.

11. What are the methods of screening for cervical cancer?

Methods for cervical cancer screening are:
- Pap smear (exfoliative cytology), sensitivity (72%), specificity (94%)
- Speculoscopy
- Microcolpohysteroscopy
- Colposcopy
- Cervicography
- VIA/VILI in poor resource areas
  VIA/VILI—Visual inspection after application of acetic acid/Lugol's iodine
- HPV DNA testing, sensitivity (88-97%), specificity (73-93%).

12. What are the screening guidelines?

ACOG 2009 recommends:
- Begin screening at the age of 21 years
- Screen 2 yearly till age of 30 year
- Screen every 3 years from age 30 year:
  if previous 3 consecutive negative smears
  - No CIN II/III, HIV infection
  - Not immunocompromised
  - No DES exposure *in utero.*
- Stop screening at 65-70 years, if previous 3 smears are negative
- No screening after hysterectomy except when performed for CIN II/III
- Conventional cytology or liquid-based cytology (LBC) can be used
- For women >30 years, combined cytology and HPV testing recommended.

13. What are the precautions to be taken before collection of Pap smear?

Precautions to be taken are:
- Smear collection before bimanual examination
- No antiseptic application
- No vaginal douching.

14. Collection of Pap smear is done with: How collection of pap smear is done?:

- Ayre's spatula
- Cotton swab stick
- Cytobrush.

15. What is the fixative used for pap smear?

95% absolute alcohol and ether and fixative sprays are available.

16. What are the reports/grade of pap smear?

- Grade I—Normal cells
- Grade II—Inflammatory cells
- Grade III—Suspicious abnormality in cells
- Grade IV—Distinctly abnormal, possibly malignant
- Grade V—Malignant cells.

17. What is newer classification of pap smear?

a. Normal cytology
b. Inflammatory smear
c. CIN-I (Mild dysplasia)
d. CIN-II, III and carcinoma *in situ*
e. Malignant cells seen.

18. How much is the incidence of dysplasia in India?

16/1000 patients.

19. What are reasons for false negative pap smear reports?

- Improper smear taking
- No access to squamocolumnar junction (menopausal woman)
- Laboratory error.

20. What are the uses of colposcopy?

- Localization of lesion
- Making the diagnosis
- Taking directed biopsy
- Guiding ablative procedures.

21. What are the indications for colposcopy?

Indications for colposcopy are:
- Abnormal cytology
- Diagnosis of suspicious invasive lesion
- Diagnostic directed biopsy
- Conservative therapy under colposcopic guidance
- Follow-up cases treated conservatively.

22. What is cervicography?

New technique of screening for cervical cancer involving taking the photograph of the entire cervical os after applying 5% acetic acid to the cervix and sent for evaluation to colposcopist.

23. What are the types of biopsy that can diagnose cervical malignancy?

Following types of biopsy can diagnose cervical malignancy:
- Punch biopsy
- Colposcopic directed biopsy
- Endocervical curettage
- Cone biopsy
- Large loop excision of the transformation zone.

24. How will you treat CIN I?

CIN I is inflammatory in nature so treatment of infection is done with repeat smear after 3-6 months.

25. What are the treatment modalities for CIN II and III?

CIN II and III treatment modalities are:
- Local destructive methods
- Excision of local tissue
- Surgery.

26. What are the local destructive methods for treating CIN II and III?

Local destructive methods used are:
- Cryosurgery
- Fulguration/coagulation
- Laser ablation.

27. What are the methods of local tissue excision for CIN II, III?

Methods for local tissue excision are:
- Conization by cold knife
- Laser conization
- Large loop excision of the transformation zone (LLETZ).

28. How will you treat CIN II and III in woman over 40 years of age?

CIN II and III in 40 years of woman is treated by—hysterectomy.

29. What are the indications for hysterectomy in severe dysplasia (CIN II, III)?

Indications are:
- Women over 40 years of age
- Family completed
- Associated problem like DUB, fibroids
- Not able to do regular follow-up.

30. What type of cervix biopsy you take from cauliflower-like lesion?

Punch biopsy from the margin of lesion including same normal tissue.

31. What are the histopathological types of cervical cancer?

- Squamous cell carcinoma
  - Large cell keratinizing
  - Large cell nonkeratinizing
  - Small cell type
  - Verrucous carcinoma
  - Papillary carcinoma
- Adenocarcinoma.
  - Adenosquamous carcinoma
  - Sarcoma – Embryonal rhabdomyosarcoma
  - Malignant melanoma.

32. What predisposes younger women for endocervical cancer?

Prolonged used of oral contraceptives pills for >8 years.

33. What are the types of lesion in cervical cancer?

- Ulcerative growth
- Cauliflower-like lesion
- Flat raised induration
- Endocervical cancer shows barred shaped bulky cervix.

34. What are the modes of spread in cervical cancer?

Cancer cervix spreads by:
- Direct spread locally
- Lymphatic spread
- Blood spread
- Intraperitoneal implantation.

35. What are the commonly involved structures with direct spread of cancer cervix?

Direct spread of cervical cancer occurs to:
- The parametria on both side
- Upper part of cervix
- Endometrium, myometrium and body of uterus
- Anterior vaginal wall
- Bladder
- Rarely Fallopian tubes and ovaries.

36. What group of lymph nodes is involved in cancer cervix?

- Lymph nodes in parametrium
- Obturator
- External iliac
- Hypogastric glands
- Rarely aortic and lumbar glands.

37. What are the cardinal symptoms of cancer cervix?

There are four main symptoms of cancer cervix:
i. Hemorrhage (postcoital/intermenstrual bleeding)
ii. Discharge (foul smelling discharge sometimes blood mixed)
iii. Cachexia
iv. Pain.

38. What type of bleeding pattern exists in carcinoma cervix?

- Postmenopausal bleeding
- Metrorrhagia (intermenstrual irregular bleeding)
- Postcoital bleeding
- Blood-stained vaginal discharge.

39. What are the causes of pain in cancer cervix?

Causes of pain in cancer cervix are:
- Parametritis
- Lymph nodes involvement at bifurcation of common iliac

- Involvement of obturator nerve
- Involvement of bladder
- Sacral plexus involvement by growth
- Pyometra.

40. What are the four main cardinal signs of cancer cervix?

Four main (cardinal) signs are:
i. Growth bleeds on touch
ii. Growth is friable
iii. Fixed cervix
iv. Induration of cervix.

41. Write differential diagnosis of vaginal bleeding following digital examination of cervix.

- Carcinoma cervix
- Vascular erosion ectropion
- Mucus polyp
- Myomatous polyp
- Retained products of conception.

42. Enumerate the list of investigations in a patient of carcinoma cervix.

Investigations to be done in carcinoma cervix are:
- Pelvic examination under anesthesia
- Chest X-ray
- IVP barium enema
- Cystoscopy proctoscopy
- Proctosigmoidoscopy
- Colposcopy biopsy
- Endocervical curettage
- Bone survey
- CT scan USG
- Bone scan MRI, PET Scan
- Retroperitoneal periaortic nodes sampling
- Scalene fat pad biopsy.

43. What is preinvasive carcinoma stage?

Carcinoma *in situ* cases of stage 0 (zero) should not be included in any therapeutic statistics.

44. What are the treatment modalities for cancer cervix?

Treatment modalities are:
- Surgery
- Radiotherapy
- Combined therapy
- Chemotherapy.

45. Describe FIGO staging 2014.

Stage 0: The carcinoma is confined to the surface layer (cells lining) of the cervix. Also called carcinoma *in situ* (CIS).

Stage I: The carcinoma has grown deeper into the cervix, but has not spread beyond it (extension to the corpus would be disregarded).

IA Invasive carcinoma which can be diagnosed only by microscopy, with deepest invasion <5 mm and the largest extension <7 mm
IA1 Measured stromal invasion of <3.0 mm in depth and extension of <7.0 mm
IA2 Measured stromal invasion of >3.0 mm and not >5.0 mm with an extension of not >7.0 mm
IB Clinically visible lesions limited to the cervix uteri or pre-clinical cancers greater than stage IA
IB1 Clinically visible lesion <4.0 cm in greatest dimension
IB2 Clinically visible lesion >4.0 cm in greatest dimension.

Stage II: Cervical carcinoma invades beyond the uterus, but not to the pelvic wall or to the lower third of the vagina.
IIA Without parametrial invasion.
IIA1 Clinically visible lesion <4.0 cm in greatest dimension.
IIA2 Clinically visible lesion >4.0 cm in greatest dimension.

Stage II: Cervical carcinoma invades beyond the cervix, but does not extend into the pelvic wall. The carcinoma involves vagina but not as far as the lower third.
IIA1 Without parametrial involvement. Involvement up to upper 2/3rd vagina with lesion <4.0 cm in greatest dimension
IIA2 Clinically visible lesion >4.0 cm in greatest dimension.
IIB With obvious parametrial invasion.

Stage III: The tumor extends to the pelvic wall and/or involves lower third of the vagina and/or causes hydronephrosis or nonfunctioning kidney.
IIIA Tumor involves lower third of the vagina, with no extension to the pelvic wall.
IIIB Extension to the pelvic wall and/or hydronephrosis or nonfunctioning kidney.

Stage IV: The carcinoma has extended beyond the true pelvis or has involved (biopsy proven) the mucosa of the bladder or rectum. A bullous edema, as such, does not permit a case to be allotted to Stage IV.
IVA Spread of the growth to adjacent organs.
IVB Spread to distant organs.

46. What are the indications for Wertheim's hysterectomy?

Stage Ia1 with lymphovascular space invasion and Ia2 removal of total uterus along with upper 3rd of vaginal cuff and bilateral salpingo-oophorectomy with pelvic lymphadenectomy. Cervix/uterus can be conserved in young women.

47. How much is mortality with Wertheim's hysterectomy?

One percent mortality.

48. What are the complications of Wertheim's hysterectomy?

Hemorrhage, bladder injury, ureter injury, causing ureteric fistula, sepsis, thrombophlebitis, embolism, paralytic ileus, chest infection, wound sepsis, burst abdomen, scar hernia and mortality.

49. Radiotherapy is indicated in which stages of cervix cancer?

Stage IIB to stage IV radiotherapy is given.

50. What are the techniques of radiotherapy?

Brachytherapy and teletherapy.

51. What is brachytherapy?

It consists of intracavitary radiation using high activity "after loading" remote controlled system.

52. What are the sources of radiation?

Cobalt, cesium or selectron is the source of radiation.

53. What are indications for chemotherapy in cancer cervix?

- Recurrence of lesion with no history of prior radiotherapy stage II onwards
  Stage I with high-risk factors for recurrence
- Adenocarcinoma of endocervix.

54. What are the drugs used for chemotherapy?

Cisplatin, ifosfamide, cyclophosphamide, vincristine, methotrexate, thiotepa, doxorubicin, epirubicin, paclitaxel, topotecan, gemcitabine.

55. Write treatments modalities for cervical dysplasia.

- Cone biopsy
- LEEP
- Cryosurgery (freezing)
- Electrocauterization
- Laser surgery
- Traditional surgery.

56. What is the most common causative pathogen for carcinoma cervix.

HPV.

57. What are the HPV strains for highest risk factor for cancer cervix?

HPV type 16, 18, 31, 45, (16 and 18 are responsible for 70% of cases).

58. What are the vaccines available for prevention of precancerous and cancerous lesions of cervix?

- Two vaccines are available—Cervarix (gsk) and Gardasil (merck)
- Both are US FDA approved
- They reduce the risk by 93%
- Cervarix is bivalent for HPV 16,18
- Gardasil is quadrivalent for HPV 6,11,16,18. Gardasil also helps protect girls and young women aged 9–26 against 70% of vaginal cancer cases and up to 50% of vulvar cancer cases
- Gardasil also protects against genital warts and has been shown to protect against cancers of the anus, vagina and vulva. Both vaccines are available for females. Only Gardasil is available for males.
- Active component is L1 protein of HPV capsid.

Contraindications:
- Allergic to yeast
- Pregnancy.

Side effects:

Pain, swelling, itching, bruising, and redness at the injection site, headache, fever, nausea, dizziness, vomiting, and fainting.

59. Girls/women who have been vaccinated still need cervical cancer screening?

Yes, vaccinated women will still need regular cervical cancer screening (Pap tests) because the vaccines protect against most but not all HPV types that cause cervical cancer. Also, women who got the vaccine after becoming sexually active may not get the full benefit of the vaccine if they had already been exposed to HPV.

60. Are there other ways to prevent HPV?

Only sure way to prevent HPV is to avoid all sexual activity.

61. Which girls/women should receive HPV vaccination?

Ideally females should get the vaccine before they become sexually active and exposed to HPV in three doses over 6 months as 0, 1, 6/0, 2, 6. HPV vaccination is recommended with either vaccine for 11 and 12 years old girls. It is also recommended for girls and women aged 13 through 26 years of age who have not yet been vaccinated or completed the vaccine series; HPV vaccine can also be given to girls beginning at age 9 years.

62. Should endocervical curettage/brushing be the part of colposcopic examination?

As per ASCCP (American Society for Colposcopy and Cervical Pathology) guidelines, endocervical curettage is not required, cytobrush is sufficient for sampling the endocervical canal, if needed.

63. What is the most common type of cervical carcinoma?

Squamous cell carcinoma.

64. What are prognostic variables for early stage carcinoma cervix (Ia–IIa)

Intermediate risk factors:
i. Large tumor size
ii. Cervical stromal invasion to middle or deep third
iii. Lymph-vascular space invasion.

High-risk factors:
- Positive or close margins
- Positive lymph nodes
- Microscopic parametrial involvement.

65. Write treatment of cancer cervix by stage.

Ia_1	LVSI −ve : Conization/type I hysterectomy
	LVSI +ve : Type II hysterectomy
Ia_2	Radical Trachelectomy/type II Wertheim's hysterectomy. Adjuvant radiation with intermediate risk factors. Chemoradiation with high-risk factors.
Ib_1 Ib_2 $IIIa_1$	Radical trachelectomy (If with low risk, i.e. no LVSI and <2 cm)
Type III	Radical hysterectomy
	Adjuvant radiation with intermediate risk factors.
	Chemoradiation with high-risk factors.
Bulky Ib_2 and IIa_2	Primary chemoradiation
Type III	Radical hysterectomy with adjuvant chemoradiation.
IIb to IIIb	Chemoradiation, cisplatin is agent of choice.
IVa and IVb IVa	Chemoradiation, primary exenteration, if, VVF or RVF
IVb	Chemotherapy and palliative pelvic radiation

66. What is the incidence of carcinoma cervix with pregnancy?

1.2 in 10000

67. What is sentinel lymph node?

Sentinel lymph node is specific lymph node/nodes that is the first to receive drainage from a malignancy and is a primary site for nodal metastasis. Negative sentinel lymph node would allow omission of lymphadenectomy of the involved nodal basin.

It can be detected by perilesional injection of radiolabeled Tc^{99} or blue dye, intraoperative identification of the sentinel lymph nodes using gamma probes or visual identification of blue stained nodes.

It is useful in early stage disease. Its role in cancer cervix is purely investigational.

MUST REMEMBER

- Almost all squamous cell cancers arise from transformation zone which is area between original and new squamo-columnar junction.
- HPV 16 and 18 are associated with most of invasive cancers.
- Squamous cell cancer comprises 80–85% adenocarcinoma comprises 10–15% of all cervical cancers.
- *Risk factors:* High parity, early sexual activity, multiple sexual partners, STIs.
- Cytology is most popular screening test used.
- Colposcopy is visualization of cervix under magnification
- Cervical cancer spreads by direct, lymphatic and hematogeneous spread.
- FIGO staging is recommended.
- Surgery and radiochemotherapy are the options in management.

Endometrial Carcinoma

Kavita N Singh

HISTORY
Age >50 years, nullipara.

Symptoms
Abnormal uterine/postmenopausal bleeding.

Past History
- Anovulatory cycles, early menarche, late menopause, family history of hereditary nonpolyposis colon cancer (HNPCC). Medical disorders—Diabetes mellitus, hypertension medications—HRT, tamoxifene.
- Physical examination:
  - BMI > 25, hypertension, lymphadenopathy
  - PA organomegaly, uterine enlargement
  - PS examination for bleeding
  - PV examination for uterine enlargement, tenderness or adnexal mass.

1. What are the causes of postmenopausal bleeding (PMB)?
The causes of postmenopausal bleeding are:
- Organic lesions of the female genital tract, e.g. mainly malignant lesions of vulva, vagina, cervix, uterus, Fallopian tubes and ovary
- Benign lesions, which cause of postmenopausal bleeding are atrophic endometritis, and senile vaginitis
- Other uterine lesions which cause postmenopausal bleeding are:
  - Polyps—2–12%, hyperplasia—15–25% cases.
  - Some iatrogenic conditions are tamoxifen given for breast cancer and estrogen replacement therapy for menopausal symptoms also known as 'the youth pill.'

2. Which are the 'high-risk factors for the carcinoma of endometrium'?
a. Genetic predisposition, e.g. history of hereditary non-polyposis colon cancer (HNPCC)
b. Late menopause >52 years risk 2.4 times higher
c. Obesity weight >10–25 kg, risk 3 times and >25 kg that expected risk 10 times
d. Diabetes mellitus
e. Hypertension (c, d and e together are called as corpus cancer syndrome)
f. Low parity
g. Unopposed estrogen activity
   - Endogeneous, e.g. feminizing tumors of ovary, i.e. granulosa or theca cell tumors of ovary
   - Exogeneous, e.g. estrogen replacement therapy for menopausal symptoms
h. Tamoxifen therapy for breast cancer.

3. What is the histopathological nature of carcinoma of endometrium?
The histopathological nature of carcinoma of endometrium is adenocarcinoma, occasionally adenosquamous and very rarely pure-squamous variety.

4. What are the endometrial carcinoma precursors?
Different types of endometrial hyperplasia are known and their relative risks of developing into endometrial carcinoma are as follows:
- Simple hyperplasia without atypia—1%
- Complex hyperplasia without atypia—3%
- Simple hyperplasia with atypia—8%
- Complex hyperplasia with atypia—29%, very important.

5. Can you prevent progression of hyperplastic endometrium developing into endometrial carcinoma?
Progestin therapy is more effective in preventing progression of hyperplastic endometrium without atypia developing into endometrial carcinoma than hyperplastic endometrium with atypia.

6. Are there any 'screening tests' for the diagnosis of endometrial carcinoma in early stages? Like carcinoma of cervix?
'Screening tests' for the diagnosis of endometrial carcinoma are neither warranted nor they are cost-effective. However in high-risk cases:
- Pap smear is not very much useful to diagnose endometrial carcinoma in early stages as is useful to diagnose carcinoma of cervix.

- Transvaginal ultrasonography (TVS) endometrial thickness >4 mm or polypoidal mass in the uterine cavity needs further evaluation and progesterone challenge test have been recommended in postmenopausal cases, but they do not have the cost benefit as the 'screening tests'.

However, patients on estrogen replacement therapy for menopausal symptoms and tamoxifen therapy for breast cancer form a high-risk group for the carcinoma of endometrium' and these cases must be vigilantly kept under follow-up.

7. What are the main symptoms of endometrial carcinoma?

Pervaginal bleeding is the main symptom.
- In premenopausal age group, the patient may complain of menometrorrhagia mainly
- All cases of postmenopausal bleeding be considered as carcinoma of endometrium unless proved otherwise
- Pain because of colicky uterine contractions (Simpson's pain) in suprapubic region occurring at fixed time of the day lasting for 1–2 hours
- With pyometra, patient can have pain and fever.

8. What are the main signs of endometrial carcinoma?

Try to know the risk factors.
- Patient may have undergone D and C for menstrual abnormality. Review the report
- In general examination, mention built (obesity) and record her blood pressure. Palpate for lymphadenopathy
- Do not forget to examine breasts (also in cases of ovarian carcinoma)
- Pervaginal and rectal examination to confirm the size of the uterus, to know mobility of the uterus, parametrial induration and nodularity of the cul-de-sac
- Positive Clarke's test (negative Clarke's test does not rule out endometrial carcinoma).

9. How will you confirm the diagnosis of endometrial carcinoma?

- All cases of peri- and postmenopausal bleeding must be subjected to endometrial sampling to confirm/rule out carcinoma of endometrium
- Aspiration biopsy has the diagnostic accuracy of about 90–98%
- Endometrial lavage/brush, vabra aspirator, Tis-U trap, Pipelle suction curette
- However, if patient tolerance or cervical stenosis does not permit aspiration biopsy or recurrence of pervaginal bleeding after previous negative/inadequate biopsy D and C along with (if available) hysteroscopy (gold standard) should be done
- TVS acts as an adjunct to endometrial sampling.

10. What is G1, G2 or G3 in endometrial carcinoma?

It refers to the histopathological feature of carcinoma of endometrium as follows:
- G1 < 5%: Solid nonsquamous growth pattern
- G2 6–50%: Solid nonsquamous growth pattern
- G3 > 50%: Solid nonsquamous growth pattern.

11. What is squamous differentiation of carcinoma of endometrium'?

- About 15–25% endometrial carcinoma have areas of squamous differentiation. Benign squamous differentiation is called as adenoacanthoma and malignant adenosquamous carcinoma.
- Today both these terms are replaced by the term carcinoma of endometrium with squamous differentiation, irrespective of the nature of the squamous component.

12. What is FIGO staging of endometrial carcinoma?

	FIGO 2010 staging for endometrial cancer
IA	Tumor confined to the uterus, no or <½ myometrial invasion
IB	Tumor confined to the uterus, >½ myometrial invasion
II	Cervical stromal invasion, but not beyond uterus
Stage III locoregional spread	
IIIA	Tumor invades serosa or adnexa
IIIB	Vaginal and/or parametrial involvement
IIIC1	Pelvic lymph node involvement
IIIC2	Para-aortic lymph node involvement, with or without pelvic node involvement
Stage IV	Tumor invasion bladder and/or bowel, with/without distant metastasis
IVA	Tumor invasion bladder and/or bowel mucosa
IVB	Distant metastases including abdominal metastases and/or inguinal lymph nodes.

13. Describe briefly fractional curettage.

Total six specimens endocervical (2) and endometrial (4) are obtained in fractional curettage as follows. Specimens must be meticulously labeled.
a. Endocervical specimen no. 1 from endocervical canal before uterine sounding and cervical dilatation
b. Endocervical specimen no. 2 from isthmus 1 cm beyond the internal os after cervical dilatation
c. Four endometrial specimens are obtained after cervical dilatation as follows:
   - Right and left cornual specimen one each (Total 2)
   - Anterior and posterior wall of the uterus one each (Total 2).

14. What is the pretreatment evaluation of a case of endometrial carcinoma?

- Review of detailed history and thorough physical examination as discussed earlier
- High-risk factors, associated systemic problem
- CBC, chest X-ray, ECG for cardiorespiratory status
- Liver and renal function tests
- Stools for occult blood
- Hysteroscopy (risk of spillage)
- IVP, cystoscopy, rectosigmoidoscopy, Ba enema
- CT abdomen and pelvis to be done as per the merit of the case
- USG and MRI to know the extent of myometrial invasion
- CA-125 to know the extent of extrauterine disease.

15. What are the prognostic variables?

	Variables	Good prognosis	Bad prognosis
1.	Age group	Younger	Older
2.	Histological variety	Endometroid	Non-endometroid
3.	Grade	G1, G2	G3
4.	LVSI	Absent	Present
5.	Cervix involvement	Cx extension absent	Cx extension present
6.	Tumor Size	<2cm	Tumor size >2 cm
7.	Receptor positively	Receptor positive	Receptor negative
8.	Gytogenetics	Diploidy	Nonploidy
9.	Gene expression	Oncogene absent	Her 2 new, K-ras, poor prognosis

16. What are the different treatment options for endometrial carcinoma?

Surgery is the mainstay.
a. Total abdominal hysterectomy with bilateral salpingo-oophorectomy along with peritoneal cytology and omentectomy and lymph node sampling.
b. Today laparoscopically-assisted vaginal hysterectomy is one more option
c. Vaginal hysterectomy has a limited scope as lymph node sampling and adnexectomy is not possible (very high surgical risks with well-differentiated stage I cases).

17. What is adjuvant therapy for endometrial carcinoma?

- Radiotherapy with external beam irradiation or intracavitary
- Intraperitoneal phosphorus.

18. What are the different drugs used in the treatment of endometrial carcinoma?

- Hormones progestins for peritoneal cytology positive cases.
- Chemotherapeutic agents as doxorubicin, cisplatin, carboplatin and paclitaxel.

19. Can endometrial carcinoma be prevented?

Screening for high-risk factors including endometrial sampling before:

- Estrogen replacement therapy for menopausal symptoms
- Patients on tamoxifen therapy for breast cancer form a high-risk group for the carcinoma of endometrium and these cases must be vigilantly kept under follow-up.
- Premalignant lesions followed and treated
- Estrogen replacement therapy for menopausal symptoms should be combined with progestogens to counteract unopposed estrogen activity.

The revised FIGO staging system 2010 for carcinoma of the endometrium, there are four major changes, which are as follows.

- First, the previous stages IA and IB have been combined as stage IA because there was no significant difference in a 5-year survival among previous stage IA G1, IB G1, IA G2 and IB G2, as stated in volumes 23–26 of the FIGO annual report. Moreover, stage IB is now equal to or greater than the outer one-half of the myometrium.
- Second, stage II no longer has a subset A and B, and involvement of the endocervical gland of the cervix is now considered stage I.
- Third, pelvic and para-aortic lymph node involvement in previous stage IIIC has been separated because many previous studies have suggested that the prognosis may be worse if para-aortic lymph nodes are involved. Thus, the previous stage IIIC is now categorized as IIIC1 (indicating positive pelvic lymph nodes) and IIIC2 (indicating positive para-aortic lymph nodes with or without positive pelvic lymph nodes).
- Fourth, positive cytology has been excluded as factors for defining the new surgical staging.

Plan after surgical management

- Low risk—G1/2, no MI/LVSI, tumor <2 cm—no treatment
- Intermediate risk—G1/2 <50 percent MI, no LVSI/cervical stromal invasion—Brachytherapy
- High risk—G3, >50 percent MI, cervical invasion, LVSI, metastases, whole pelvic RT/External field RT, CT.

MUST REMEMBER

- Young women with hyperplasia present with prolonged bleeding after periods of amenorrhea. Older women present with perimenopausal or postmenopausal bleeding.
- Endometrial cancer is the most common gynecological cancer in developed countries, but not in developing countries.
- It spreads by lymphatic, hematogeneous and direct spread.
- Most common symptom is abnormal uterine bleeding, perimenopausal/postmenopausal bleeding, vaginal discharge. Uterus may be enlarged or normal. Diagnosis is by histopathology.

MULTIPLE CHOICE QUESTIONS

1. Only one of the following triads is true for endometrial carcinoma.
A. Obesity + Hypertension + Diabetes mellitus
B. Obesity + Nulliparity + Diabetes mellitus
C. Obesity + Nulliparity + Hypertension
D. Diabetes mellitus + Nulliparity + Hypertension.

2. Only one of the following is a cause and treatment for endometrial carcinoma.
A. Estrogen replacement therapy for menopausal symptoms
B. Tamoxifen
C. Progestogens
D. GnRH analogs.

3. Only one of the following predisposes to endometrial carcinoma.
A. Combined oral contraceptive pill
B. Sequential pills
C. Minipills
D. None of these.

4. Endometrial carcinoma is commonly associated with.
A. Feminizing tumors of ovary
B. Masculinizing tumors of ovary
C. Endometroid tumors of ovary
D. Germ cell tumors of ovary.

5. Only one of the following ovarian tumors predisposes to endometrial carcinoma.
A. Sertoli cell tumor
B. Leydig cell tumor
C. Sertoli–Leydig cell tumor
D. Granulosa cell tumor.

6. All of the following are commonly associated with endometrial carcinoma, except:
A. Obesity
B. Nulliparity
C. Estrogen replacement therapy for menopausal symptoms
D. HSV II infection.

7. Pain occurring at regular time of the day in a case of endometrial carcinoma is known as:
A. Sim's pain
B. Sam's pain
C. Simpson's pain
D. Sampson's pain.

8. Bleeding after uterine sounding in a case of endometrial carcinoma is known as:
A. Clarke's test
B. Clement's test
C. Cullen's test
D. Cunningham's test.

ANSWERS

(1) A; (2) B; (3) D; (4) A; (5) D; (6) D; (7) C; (8) A

Endoscopy

Ashish R Kale, Rajesh Darade

INTRODUCTION

Laparoscopy is visualization of interior of body cavities by endoscopes. This is called keyhole surgery.

Telescope with fiberoptic cable introduced through a port is used to visualize the abdominal and pelvic contents. Operating instruments are introduced through separate ports. Hysteroscopy is the visualization of the endocervical canal and uterine cavity.

Hysteroscopy can be used for diagnostic and therapeutic procedures. Diagnostic and operative hysteroscopy have been considered separate entities, as they require different instruments and a different approach to the patient.

1. What are the indications for laparoscopy?

Indications for diagnostic laparoscopy are:
- Evaluation of a patient with infertility; to look at pelvic pathology, tubal status, patency, adhesions, endometriotic spots, tubercles
- Acute or chronic pelvic pain
- Ectopic pregnancy
- Endometriosis
- Ovarian cysts
- Acute adnexal torsion
- Pelvic inflammatory disease; when diagnosis is not clear
- To diagnose and treat Müllerian duct anomalies.

2. What are the indications for therapeutic laparoscopy?

Tuboplasty, tubal sterilization, adhesiolysis, aspiration of simple ovarian cysts, ectopic pregnancy, ablation/fulguration of endometriotic lesions, myomectomy, correction of urinary incontinence, repair of pelvic organ prolapse, hysterectomy for various indications like fibroid and adenomyosis.

3. What are the advantages of laparoscopy?

Less adhesion formation, rapid postoperative recovery, less postoperative pain, hence less analgesia required, less hospital stay, minimal scar, quick resumption of day-to-day activity.

4. What are the contraindications for laparoscopy?

- Severe cardiorespiratory disease
- Large diaphragmatic hernia
- Generalized peritonitis
- Ileus/intestinal obstruction
- Inexperienced surgeon
- Hemodynamic compromise/instability
- Large abdominal masses/advanced pregnancy.
- Advanced malignancy.

5. What are the precautions to be taken at abdominal entry of Veress needle?

- Veress needle patency should be checked
- The abdomen is lifted up; this elevates the umbilicus and puts the peritoneum at stretch
- The intra-abdominal pressure is kept at 10–12 mm Hg
- The Veress needle is inserted at right angles to the skin directed into the axis of the true pelvis (30 degrees towards pelvis)
- In obese patients, the needle may have to be inserted more vertically.

6. What are the tests done to check peritoneal entry?

- *Hanging drop test:* This observes a hanging drop of fluid in the Veress needle that flows downward freely if the needle is in the peritoneal cavity. Lifting of the abdominal wall decreases intra-abdominal pressure and enhances the free flow.
- A syringe barrel is attached to the Veress needle and 1–2 mL saline poured into it; if the needle is intraperitoneal, the fluid will flow freely into the abdomen.
- Aspiration can be done with a syringe to make sure that the four B's should be absent—blood, bile, bladder and bowel
- Gas is insufflated at a low flow rate of 1 L/min, with the pressure below 10 mm Hg. With patient's respiratory efforts, there should be slight elevation in the pressure if the needle is intraperitoneal. If gas is insufflated and the pressure is persistently >10 mm Hg, the needle is probably preperitoneal or has entered the viscous or the omentum.

- At flow rate of 1 L/min, in 45–60 sec, there should be loss of liver dullness.

7. In difficult cases, what are the alternate points of entry?
- *Supraumbilical:* Large pelvic masses or previous scar
- Left/right lower quadrant; lateral border of the rectus at left or right McBurney's point
- *Palmer's point:* Left upper quadrant at the lateral border of the rectus, left midclavicular line 2 finger breadths below the left costal margin.

8. Which is the most dangerous part of the laparoscopic surgery?
Primary trocar entry.

9. What will happen if actual intra-abdominal pressure exceeds 25 mm Hg?
This pressure results in compression of inferior vena cava compromising venous return to heart leading to increased risk of deep vein thrombosis (DVT) and reduced cardiac output risk of air embolism is increased due to venous intravasation. There is increased risk of surgical emphysema.

10. What measures are taken if on insertion of Veress needle fresh blood or fecal matter is aspirated?
Do not remove Veress needle and immediately proceed laparotomy, as leaving needle in position helps to localize the punctured area after laparotomy.

11. What should be the maximum flow rate of CO_2 insufflation and why?
Normal caliber Veress needle can deliver CO_2 at maximum 2.5 L/min. If flow rate exceeds 7L/min, there is a risk of hypothermia to the patient.

12. What lamps are commonly used in light source?
Halogen and xenon lamps are commonly used.

13. What is open laparoscopy?
- This technique is used to minimize risk of large vessel and bowel injury during entry
- Useful in patients with previous abdominal surgeries
- *Procedure:*
  - A vertical skin incision is given over the umbilicus (intraumbilical)
  - Two strong sutures are placed on both the edges of the fascial entry
  - The sutures are lifted to elevate the abdominal wall for blunt or sharp entry into peritoneum
  - A smooth tipped Hasson's trocar and sleeve are inserted with an acorn-shaped metal obturator.

14. What are the various laparoscopic methods of sterilization?
- Silastic ring (Bands)
- Filshie clip
- Unipolar coagulation
- Bipolar coagulation
- Hulka clip.

15. Why does laparoscopy result in fewer adhesions compared to laparotomy?
- Absence of retraction and packing that can damage peritoneum
- Gentle handling of the tissue
- Lack of drying in room air
- Absence of foreign bodies.

16. Which type of coagulation has lesser peripheral damage?
Bipolar coagulation.

17. Why is CO_2 the preferred gas for creating pneumoperitoneum?
- Rapidly absorbed by blood
- Less-likely to lead to embolism
- Does not support combustion.

18. What is the maximum pressure setting during the laparoscopic procedure?
The pressure should not exceed 15 mm Hg.

19. What is gasless laparoscopy and what are its disadvantages?
- It is a method that has been introduced in an attempt to provide space in which to operate without the need for continuous gas replacement
- The anterior abdominal wall is elevated mechanically with a special device
- *Disadvantages:*
  - Pneumoperitoneum causes a dome-like elevation of the abdominal wall; the devices used here lift the abdominal wall only in the midline and not in the flanks
  - Access to the upper abdomen and POD is restricted
  - There is no increased intra-abdominal pressure to push the bowel away
  - The hemostatic effect of pneumoperitoneum does not exist
  - CO_2 gas enters in a plane and helps for the dissection which is not possible with gasless laparoscopy.

20. What are the complications of laparoscopy?

- *Due to anesthesia:*
  - Metabolic disturbances
  - Absorption of CO_2—arrhythmias
  - Inadequate oxygenation due to overdistention of the abdomen/steep Trendelenburg.
- *Hemorrhage:*
  - Superficial
  - *Major vessels:* Inferior epigastric arteries, aorta, iliac vessels.
- *Perforation of viscus:* Small bowel, large bowel, stomach
- Perforation of the uterus
- Extravasation of the gas into extraperitoneal space
  - Subcutaneous emphysema
  - Mediastinal emphysema.
- Gas embolism.
- Intra-abdominal burns/explosion
  - Release of methane gas from bowel perforation
  - Electrocautery injuries.
- Injury to the bladder, ureter.

21. What are the various methods of controlling hemorrhage from an injured inferior epigastric artery?

- Incision can be widened and the artery ligated under vision
- A figure of 8 suture placed on either sides of the trocar.
- From another trocar entry, bipolar coagulation of the vessel or laparoscopic suturing can be done
- A Foley's catheter can be inserted and the bulb inflated. This can be then pulled and traction applied.

22. Which laparoscopic procedures have highest incidence of ureteric injury?

- Infundibulopelvic ligament
  - Oophorectomy
  - *Adhesiolysis:* In ovarian fossa and lateral pelvic wall
  - Presacral neurectomy
  - Endometriosis–ablation
- Laparascopic uterine nerve ablations (LUNA)—uterosacral plication
- Hysterectomy—closure of vaginal cuff.

23. What are the indications for laparoscopic hysterectomy?

To transform an abdominal hysterectomy into a vaginal one. Avoid abdominal hysterectomy.

Traditional contraindications for vaginal hysterectomy (and hence indications for laparoscopic assistance) include:

- Poor access to ovaries
- Nulliparity without descent
- Previous pelvic surgery
- History of pelvic inflammatory disease
- Moderate-to-severe endometriosis
- Adnexal masses
- Known pelvic adhesions
- No mobility of the uterus
- Stage I endometrial cancer
- Uterine size >280 g
- Needing adnexectomy.

24. Define laparoscopic hysterectomy.

- Division of all major uterine pedicles and supports by laparoscopy
- Prof Harry Reich's definition: "Ligation of uterine arteries laparoscopically."

25. Which instrument is used to decrease size of tumor mass to be removed through small hole?

Morcellator is used.

26. Name distending media used in hysteroscopic surgery.

Hyskon, normal saline, CO_2, glycine 1.5 percent, sorbitol 3 percent.

27. What properties should distention media have for operative hysteroscopy?

Media should be isotonic, nonhemolytic, non-electrolytic, nontoxic when absorbed, should not influence osmolarity of blood, should be rapidly excreted and should be an osmotic diuretic.

28. What are the indications for diagnostic hysteroscopy?

- *Infertility:* To rule out any polyps, adhesions, fibroids in uterine cavity
- Postmenopausal bleeding
- Fibroid uterus; diagnose submucous fibroids
- Abnormal uterine bleeding not responding to medical management
- *Bad obstetric history:* Uterine anomalies, submucous fibroids, intrauterine adhesions
- Misplaced intrauterine device.

Polypectomy, myomectomy, synechiolysis, endometrial resection/ablation, metroplasty, biopsy of suspected endometrium, tubal cannulation, sterilization-insertion of Essure/electrocoagulation or laser destruction.

29. What are the contraindications of hysteroscopy?

Cervical stenosis, pregnancy, pelvic infection, cancer cervix, cardiopulmonary disorder.

30. What are the complications of hysteroscopy?
- Fluid overload due to absorption of the media
- Hyponatremia (absorption of hypo-osmolar media)
- Intra- and postoperative bleeding
- Uterine perforation and possible bowel injury
- Poor visibility
- Gas embolism (CO_2)
- Infection.

31. What are the methods of controlling bleeding complicating hysteroscopy?
- Aspirate the blood and increase the pressure of the distending medium
- The bleeding vessel can be coagulated with electrocautery
- Intrauterine balloon can be inflated and left *in situ* for 6–12 hours.

32. What are the precautions taken to avoid gas embolism in hysteroscopy?
- Use of pressure bag in hysteroscopy with proper care, i.e. avoid air in tubing of pressure bag, change the normal saline immediately once it gets over, surgeon and assistant should be alert during hysteroscopy
- Use of hysterometer with proper monitoring of intrauterine pressure
- Avoid Trendelenburg positioning
- Remove last dilator just before inserting the resectoscope.
- Limit repeated removal-insertion of the resectoscope.

33. What are guidelines for distension media in hysteroscopy?
- Keep distension media at body temperature and monitor the patient's core temperature continuously
- Use bipolar resectoscope, where isotonic electrolyte fluid, Ringer's lactate or 0.9% saline can be used
- Continuously record inflow and outflow using the electronic monitor with deficit alarm at 500 mL
- Do preoperative serum electrolytes for a baseline in all patients undergoing major monopolar resectoscopic surgery and evaluate electrolytes (Na⁺) status of procedure and patient's condition, if deficit is more than 1000 mL. If fluid deficit reaches 750 mL, immediately give 20 to 40 mg of intravenous frusemide and draw serum sodium
- Discontinue the procedure if the fluid deficit reaches 1,500 mL or serum Na level is below 125 mEq/L
- Consider spinal or epidural anesthesia for operative hysteroscopy or in high-risk patients
- Interrupt the procedure for 5–10 minutes to allow the uterus to contract and to seal off small blood vessels.

34. What are do's in hysteroscopic surgery?
- Always select the patient properly
- Counsel the patient properly, regarding the procedure
- Get all the investigations necessary
- Keep all the equipment and instruments ready, before the surgery
- Follow all the safety precautions recommended, like the inflow pressure, current setting, etc
- Try to use isotonic electrolyte containing solutions for all hysteroscopic surgeries
- Switch over to bipolar current as a modality of choice in resectoscopic surgeries
- In the event of fluid overload or any other complications, abandon the procedure, identify the complications and rectify them
- Always remember that surgery can be completed at a second sitting
- Keep proper record of all the procedures done and document all steps.

35. What are don'ts in hysteroscopic surgery?
- Do not start surgery if instruments are malfunctioning
- Do not use unsafe pressure devices for delivering fluid
- Do not give deep head low positions
- Do not over dilate the cervix
- Do not begin or continue surgery if the anatomy is not clear
- Do not use electrolyte containing solutions for monopolar resectoscopic surgeries
- Do not exceed the recommended fluid, the deficit during hysteroscopic surgeries.

36. What is an optical trocar?
Trocars that contain a window at the tip and are designed to handle a laparoscope to look through the window to enable surgeons to view the tissue layers during penetration and to see the abdominal cavity after penetration.

37. What are the indications and contraindications for laparoscopic myomectomy?
- *Indications*
  - Pedunculated myomas
  - Intramural myomas <10 cm. In infertility, if > 5 cm.
- *Contraindications*
  - Diffused, multiple myomas
  - Large uterus >18 weeks
  - Myomas >10 cm
  - Inexperienced surgeon unfamiliar with endosuturing
  - Submucous >50 percent extension into cavity.

38. What are the causes of intrauterine adhesions?
Vigorous curettage postabortal or postpartum sepsis, Asherman's syndrome secondary to PPH, endometrial

tuberculosis, IUCD use, postsubmucous myomectomy or metroplasty.

39. What is a microhysteroscope and what are its uses?
- This contains a magnifying lens built into the telescope
- Magnification up to 150 × can be achieved
- Used for studying vascular and glandular structures of the cervix, endometrial lining and tubal mucosa.

40. What are the various methods of laparoscopic management of distal tubal disease?
- *Fimbriolysis:* Adhesiolysis around the fimbria, tube patent following procedure
- *Fimbrioplasty:* Adhesiolysis followed by dilatation of fimbrial phimosis by dilator or atraumatic forceps (Maryland forceps)
- *Salpingostomy:* Terminal hydrosalpinx with a star-shaped occluded infundibulum; radial incisions made at ostia and edges everted.

41. What is the technique of ovarian drilling?
The ovarian surface inspected and intestines are kept at a distance. A bipolar or unipolar needle or a versapoint probe is used. The needle is inserted into the ovarian capsule 0.8 cm deep. Small needle diameter is used to decrease complication rates. No consensus about the number of holes to be made. About 10–15 holes can be made in each ovary which depends upon the severity of PCOS.

42. What is preoperative bowel preparation for laparoscopic surgery?
Liquids orally for 24 hours prior to surgery are sufficient for bowel preparation.

If any complicated case involving bowel surgery, we can give exelyte solution or colowash day prior to surgery.

MUST REMEMBER
- Laparoscopic surgery is known as keyhole surgery. It has several advantages like no large incision, short hospital stay, early return to work, less postoperative pain and minimal risk of incisional hernia.
- Laparoscopic procedures may be diagnostic or therapeutic.
- Indications include evaluation of infertility, endometriosis, ectopic pregnancy, chronic pelvic pain, tubal sterilization, ovarian cystectomy, oophorectomy and hysterectomy.
- Hysteroscopy can also be used for diagnostic and therapeutic procedures. Visualization of endometrial cavity and surgical procedures within the endometrial cavity are performed using hysteroscopy.

Index

Page numbers followed by *t* refer to table and *f* refer to figure

A

Abdominal compartment syndrome 85
Abdominal pain 166
Abortion 1, 2
   incidence of 1
   incomplete and complete 1
   missed 2
   septic 2
   threatened 1, 58
Abruptio placentae 16, 17
   treatment of 16
Adenomyosis 161, 170
Amenorrhea 166-168
   athletic 167
   causes of 166, 167
Amniocentesis, role of 62
Anemia 18, 22, 23
   blood transfusion in 19
   in pregnancy, classification of 21
   on pregnancy, impact of 18
Anovulatory endometrium, type of 164*t*
Antiandrogens 188
Antiestrogens 186
Antihypertensives in pre-eclampsia, role of 8
Antiphospholipid antibody syndrome 3
Antiprogesterones 187
APH, causes of 14
Artificial rupture of membrane, role of 35
Asherman's syndrome 209
Assisted vaginal delivery 103, 103*f*

B

Bacterial vaginosis 62, 145, 146, 151
Bandl's ring 82
Benign ovarian cyst 217
Betamethasone 94
Biopsy, type of 220
Biphosphonates 182
Bishop's score 100
Blade, curves of 105*f*
Bleeding pattern exists in carcinoma cervix, type of 221
Blighted ovum 1
Blood sugar estimation, role of 145

Brachytherapy 223
Breastfeeding 70
Breech delivery
   fetal dangers in 77
   principles of 77
Breech extraction 79
Breech presentation, postural management of 79
Broad ligament fibroid 200
Bromocriptine 189
   uses of 189

C

Cancer cervix 219, 221-223
   cardinal symptoms of 221
   treatment of 224
Candida albicans 145
Candida vaginitis 145
Candidiasis 154
Caput succedaneum 35
Carcinoma cervix with pregnancy 224
Cardiomyopathy 25
   causes of 159*t*
Cefotaxime 94
Cephalhematoma 35
   treatment of 35
Cervical cancer 219-221
   type of 221
Cervical carcinoma, type of 223
Cervical dysplasia 219, 223
   type of 219
Cervical epithelium 219
Cervical fibroid 200
Cervical incompetence 3
   treatment of 3
Cervical intraepithelial neoplasia 219
Cervical malignancy 220
Cervicography 220
Cervix biopsy, type of 221
Cervix cancer, stages of 223
Cervix, carcinoma of 222, 223, 225
Cervix, precancerous and cancerous lesions of 223
Cesarean section 51, 70
   type of 52
Chancroid 154, 155
Chemotherapeutic drugs, combination of 217
Chemotherapy 137223

Chlamydia infection 151
   treatment of 145
Chlamydia trachomatis 151
Chocolate cysts 171
Chorioamnionitis 46
Choriocarcinoma 139
Ciprofloxacin 95
Clifford's classification of postdated infant 49
Clindamycin 95
Clomiphene citrate 186
Clotrimazole 95
Clue cell 146
Colposcopy 220
   uses of 220
Combined oral pills 116
Condom
   advantages and disadvantages of 111
   failure rate of 111
   female 111
   male 111
   uses of 111
Congenital syphilis 42, 149
Conjugated steroidal estrogens 97
Constriction ring 82
Contraception 110, 121
Contraction stress test 32
Corticosteroids 94
   in preterm labor, role of 65
Couvelaire uterus 16
Culdocentesis 142
Cu-T, uses of 114
Cyproterone acetate 188
   uses of 188
Cytoreduction, advantages of 216

D

Danazol 173, 186
   uses of 186
Dexamethasone 94
   role of 126
Diabetes 27, 28
   after delivery, management of 29
   management of 28
   mellitus in pregnancy 27
Dietary iron, sources of 19
Digitalization 25
Dilutional coagulopathy 85

Dimorphic anemia 23
Disseminated gonococcal infection 150
Distal tubal disease, management of 233
Donor insemination 211
Drug resistant disease, management of 138
Dysfunction of systems 134*t*
Dysfunctional uterine bleeding 159
Dysplasia 219-221
Dysplastic cells 219

E

Early stage carcinoma cervix 224
Eclampsia 9
    management of 12
Ectopic pregnancy 123, 140, 142
    acute 142
    chronic 142
    treatment of 141
Edema feet in pregnancy, causes of 31
Emergency 52
    contraception, methods of 120
Endocervical cancer 221
Endometrial ablation 164
Endometrial carcinoma 163, 164t, 225-228
    FIGO staging of 226
    symptoms of 226
    treatment of 227
Endometrial cells 170
Endometrial hyperplasia 161
Endometriomas 171, 174
Endometriosis 170-175, 210
    pathogenesis of 171
    pathology of 171
    treatment of 173, 175
Endometrium
    carcinoma of 225
    squamous differentiation of carcinoma of 226
    type of 163
Endoscopy 229
Enumerate neonatal complications 29
Epigastric artery 231
Episiotomy 36
    role of 109
    type of 36
Erythroblastosis fetalis 56
Estrogen 97, 184
    analogs 97
    role of 179
    synthesis of 97
    uses of 184, 185
Ethacridine lactate 93
Excessive vaginal discharge 144
Expectant management in severe pre-eclampsia, role of 8
Expected date of delivery 34
Exteriorization of uterus, role of 54

F

Face to pubis delivery 75
Fallopian tubes 209
Fetal complications 46
Fetal distress 35
Fetal fibronectin 66
Fetal head, hyperextension of 78
Fetal well-being test 51
Fetomaternal hemorrhage 56
Fetus papyraceous 89
Fibroid 197-200, 203
    management of 201, 204
FIGO classification system 161
FIGO staging 222
Fitz-Hugh-Curtis syndrome 150, 209
Fluconazole 95
Folate deficiency anemia, treatment of 21
Folic acid 93
    deficiency anemia in pregnancy 20
    in pregnancy 32
Forceps 104
    application 104, 105, 107
        technique of 106, 106*f*
        type of 105
    assisted birth 103*f*
    delivery 104
    functions of 104
    in modern obstetrics, role of 107
    over vacuum, advantages of 107
    type of 103

G

Gasless laparoscopy 230
Genital tract 209
Genital warts 152, 153
    treatment of 153
Gestational diabetes mellitus 27, 29, 31
Gestational hypertension 5
Gestational trophoblastic neoplasia 136
Gestrinone 186
Glucose challenge test 27
Glucose metabolism 29
Gonadotropin 176
    therapy, role of 212
Gonococcal infection 150, 151
Gonorrhea 150, 151
    infection of 150
    symptoms and signs of 150
Gonorrheal infection 150
Gonorrhea 150
    treatment of 145
Grand multipara 41, 72
Granuloma inguinale 156
Growth restriction, type of 125
GTN, FIGO staining of 138
Gynecological cancers 148

H

Heart disease 24, 25
    fetal prognosis in 26
    in pregnancy 24
    MTP in 25
Hellin's law 87

HELLP syndrome 10
Hemorrhage 14, 15
Hemostatic resuscitation 85
Hepatitis infection 156, 156, 156*t*, 157
Herpes genitalis 152
Herpes virus infection 152
HIV and tuberculosis, association of 68
HIV infection
    during pregnancy 67
    impact of 150
HIV spread, prevalent mode of 68
HIV transmission rate from mother-to-child 69
HIV viruses, type of 67
HSV disease 152
HSV infection 152
    type of 152
Human papillomavirus infection 152, 153
Hydrops fetalis 56
Hyperplastic endometrium 225
Hyperprolactinemia 167
Hypertension 6
Hypertensive disorders in pregnancy 5
Hypochromic anemia 19
Hysterectomy 139, 163, 221
Hysteroscopic myomectomy 202
Hysteroscopic surgery 231, 232
Hysteroscopy 231, 232

I

Iatrogenic preterm labor 66
Immunized mother, management of 59
Incubation period 151
Induction, methods of 101
Infertile couple 207
Infertility 208
    anovulatory 208
    causes of 207, 208
    evaluation of 207
    type of 208
    unexplained 211
Instrumental vaginal delivery 103
Internal podalic version 81
Intrapartum maternal blood sugar level 29
Intrauterine adhesions, causes of 232
Intrauterine blood transfusion 57
Intrauterine growth retardation 125
Intrauterine insemination 213
Intrauterine therapy 57
Intrauterine transfusion 57
Intravenous leiomyomatosis 204
Invasive cervical cancer 219
Invasive mole 139
Inversion 85
    of uterus, causes of 85
Inverted uterus, management of 85
Iron deficiency
    anemia 22
    development of 22
Iron sucrose complex, advantages of 22
Iron therapy 19

Isoimmunization 56
Isoxsuprine 94
IUCD insertion 113
　technique of 112
IUGR
　causes of 125
　management of 126

J

Jarisch-Herxheimer reaction 149

K

Kallmann's syndrome 166
Keilland's forceps 104
Kleihauer count 56
Krukenberg's tumor 217
Kurzrok-Miller test 213

L

Labetalol 90
　in treatment of pre-eclampsia, role of 9
Labor 24, 34
　augmentation of 102
　induction of 100, 101, 102
　management of 35
　pain 35
　stages of 34
Laparoscopic hysterectomy 231
Laparoscopic myomectomy 232
Laparoscopy 229, 231
　in management of fibroid, role of 202
Laparotomy 216
Leiomyoma 161, 161f
Leiomyosarcoma 203
Lesion in cervical cancer, type of 221
Letrozole 187
Lower segment cesarean section 52
LSCS, technique of 54
Lymphogranuloma venereum 155

M

Macrocytic anemia 20
Macrosomia, pathogenesis of 29
Magnesium sulfate 90, 90t
Magpie trial 12
Malignancy index 215
Malignant ovarian tumor, treatment of 216
Manning score 32
Maternal corticosteroids 94
Maternal death 130
　causes of 129
　in eclampsia, causes of 11
Maternal mortality 128
　causes of 30
Mauriceau-Smellie-Veit maneuver 79
McDonalds vs Shirodkar operation 3
Medical management in fibroid, principles of 201

Medical Termination of Pregnancy Act 4
Megaloblastic anemia 20
Meigs' syndrome 217
Membranes
　prelabor rupture of 45, 47
　sweeping of 101
Menopausal irregular uterine bleeding 176
Menopausal syndrome 176
Menopause 176, 183
　stages of 182t
　symptoms of 176
Menorrhagia 159
Metformin 96
Methotrexate 96
　in management of GTD, role of 139
Methylergometrine 91
Metronidazole 94
Midepigastric pain, causes of 10
Misoprostol 92
Mitral stenosis 25
Modified Bishop's score 100
Molar pregnancy 58, 136
　treatment of 137
Monitoring blood coagulation disorders 16
Multiple pregnancy 87, 88
Murmur, grades of 25
Myoma resection 203f
Myomectomy 202
　principles of 201

N

Neonatal prophylaxis 156
Nevirapine 95
New York Health Association classification 25
Newborn, hemolytic disease of 56
Nifedepine 91
Nitrazine paper test 46
Nonconjugated synthetic estrogens 97
Nonsteroidal oral contraceptive pill 118
Nonstress test 32
Normal fetal
　growth 125
　heart rate 35
Normal labor 34, 35
Normal vaginal flora 148
Nuchal translucency 43

O

Obstructed labor 73, 82
　causes of 82
　complications of 82
　treatment of 82
OC pills 173
Oligohydramnios 126
　in post-term pregnancy, causes of 50
Open laparoscopy 230
Operative vaginal delivery 107
Optical trocar 232

Oral glucose tolerance test 27
Osteoporosis 180, 181
　treatment of 181
Ovarian cyst 217
　causes of 217
Ovarian drilling, technique of 233
Ovarian malignancy 215, 216
Ovarian mass 215
Ovarian pedicle 218
Ovarian reserve 213
Ovarian tumor 214, 217
　classification of 217
Ovulation induction 187, 188, 213
Ovulation, disorders of 213
Oxytocin 91

P

Pain in cancer cervix, causes of 221
Pain in endometriosis, causes of 175
Painful genital ulcer, causes of 148
Pap smear, grades of 220
Paraovarian cyst 217
Parenteral iron therapy 20
Partial hydatidiform mole 136
Partogram 37-39
PCOS 209
PCPNDT Act 31
Perinatal death 14
Perinatal mortality in eclampsia, causes of 11
Peripartum cardiomyopathy 25
Persistent vaginitis 145
Phytoestrogens 182
Pills
　beneficial side effects of 118
　uses of 117
Pinard's maneuver 79
Pituitary gonadotropins 188
Pivot point 108f
Placenta
　accreta 85
　previa, type of 14
　migration of 15
　separation of 35
　previa 14, 15
Placental insufficiency 126
Placental site trophoblastic tumor 138
Polycythemia 204
Ponderal index 126
Post molar pregnancy 137
Postcoital test 213
Postdate pregnancy 51, 58
Postmaturity/dysmaturity syndrome 49
Postmenopausal bleeding, causes of 225
Postmenopausal osteoporosis 179
Postmyomectomy adhesions 206
Postpartum hemorrhage 15, 83
Postpartum period 133
Postpartum shock 85
Post-pill amenorrhea 167

Post-term pregnancy 49, 50
    labor management of 51
PPH
    causes of 83
    type of 83
Prague maneuver 79
Preconception and Prenatal Diagnostic Techniques Act, 1994 4
Pre-eclampsia 6
    causes of 6
    management of 7
Pregnancy 19
    anemia in 18, 21
    high-risk 41, 44
    induced hypertension 5
    prolongation of 50
Premature ovarian failure 168
Premenopausal ovarian tumor 216
Preterm labor 60, 62, 63, 65, 66
    management of 62
    pathophysiology of 60, 61
    signs of 60
Previous cesarean section 52
Progesterone
    challenge test 169
    type of 185
Progestins 98
Progestogens 185
    contraceptive use of 185
Prolonged labor 39
Prolonged pregnancy, management of 51
Prolonged second stage of labor, causes of 34
PROM, pathophysiology of 46
Prophylactic chemotherapy 137
Prophylactic forceps delivery 105
Prophylaxis
    against nutritional anemia 22
    antepartum 57
    choice of 57
Pruritus vulvae 144
Pseudomenopause treatment 173
Pseudomyxoma peritonea 218
Pulmonary edema 25

R

Radiotherapy, technique of 223
Recurrent endometriosis 173
Recurrent pregnancy loss 2
Recurrent vaginitis 145
    treatment of 145
Rein's hypothesis 197
Retained placenta 84
    management of 84
Retraction ring 82

Rh disease in fetus, pathogenesis of 56
Rh-negative mother, management of 58
Robotic myomectomy 202
Robotic surgery team and set-up 203f
Rule of 3 109
Rule of five 24

S

Selective reduction in multiple pregnancy, role of 89
Semen analysis 213
Senile vaginitis, treatment of 145
Sensitized pregnancy, management of 58
Sentinel lymph node 224
Severe abdominal pain, causes of 17
Sexually transmitted infections 147, 148
Shoulder dystocia 29, 51
    management of 29
Sickle cell crisis 22
Sickle cell disease 22
Sickle cell disorder 22
Single gene disorders 42
Soft and hard chancre 148
Sperm penetration test 213
Spironolactone 188
Stabilizing induction 100
Stallworthy's sign 15
Sterilization, laparoscopic methods of 230
Steroidal contraceptives, type of 115
Strawberry sign 146
Surrogacy 212
Syphilis 148, 149, 149t

T

Tamoxifen 187
    uses of 187
Teenage pregnancy 41
Terbutaline 93
Termination of pregnancy, methods of 4
Testosterone 186
    uses of 186
Tetanus vaccine 96
Thalassemia 22
Therapeutic laparoscopy 229
Tocolytic therapy 63
Tranexamic acid 97
Transverse lie 81
Trial forceps 105
Trichomonas infection 145
Trichomonas vaginalis 154
    infection, asymptomatic 148
    treatment of 154
Trichomonas vaginitis 145
Trichomoniasis 153

Triple test 31
Tubal pregnancy 142
Twin
    development of 87
    pregnancy in labor 88
Twin-to-twin transfusion syndrome 89

U

Urinary incontinence 177
Urinary tract infection 177
USG in abruptio placentae, role of 16
Uterine bleeding, abnormal 158, 159, 176
Uterine contractions, complications of 102
Uterine fibroids 197
Uterus
    inversion of 85
    rupture of 53, 73

V

Vacuum assisted birth 103f
Vacuum cups 108
    type of 108
Vacuum delivery 109
Vacuum extraction 107
    procedure of 108
Vacuum extractor, indications of 107
Vacuum over forceps 107
Vaginal candidiasis 145
Vaginal delivery 78, 126
Vaginal diaphragm, advantages and disadvantages of 112
Vaginal discharge 144, 145
    color of 148
Vaginal infection, type of 219
Vaginitis 144, 145
    classification of 145
    type of 144
Vanishing twin syndrome 89
VDRL test 148
Ventouse delivery 109
Viral hepatitis 156
Vitamin B_{12} deficiency 20
    anemia, treatment of 21

W

Wertheim's hysterectomy 222, 223
Whiff's amine test 146
Wrigley's outlet forceps 104

Z

Zatuchni and Andros scoring system 77
Zatuchni-Andros breech scoring 77t